Effective Helping

Effective Helping

Interviewing and Counseling Techniques

SEVENTH EDITION

BARBARA F. OKUN
Northeastern University

RICKI E. KANTROWITZ
Westfield State College

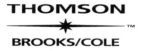

THOMSON

™

BROOKS/COLE

Australia • Brazil • Canada • Mexico • Singapore • Spain • United Kingdom • United States

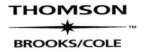

THOMSON
™
BROOKS/COLE

Effective Helping: Interviewing and Counseling Techniques, **Seventh Edition**
Barbara F. Okun, Ricki E. Kantrowitz

Senior Acquisitions Editor: *Marquita Flemming*
Assistant Editor: *Samantha Shook*
Editorial Assistant: *Meaghan Banks*
Technology Project Manager: *Julie Aguilar*
Marketing Manager: *Meghan McCullough*
Marketing Communications Manager: *Shemika Britt*
Project Manager, Editorial Production: *Rita Jaramillo*
Creative Director: *Rob Hugel*
Art Director: *Vernon Boes*
Print Buyer: *Nora Massuda*
Permissions Editor: *Roberta Broyer*
Production Service: *Anne Draus, Scratchgravel Publishing Services*
Copy Editor: *Margaret C. Tropp*
Cover Designer: *Lisa Devenish*
Cover Image: *Stuart Westmorland / Corbis*
Cover and Text Printer: *West Group*
Compositor: *International Typesetting and Composition*

Thomson Higher Education
10 Davis Drive
Belmont, CA 94002-3098
USA

For more information about our products, contact us at:
Thomson Learning Academic Resource Center
1-800-423-0563

For permission to use material from this text or product, submit a request online at
http://www.thomsonrights.com.
Any additional questions about permissions can be submitted by e-mail to
thomsonrights@thomson.com.

Printed in the United States of America.
1 2 3 4 5 6 7 11 10 09 08 07

Library of Congress Control Number:
2006936557

ISBN-13: 978-0-495-00625-1
ISBN-10: 0-495-00625-4

In Memoriam
Catherine A. Brenner
Katherine M. Newman
Henry G. Altman
Eunice S. Kantrowitz

Contents

Preface

The seventh edition of *Effective Helping: Interviewing and Counseling Techniques* is coauthored with an experienced colleague and friend who developed the Instructor's Manual for the sixth edition. In this edition, we refer to significant changes that are occurring in the 21st century, including the impact of globalization, war, and the spread of terrorism, as well as an apparent increase in natural disasters. Within the United States, there continue to be significant changes: rising immigration leading to shifting demographics; further emergence of nontraditional family systems and lifestyles; accelerated use of computers and the Internet by more and more people, leading to further globalization; an alternately expanding and shrinking economy; and significant advances in health sciences. These changes affect each of us: our lifestyle choices, our personal and work identities, the composition and meaning of family, and the restricted availability of and access to community and health resources and services, which in turn affect health status.

In our increasingly complex, multicultural society, there is a significant incidence of family disharmony, substance abuse, anxiety, and depression, as well as serious mental illness, in people of all ages. There is a critical need for culturally sensitive mental health and human services workers and programs. Yet, in the current economic and political environment, there is a tension between the need for expanded quality services and the need for cost containment. Health care payers often want helping professionals to rely on psychopharmacology, as well as short-term, solution-focused, action-oriented helping assessment and interventions, for emotional and mental health difficulties. Many mental health professionals believe in the efficacy of counseling alone or combined with medication and continue to practice longer-term interventions.

Mental health and human services workers are being increasingly asked to provide evidence to support their claims of treatment effectiveness. An important and consistent finding has been that, no matter what the theory or strategy, a positive outcome is often enhanced by the presence of an effective helping relationship. There is agreement that helpers must know how to build an effective relationship with helpees. Whatever treatment or strategy is used, helpers must have not only *knowledge* about culturally diverse human behavior and development and the process of change, but also helping and communication *skills*.

This book is intended for undergraduate and graduate students in professional disciplines—as well as human services trainees, instructors, supervisors, trainers, managers, and administrators at all levels. With the use of the material in this book, helpers-in-training will develop skills and a knowledge base that will enhance the success of helping strategies and will apply to both professional and personal relationships.

New to This Edition

This seventh edition is shaped by the sociocultural and professional changes of the new millennium and the economic pressures on the nature of counseling and treatment in today's service delivery. While retaining the successful format and content of the previous editions, we have discarded outdated material and added and elaborated on more contemporary material as well as new exercises. Chapter 1 elaborates on these changes from an ecological perspective, focusing on how the helping relationship is embedded in a treatment context that, in turn, is embedded in larger social systems. Chapters 1 through 4 include updates of the research on which the human relations counseling model is based. Chapter 5 presents the major theories of helping. Chapter 6 expands the contemporary theoretical models of constructivism, feminist therapies, multicultural models, integrative therapies, and ecological systems. Chapters 7 and 8 include the strategies of the models discussed in Chapter 6. A new case is included in Chapter 8. Chapter 9 presents crisis and disaster theory and interventions for individual, family, and larger systems. Particular attention is paid to a systems perspective used to address the global effects of the increasing incidence of national catastrophes and disasters. Chapter 10 highlights current ethical issues, such as online confidentiality, requests for information by third-party payers, multiple-role relationships, misrepresentation, conflict of interest, and financial constraints on the availability of helping services. This edition includes updated citations, cases, and examples reflecting multicultural issues.

The updated *Instructor's Manual with Test Bank* contains Internet exercises and sample class assignments and activities. There is also a book companion website, where students can access tutorial quizzes and Internet activities.

The Human Relations Counseling Model

The human relations counseling model brings together the skills, helping stages, and issues involved in the helping process. Communication skills include the ability to hear and understand verbal and nonverbal messages and to listen responsively to both kinds of messages within an empathic context. They allow one to tune into another's cultural framework by focusing on the helpee's meanings. These skills enable helpers to progress through the two stages of helping: the relationship stage, during which rapport and trust develop and problems are clarified; and the strategy stage, which involves selecting and applying appropriate helping methods. Contextual issues that may arise during the counseling process include values clarification, ethics, sexism, ethnocentrism, racism, classism, ageism, heterosexism, and other social and professional topics that can have either a positive or a negative impact on a helping relationship. Knowledge of the major aspects of the human relations counseling model is crucial to a helper's effectiveness in all types of settings and with all kinds of people.

Acknowledgments

Although many students, colleagues, and trainees have provided invaluable feedback to us with regard to the seventh edition, we want to express particular appreciation to our good friend and colleague, Marsha M. Mirkin, a faculty member at LaSalle College in Newton, Massachusetts who has painstakingly supported and constructively contributed to this endeavor. We want to express appreciation to Lisa Gebo, our former editor at Thomson, for her ongoing encouragement and support over many years. We also want to acknowledge the detailed pre-revision reviews of the following: Dorothy Bagwell, Texas Tech University; John Bourdette, Western New Mexico University; Keith Britany, San Jose City College; Louis Downs, California State University, Sacramento; Jane Fried, Central Connecticut State University; Marsha Mirkin, Lasell College; Chester Robinson, Texas A&M University–Commerce; Daniel Stern, CUNY–York College; and Noreen Smith, Northern College of Applied Arts and Technology.

Effective Helping

1

Introduction

Since the sixth edition of *Effective Helping* was published in 2002, the climate in which people are helped has continued to change significantly. These changes occur in two major areas: (1) the nature, process, and scope of counseling and therapy; and (2) the settings and environments in which counseling and therapy are conducted. The two areas are intertwined: a change in context (setting and sociocultural environment) requires corresponding changes in how counselors and therapists function. (In this text, the terms *counselor* and *helper* will be used interchangeably, as will the terms *counseling, psychotherapy,* and *helping.*)

Over the past several decades, counseling and therapy models have evolved from (1) traditional psychodynamic approaches, which assumed an intrapsychic, individual perspective, to (2) integrated cognitive-behavioral approaches developed in the 1970s and 1980s, which took an individual problem-solving perspective, to (3) systemic approaches, which focus on family interactions, and, most recently, to (4) outcome-oriented brief therapies within a multicultural systems/ecological perspective. Figure 1.1 illustrates the **ecological*** model, in which the individual is viewed as an element of the primary family, which is an element within larger systems. The individual cannot be fully understood as a person unless one understands the influences of these larger systems. A person is embedded in the context of his or her primary family, which is embedded in the contexts of larger social systems such as school, work, and community.

***Boldface** terms in the text are defined in the glossary at the end of the book.

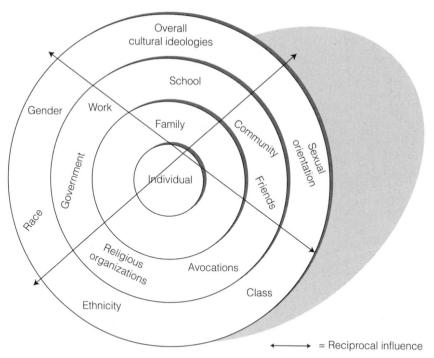

FIGURE 1.1 The interface of individual, family, sociocultural systems, and overall cultural ideologies (adapted from Knoff, 1986, p. 16)

These social systems, in turn, are embedded in a macrosystem comprised of cultural attitudes and ideologies, gender, race, class, ethnicity, religion, sexual orientation, geographical region, and other factors. All these systems and factors mutually interact, creating reciprocal influence—each system influences and is influenced by each of the others.

The professional helper needs to have more skills and knowledge than ever before. Like a driver, one cannot take effective shortcuts unless one is thoroughly familiar with the terrain. In order to adhere to today's model of outcome-oriented brief therapy from a multicultural systems/ecological perspective, the helper must be knowledgeable and skilled in relationship building and strategy application so that the pace of the sessions and progress are not impeded. The helper must also be educated about physiological functioning and understand the impact of race, ethnicity, class, gender, religion, geography, generation, and sexual orientation on his/her own development and identities as well as on those of clients (Comas-Diaz & Greene, 1994; Mirkin, Suyemoto, & Okun, 2005; Okun, 2005).

THE TWENTY-FIRST CENTURY

Many shifts created by changing society are apparent in the 21st century. These issues affect communities, dominant and nondominant populations, families, and individuals differently. They also affect political, economic, and social policies, such as people's access to and the availability of human services. A brief overview of these major shifts will help us understand the changing roles and functions of professional, generalist, and nonprofessional helpers.

In the first years of the 21st century, the economy appears to be slowing down. A growing segment of the middle-class population is struggling with employment instability as a result of layoffs, corporate mergers, high-technology skill requirements, and the shifting of jobs to other countries; adding to this instability is the loss of employment benefits, which can limit access to health care, education, and pensions. U.S. military involvement in the Mideast has had a major impact on the well-being of reservists and enlistees, as well as their families. Terrorism and natural disasters, such as Hurricanes Katrina and Rita, have had an impact on our society on many levels. Financial stress, in addition to many other uncertainties in people's lives, may impair their physical and mental health.

A significant portion of the U.S. population lives at or below the poverty line, and a disproportionate number suffer from physical and mental illness, societal discrimination, and lack of training or education. This growing underclass is unable to obtain or maintain jobs, is often dependent on social welfare, and is frequently ill, homeless, or involved in crime. Not only are they underserved by health and other helping professions, but the cycle of poverty in which they are caught often repeats itself generationally. Increasing levels and incidence of domestic violence, substance abuse, crime, homelessness, and severe emotional distress indicate a breakdown in social values and structures. There is a serious erosion of trust and confidence in our business, educational, health, and political institutions. The dichotomies of the "haves" and "have-nots," the employed and the un- or underemployed, are undermining the spirit of unity and collaboration that many assumed to be an integral component of North American culture.

The demographics of U.S. society are changing. The influx of immigrants and refugees from Third World countries continues, birthrates among ethnic groups vary, and before long the dominant European American population will be a minority in a multicultural country (Carter, 1995; Comas-Diaz & Greene, 1994; Sue, 2002, 2005; Suyemoto & Kim, 2005). Although some immigrants and refugees are eager to assimilate into the dominant culture, others wish to maintain their separate ethnic identities and communities, and still others strive to be fully bicultural. Many of the controversies about bilingual education and affirmative action are related to differences in the needs, assumptions, and values of various groups.

Another dichotomy arises from the growing acceptance of diversity in some parts of the population and country and increasing resistance to diversity in other parts. This diversity refers not only to national/ethnic origin, but to religious beliefs and sexual orientation as well. The resistance threatens some of the inclusive societal gains and programs already achieved. The very notions of who constitutes a "family" and what is an "acceptable lifestyle," and how these are defined legally, are controversial; the answers affect one's access to tax, welfare, unemployment, family leave, and health benefits. (See Okun, Fried, & Okun, 1999, for a more complete discussion of cultural diversity with accompanying exercises; Okun, 2004.)

Another change is the rapid development of information technology. On the one hand, it extends our scope of contact and gives us greater access to information more rapidly. On the other hand, these tools are often very invasive, creating difficulties such as maintaining privacy and involuntarily disclosing more than intended.

The amount of psychosocial stress accompanying economic and sociocultural changes underscores the need for helping services; however, the privatization and restructuring of health care delivery systems require minimal, symptom-reducing, brief treatments and control of services by the payers rather than the providers. This dichotomy between the need for and the lack of availability of helping services creates a dilemma for those in the helping professions.

The Helper's Changing Roles/Functions

Since the first edition of this book 30 years ago, some characteristics of effective helping have remained the same, some have shifted, and some have dramatically changed. A core concept about effective helping remains constant: a "working alliance"—an authentic, warm, empathic relationship between the helper and the helpee—is a necessary framework for any kind of psychological change. Along with development of this rapport, accurate assessment, individualized treatment formulation and planning, and short- and long-term outcome evaluations are essential elements of professional helping. Ongoing dilemmas for professional helpers in today's world include keeping confidentiality and focusing on the client's rather than the helper's, agency's, or third-party payer's needs.

Our present era of cost-contained managed health care has necessitated a shift toward primarily short-term, outcome-oriented counseling and therapy. In fact, the third-party payer's criterion of "medical necessity" is increasingly required for clients to be eligible for treatment, and less and less attention is paid to prevention and early intervention. Yet, according to a recent survey, almost half of all Americans will have a diagnosable mental disorder at some point in their lifetime (Kessler, 2005). These disorders cannot be addressed outside the contexts of family, community, and larger systems variables.

The shift to brief treatment may work well for many people experiencing adjustment and developmental difficulties—the "worried well." However, it may not be very useful for an increasing number of people coming to helpers with severe physical and mental health difficulties. Today's helper, restricted by insurance regulations, is often not able to differentiate between the number of sessions and types of treatment needed for the "worried well" and the seriously disturbed population. The focus of managed care is on directive, action-oriented resolution of clients' presenting problems, along with a reduction of symptoms. Identification and exploration of underlying difficulties is unlikely to be achieved in six to eight sessions—the typical number initially allowed per year for any one client. Even so, this mandate has some positive results: people do not remain in endless counseling without measured outcomes; a team approach by interdisciplinary helpers, which can include individual, group, family, and larger organizational strategies, is often utilized; and helpees' strengths rather than weaknesses are frequently highlighted. Competent communication skills are essential so as to develop the necessary helping relationship quickly and effectively. Rapport building, assessment, empowering interventions, and outcome evaluation are intertwined in a limited treatment package.

Effective helpers must expand their knowledge base to include the biopsychosocial model. The increases in societal complexity make it essential for helpers to consider individuals and their behaviors within the psychosocial contexts of their relevant social and cultural systems: varying styles of immediate and extended families, ever-changing neighborhood and communities, and both conventional and alternative work and school settings. Not only is it important to differentiate among the particular personal, interpersonal, cultural, and societal variables contributing to an individual's stress level, but it is also necessary to understand the interrelationship of those variables. For example, fear of losing one's job in a constricted economy or dissatisfaction with one's job may result in a person feeling trapped and frustrated. That frustration may surface in marital arguments or in physical symptoms such as headaches, ulcers, or hypertension.

In addition to learning the intricacies of the multicultural systems/ecological perspective, counselors must be aware of the individual's physiological functioning. Recent cognitive and neuroscience (genetic, neuroendocrinological, and brain function) research has led to a greater understanding and appreciation of the powerful influences of biology on our psychological development and functioning (Lewis, Amini, & Lannon, 2000; Ratey, 2001). Today, mind and body are considered to be one system; physical and mental health comprise our concept of health (Stewart & Okun, 2005). The current concept of embodied mind recognizes the role of body and brain in human reason and language (Lakoff, 2004).

Another change is the broadening range of resources and techniques available to counselors and therapists. We have more refined assessment tools, computerized programs, and cognitive-behavioral strategies. We use tools such as **hypnosis, eye movement desensitization and reprocessing (EMDR), biofeedback,** and newer generations of drugs to treat moderate as well as major illnesses and anxieties. All these help people manage situational and developmental stress and improve their competencies, coping skills, and resources so they can negotiate relationships and life transitions more effectively. We encourage clients as well as helpers to utilize the tremendous knowledge base easily accessible on the Internet. For example, a helper may encourage a client to look up a particular company and learn as much as possible about its culture prior to a job interview. Further, since we are more aware of the mind/body system, we encourage helpees to maintain physical fitness through exercise using mindfulness techniques such as meditation, yoga, and appropriate nutrition. More and more people, including mainstream health care providers, are finding that alternative approaches such as herbal supplements, Eastern massage therapies, and acupuncture alleviate stress-related symptoms.

With social services severely constrained by economic and political factors, competition for limited resources among various helping professions has increased, and cutbacks among helping professionals and human services providers have become common. The environment for service delivery is economically driven, creating a tension between the service agency wanting to balance its budget and the helpers' personal and professional values, beliefs, and training. Under managed care, provision for time-limited crisis intervention services is more dependent on medications and impersonal short-term service delivery than on helping relationships that can be tailored to meet individual needs. There is a constant pull between the mission of community agencies and the need for reimbursement from third-party payers for a significant proportion of the population they serve. More and more nonprofit community agencies and hospitals are being purchased by profit-driven health care conglomerates. As a result, communities have experienced the loss of unprofitable but socially and morally necessary programs and services, particularly those geared to the disenfranchised. The disparity between the increasing need of our stressed population for human services and the decreasing availability of and support for such services is indeed paradoxical.

Helpers who work in agencies, schools, counseling centers, and health care centers are faced with increased client hours ("units of productivity"), a heavier load of paperwork, and more telephone time with collateral helpers (primary care physician, ancillary providers, schools, family, etc.). They must follow the HIPAA (Health Insurance Portability and Accountability Act of 1996) established by the federal government to protect the privacy of patients' health and medical information (see Appendix D). In many settings, the helper must scramble to fill the unbillable hours from last-minute cancellations or "no-shows" in order to receive payment. There is little time for relationship development and reflection in today's health care environment.

Yet we believe that well-trained counselors will recognize that multiple external and internal factors usually contribute to personal problems. Table 1.1 summarizes the kind of information that helpers need to consider for accurate assessment and treatment planning from a multicultural systems/ecological perspective. This information also allows helpers to identify collateral helpers from different interacting social systems.

Communication Skills

The mass media have drawn attention to the many different forms of today's social ills, and we know that personal, familial, and environmental stresses can show up in physical, psychological, and social symptoms (biopsychosocial perspective). Underlying or at the very least contributing to these symptoms are interpersonal difficulties, which affect friendships, familial and work relationships, and community, national, and international relations. Most of us feel sincere concern for others and their problems despite our own personal

TABLE 1.1 Ecological intake sheet

Individual Context	Family Context
Developmental	■ Who is included in the current family?

■ Is client at appropriate developmental task?
  Social   Work/school
  Emotional   Relationships
  Cognitive   Outside interests
                    Coping strategies
	Family members, extended family, friends?

	■ Developmental stage of current family
Medical/Health	What is current task? How does this interact with tasks of individuals within system?
■ Receiving primary care?	■ Rules/roles/norms of current family
■ Chronic health issues?	■ Rules/roles/norms of family-of-origin

■ Wellness/stress management?
  Nutrition
  Exercise
  Alcohol/tobacco/recreational drug use
  Relaxation/self-care
	Couple system
	Parent system
	Sibling system

	■ Nature of current crisis
■ Hospitalizations/surgery	■ History of past crises with current family and family-of-origin
■ Head trauma/loss of consciousness	■ Whose problem is it? Who would benefit/lose if problem were "solved"?
Client Coping Strategies/Strengths	■ Family coping strategies and family strengths
■ How does client generally manage stress? Coping skills/internal resources Defenses	
■ What strengths does client bring to therapy to aid treatment?	**Treatment/Professional Context**
Sociocultural Context	■ Context of treatment: Inpatient, outpatient, clinic, school-based, crisis?
	■ Other treatment providers: prior treatment?
Community Resources	■ Who are decision makers regarding type and length of treatment?
■ How connected/disconnected is client to community and possible resources? Are the connections different for different family members within the presenting family?	■ Whose idea was it for client to seek treatment?
	■ Therapist's individual/family/cultural background and resources
■ Community of culture	■ Therapist's level of experience
■ Community of residence	■ Supervision/consultation and availability of professional resources for therapist
■ Community of faith/religion	
■ Community of school/work	
■ Rules and roles regarding use of treatment within each community	

Prepared by G. Schmelzer and B. F. Okun, January 2000.

struggles for survival, but we still experience misunderstandings resulting from our inability to communicate that concern and our desire to help and to focus on specific problems and difficult issues. Particularly in this era of budget-constrained service delivery, helpers and helpees need to learn how to communicate their concerns clearly, effectively, and expediently. As helpers, we must assist others in developing their capacities to communicate effectively.

Ineffective or faulty communication is at the root of most interpersonal difficulties. Conversely, effective communication is necessary to develop and maintain positive interpersonal relationships. Unfortunately, our educational systems emphasize the development of written communication skills, almost to the exclusion of face-to-face or interpersonal communication skills. Although schools teach us to respond to information and content conveyed in messages, they do not really encourage or teach us to hear, perceive, and respond to the emotions in messages. Nor do they teach us awareness of the explicit and implicit cultural behaviors that influence communication (Okun, 2004; Okun et al., 1999).

Communication skills awareness and training are essential for any human relations endeavor, regardless of the agency or institutional context, and regardless of whether the helping relationship is short-term or ongoing. Within the context of short-term helping, effective communication skills are particularly necessary if helpers are to develop rapport with clients and to formulate reasonable objectives within specified time limits. *Effective Helping* is intended, in part, to provide a vehicle with which you can develop these skills in order to increase your own and others' self-awareness, understanding of the impact of social forces on human development, and capacities for problem solving.

THE PURPOSE OF THIS BOOK

The basic purpose of this book is to provide a foundation for individuals to develop the human relations skills they need to build effective helping relationships. As part of this foundation, an introductory overview of the counseling process is presented to familiarize helpers with the knowledge and skills used for immediate, short-term, and long-term helping.

The major premise of this book is that every individual can learn more effective communication skills that can be applied in personal, social, occupational, and professional settings. Effective communication is the core of the helping process and allows for more satisfying relationships of all types. Improved interpersonal relations allow people to seek and receive support as well as provide it to those experiencing personal, familial, occupational, or social distress.

Over the past 30 years, this book has been used by both groups and individuals, in both mental health professional academic and clinical programs and formal and informal human relations training. It has been adopted as a text in professional counseling and generalist human services and has been used by social service agencies, courts, nursing homes, the military, prisons, pastoral counseling programs, governments, and municipal organizations. The book focuses on the knowledge and skills needed by individuals in human services positions (such as mental health assistants, counselors, probation officers, employment service workers) or persons involved in other helping roles (ancillary health care workers, supervisors, managers, teachers, colleagues).

The material is designed for use in training either beginning students entering helping professions or those people who need or want to improve their human relations effectiveness. Because it teaches fundamental skills, this material will be useful to people continuing their professional training in counseling as well as to those in nonprofessional settings who find themselves in informal helping relationships in their day-to-day encounters. The book sometimes uses technical terms with which you may be unfamiliar. The first time each of these terms appears it will be in **boldface** type to indicate its inclusion in the glossary at the end of the book.

Overall, the book is intended to be a practical, applied skills manual rather than a theoretical treatise. However, it does include a basic overview of current major theoretical approaches to helping, as a knowledge-based background to help readers understand the strategies (applications of theories) covered. This overview also provides the groundwork for helpers to evolve an integrative personal theory based on their awareness and acknowledgment of their own values, attitudes, and belief systems. It is an introduction to applied human relations skills in which users are encouraged to employ their own knowledge, learn from their own experiences, and integrate new knowledge with their own capabilities. The accompanying Instructor's Manual provides resources, test questions, and summaries. Remember, though, that human relations—the interactions among people—is a vast subject. Only a limited understanding of this field can be gained from a book such as this. You cannot expect to become an expert from the introductory exposure to theory, skills, and practice that can be given in one book.

The approach to helping presented here is flexible and adaptable: whatever strategies or techniques are considered most reasonable and useful in a given situation will be applied, rather than utilizing one or only a few theoretical modalities for all helping situations. The strategies that work for a particular client may be modified or rejected for another client in a similar situation. Helpers and helpees from different cultural groups will need to attend to culturally based communication styles in order to achieve an effective helping relationship. Likewise, certain strategies, more than others, will be more compatible with the personal values and style of the helpee and helper.

Even though you will not be able to use the counseling strategies presented in this book without further training or assistance, you can begin to use the communication skills covered. Also, your knowledge of the strategies and their applications will help you understand the part that counseling plays in the delivery of human services and relate your work to that performed by professional counselors in the human services field. For example, if you are working as a probation officer and find that one or more of your charges has difficulty meeting the terms of probation, it could be helpful to know about behavior modification strategies and how they can help your clients gain some control over their environments and behaviors. You might need some assistance in formulating and applying those strategies, but you would at least know which areas of knowledge and training you need to pursue.

The overall view of this book is that (1) effective communication is the core of every helping relationship; (2) a warm, empathic helping relationship is the single most important ingredient in the helping process; (3) the goals of every helper include assisting the helpee to increase self-esteem and achieve self-acceptance as well as gain control over and assume responsibility for his or her behavior and decisions; (4) more than one strategy can be used with any client; (5) continual self-evaluation by the helper and evaluation of "where the helping relationship is" are necessary for effective helping; (6) the helper must be aware of his or her own values, feelings, and thoughts to be able to accept helpees with their own needs, not those of the helper; and (7) the helper must be sensitive to the gender and cultural bases of clients' beliefs, values, and behaviors.

WHO IS THE HELPER?

The helper is anyone who assists others to understand, overcome, or deal with external or internal problems. We often think of human relations helpers as professionally trained specialists: psychiatrists, psychologists, social workers, psychiatric nurses, or counselors. But an increasing variety of human services workers provide direct or indirect case management and counseling services to a broad array of clients in different private and public settings. Some of these are professional helpers; others are generalist human services workers, whose work is adjunctive to or independent of professional helpers. Included in this generalist human services worker classification are helpers in other kinds of organizations, such as nursing homes, prisons, and the military; they serve as teachers, human resource workers in government and industrial organizations, supervisors, managers, judicial workers, and ancillary health workers. Then there are informal helpers—such as friends, volunteers, relatives, and neighborhood workers—who formally or informally find themselves in helper roles. These categories of helpers are not mutually exclusive; in fact, they can and do overlap (see Table 1.2).

What distinguishes these three categories of helpers from one another is the level of skills and knowledge they possess. Because the basic communication skills involved in formal or informal helping and in professional, generalist, and nonprofessional helping relationships are the same, much of what constitutes professional training has proven to be effective for generalist human services workers and lay helpers.

TABLE 1.2 Skills and knowledge required by helpers in three categories

	Nonprofessional Helper	Generalist Human Services Worker	Professional Helper
Communication skills	X	X	X
Developmental knowledge	X	X	X
Assessment skills		X	X

Professional Helpers

Professional helpers are specialists who undergo extensive graduate-level training in the study of human behavior, learn applied helping strategies, and experience supervised clinical training while helping individuals, families, and groups. Although there may be a great deal of overlap in the services delivered by trained specialists, they have different training backgrounds and credentialing requirements.

Psychiatrists are physicians who have completed residencies in mental hospitals or on psychiatric units of general hospitals. Their unique contribution to the helping professions includes a knowledge of psychopharmacology and an ability to prescribe drugs, familiarity with medical diseases and their treatment, and case management of inpatients. Today, because of the training focus on psychopharmacology and medical consultation, many psychiatrists do not receive comprehensive psychotherapy training during their residency. They may receive specialized training at psychoanalytic and other training institutes above and beyond their formal academic and residency programs.

Psychologists, on the other hand, receive training (usually at the doctoral level) in behavioral sciences and are particularly well versed in psychological (learning, developmental, and personality) theory as opposed to the medical disease model. Their unique contribution is in the field of psychodiagnosis and in research methodology. Most psychology training programs today expose trainees to major contemporary models of psychotherapy from a multicultural perspective. Although still controversial, psychologists in some states have acquired the right, with appropriate training, to prescribe medications.

In a third professional category, mental health counselors usually complete a minimum of two years of graduate study at the master's level with an emphasis on providing preventive, developmental services as opposed to the correction of severe disturbances. They take many of the same graduate courses as do psychologists, but with a concentration in practitioner rather than methodology courses, and they are required to have a certain number of hours of supervised clinical experience. Social workers also undertake two years of graduate study; they provide unique services through their knowledge and coordination of available community organizations and social policies. Most social work programs provide two full years of supervised fieldwork and rigorous coursework on social, group, and individual interactions. Psychiatric nurses receive supervision throughout their clinical experiences and in many states are trained for prescription privileges at the graduate level.

Any of these professionals, depending on their specific areas of competence, can offer counseling or therapy to clients at the individual, family, group, or larger organizational level. A 1995 *Consumer Reports* study ("Mental Health"; see also Satcher, 1999) reported that psychologists, psychiatrists, and social workers do not differ in their effectiveness as helpers.

Professional continuing education provides a forum for interdisciplinary interaction and exposure to knowledge common to all helping professions. In fact, knowing the helper's professional identity is often not enough to distinguish what type of counseling is being offered. The similarities and differences among professional helpers may lie more in individual styles and practices than in professional identities. However, economic constraints are causing intense competition among these professional disciplines, and professional organizations often focus more on differences than on overlapping skills and knowledge. Unfortunately, this can cause unwarranted claims of specialization and work against effective interdisciplinary teamwork as helpers guard their own professional turf. For example, psychologists, who have made many inroads into treatment settings previously restricted to psychiatrists, are actively seeking prescription privileges, and mental health counselors are demanding parity with social workers.

Generalist Human Services Workers

Overlapping the professional category of helpers is the category of generalist human services workers such as psychiatric aides or technicians, youth street workers, substance abuse counselors, day-care staff, probation officers, supervisors, managers, human resource personnel, and church workers. These helpers normally receive specialized human relations training at the undergraduate college level and usually work on a team with professionals or have professionals available for consultation and supervision. Much of their training occurs on the job, both formally and informally. Generalist human services workers often pick up the slack when professional helpers must direct their focus elsewhere. In some settings, they are the day-to-day service providers, having the most continuous contact with clients.

Nonprofessional Helpers

We certainly must include the nonprofessionals in our discussion. Although they probably do not receive formal training as helpers, they may attend seminars or meetings on various issues in human relations services from time to time. This group includes people who provide important helping assistance on a formal basis, such as interviewers, supervisors, and teachers; on a semiformal basis such as volunteers; and on an informal basis, such as friends, relatives, and colleagues.

The common denominator of the three groups of helpers is that they all must use communication skills effectively to initiate and develop helping relationships with the people they are assisting. To provide support for extensive kinds of problems, helpers apply certain strategies. The application of those strategies requires formal training and experience; this book illustrates their use by professional helpers and some generalist human services workers.

THE TWO STAGES OF COUNSELING

As mentioned earlier, the term *counseling,* as used in this book, encompasses the professional, generalist, and nonprofessional forms of helping. The terms *counselor* and *helper* will be used interchangeably, as will the terms *helpee* and *client.*

Many people consider counseling to be both an art and a science. It is an art in the sense that the personality, values, and demeanor (along with the skills and knowledge) of the counselor are subjective variables in the counseling process that are difficult to define or measure. It is a science in that much of what we know about human behavior and some of the helping strategies have been synthesized into structured, measurable, objective counseling systems. The changing treatment context requires a more scientific approach to the application and evaluation of counseling strategies. Increasingly, helpers are being required to document the outcomes of their helping by measuring whether the presenting problem has been resolved, whether symptoms have been decreased, and whether the client is satisfied. These measures require scientific models of empirical validity. However, counseling can still be thought of as a process with two ongoing, intertwined parts or stages—the first stage more an art, the second more a science. And the counselor's style of delivery is perhaps an art that is practiced throughout the entire helping relationship.

The first stage of the helping process focuses on building rapport and trust between the helper and the helpee. The helper offers the helpee support for self-disclosure to uncover and explore as much information and as many feelings as possible and pertinent. This exploration enables the helper and the helpee to focus on the helpee's needs and presenting issues and to determine mutually the goals and objectives of treatment and, thus, the direction of the helping relationship. This decision making must consider the criteria and rules of the setting in which the helping relationship occurs, as well as payment and reimbursement policies.

The skills involved in relationship building on a one-to-one (that is, one helper, one helpee) basis are fundamental skills that can be used when interacting with others at home, at school, at work, or in the community. These relationship skills have been identified in the work of Carkhuff (2000a, 2000b), Gordon (2000), Ivey, D'Andrea, Ivey, and Simek-Downing (2002), Ivey and Ivey (1999), Sue (2002), Sue, Ivey, and Pedersen (1996), and others who have developed helper-training systems that derive from basic Rogerian person-centered theory (which we will discuss in Chapter 5). These systems include listening, attending, perceiving, and responding as components of communication and allow for exploration, clarification, and assessment of the helpee's problems.

As a relationship that promotes accurate problem assessment is developing, the second stage of the helping process begins. This stage comprises strategy planning, implementation, and evaluation, which lead to termination and follow-up. Normally this stage of the helping process is the province of professional helpers, although it is also of some concern to generalist human services workers. Although nonprofessional helpers are not usually involved in this stage of helping, they still need a rudimentary knowledge of the theory and application of helping strategies in professional and generalist helping relationships to understand and appropriately use human services resources. The success of the second stage depends greatly on how effective the communication skills were in establishing a positive helping relationship during the first stage.

THE HUMAN RELATIONS
COUNSELING MODEL

This book is based on the human relations counseling model. This model derives from the major formal theoretical views discussed in Chapters 5 and 6. It emphasizes a client-centered, problem-solving helping relationship in which behavior changes and action (outcomes) can result from one or both of the following: (1) the client's exploration and understanding of his or her feelings, thoughts, and actions; (2) the client's understanding of and decision to modify pertinent environmental and systemic variables. Cognitive, affective, or behavioral strategies are used alone or in concert when both the helper and the helpee determine the appropriate need and timing. And some strategies combine various aspects of several formal theories of helping adapted to a multicultural systems/ecological framework.

Assumptions and Implications of the Model

The theoretical assumptions of the human relations counseling model reflect **existential, cognitive-behavioral,** and **systems** influences. These assumptions are as follows:

1. People are responsible for and capable of making their own decisions within the framework of environmental factors.

2. People are controlled to a certain extent by their environment, but they are often able to direct their lives more than they realize. They always have some freedom to choose, even if their options are restricted by environmental variables or inherent biological or personality predispositions.

3. Behaviors are purposive and goal-directed. People are continuously striving toward meeting their own needs, from basic physiological needs to abstract self-actualization (psychological, sociological, and aesthetic) needs.

4. People want to feel good about themselves and continually need positive confirmation of their own self-worth from **significant others.** They want to feel and behave **congruently,** to reduce **dissonance** between internal and external realities.

5. People are capable of learning new behaviors and eliminating or lessening existing behaviors, and they are subject to environmental and internal consequences of their behaviors, which in turn serve as **reinforcements.** They strive for reinforcements that are meaningful and congruent with their personal values and belief systems.

6. People's personal problems may arise from unfinished business (unresolved conflicts) stemming from the past (concerning events and relationships), but although some exploration of causation may be beneficial to clarify the connection between the past and present, most problems can be worked through by focusing on the here and now—on what choices the person has now. Problems may also be caused by **incongruence**

between external and internal perceptions in the present—that is, discrepancies between a person's actual experience and his or her picture of that experience.

7. Many problems experienced by people today are societal or systemic rather than interpersonal or intrapersonal. Deprivation, limited access to resources, and chronic oppression due to gender, race, ethnicity, class, or sexual orientation can create psychological problems. People are capable of learning to effect choices and changes from within the system as well as from without.

EXERCISE 1.1 ■ Review the seven assumptions just listed. Do you find that you strongly disagree, disagree, agree, or strongly agree with each assumption? How would you change each assumption and why? What would you add? Which assumption do you have the most difficulty accepting, and how would that affect how you work with people? Which populations do you think these assumptions may or may not apply to? As people in your group share their agree/disagree statements, identify those with whom you agree or disagree. You may want to have small-group discussions of each assumption, dividing into strongly disagree, disagree, agree, and strongly agree groupings; reconvene as a whole to discuss the similarities and differences you discover.

Now let's do an exercise that will help you clarify some of your own values in relation to helping.

EXERCISE 1.2 ■ For each question, rank your response: SD (strongly disagree), D (disagree), A (agree), SA (strongly agree). When you have completed the questions, go over all of your answers and look for patterns. At the conclusion of the exercise, each member of the group can share something he or she has learned about himself or herself, without necessarily revealing all of his or her answers.

1. It would be most difficult for me to work with
    a. a person 60–80 years old
    b. a person 40–60 years old
    c. a person 20–40 years old
    d. a person 15–20 years old

2. I would most prefer to work with
    a. a high school student
    b. a middle-aged person
    c. a college student
    d. an elderly person

3. It would be most difficult for me to work with
    a. a person from a different culture
    b. a person of a different sexual orientation
    c. a person of an obviously different socioeconomic class
    d. a person with an obvious physical handicap

4. I would have difficulty working with someone who confessed to
   a. lying
   b. cheating
   c. promiscuous sexual relations
   d. heavy drug use

5. I am most comfortable working with people who are
   a. verbally articulate
   b. actively gesturing
   c. quietly attentive
   d. challengingly resistant

6. My overall helping style is probably
   a. fairly directive
   b. fairly nondirective
   c. somewhere in between directive and nondirective
   d. all of the above, depending on my mood and the context

7. I am most comfortable with people who are
   a. independent and able to take responsibility for themselves
   b. helpless and needing my direction
   c. resistant to being helped
   d. insistent on egalitarian collaboration

8. I am most comfortable talking about
   a. sexual matters
   b. money matters
   c. pain and loss
   d. death

9. I feel uncomfortable expressing feelings involving
   a. loving
   b. hating
   c. resentment
   d. failure

10. I consider myself to be
    a. self-controlled
    b. spontaneous
    c. forgiving
    d. unable to forget past slights

11. For me the most important of the following values is
    a. security
    b. freedom
    c. social recognition
    d. affiliation

12. The statement that most closely fits my own beliefs is
    a. Cleanliness is next to godliness.
    b. Honor thy father and thy mother.

    c. A stitch in time saves nine.

    d. Do unto others as you would have them do unto you.

13. For me the most important of the following values is

    a. happiness

    b. inner harmony

    c. mature love

    d. success

14. It is difficult for me to

    a. let things take their own course

    b. take action and responsibility for getting what I think is necessary

    c. let someone else take the initiative

    d. share equal responsibility with others

15. I believe

    a. there is one universal set of moral values

    b. moral values are individual

    c. moral values should be taught outside the family

    d. helpers should teach moral values

The human relations counseling model also emphasizes the mutual identification by the helper and the helpee of goals, objectives, and intervention strategies whose success can ultimately be evaluated according to the observable behavioral change in the helpee. It is understood that treatment environmental factors may restrict the achievement of all of these goals. The model represents an **eclectic** approach in that it uses a variety of counseling techniques and strategies to effect change, but the major vehicle for change remains the development and maintenance of a warm, personally involved, empathic relationship.

The helper is encouraged to learn about the systems (contexts) in which helpees live and function. In addition, the helper is encouraged to learn when and how to use different techniques and strategies and to use different approaches with the same helpee to deal with as many areas of concern as possible within the cognitive, affective, and behavioral domains. The goals of helping are to integrate those three domains, to aid the helpee to become emotionally and cognitively aware of his or her responsibilities and choices, and to see that awareness translated into action. When helpees are able to assume responsibility for their feelings, thoughts, and actions and to reduce the contradictions among them, they are able to feel good about themselves and about the world and make choices that reflect the integration of internal and external variables. They are then able to behave proactively rather than reactively in their relationship systems.

As previously stated, the helping relationship is considered to be the essential foundation of the helping process no matter how much time is allowed by the treatment organization. And it is the **process** of verbal and nonverbal communication, not the **content,** on which that relationship is based. As long as there is an effective helping relationship that communicates to the helpee the helper's capacity for understanding, humanness, and strength to resist manipulation, there is a safe, protective environment allowing flexibility in selection and use of strategies.

Strategies are secondary to the helping relationship. In fact, research indicates that client variables and counselor variables are more significant than technique variables in the helping process. (Helper and helpee variables will be elaborated in Chapter 2.) If a particular strategy does not work but the helping relationship is solid, the helping process is not likely to be negatively affected.

For example, if you have developed a trustful relationship with a helpee and you ask her to dialogue (Gestalt technique; see Chapter 7) with her mother—taking both roles to become more aware of her positive and negative feelings toward her mother—and she is unable to do it, she will not think you are weird or incompetent for having tried this strategy. If she trusts and respects you, you might explore with her the feelings that emerged as a result of her inability to complete the exercise. You then can continue to explore with her, seeking strategies that will be more helpful. This type of helping relationship is reciprocal, in that the helper is considered an equal of the helpee rather than an expert or a magician.

"Equal" in this sense means that social distance is minimal and the responsibility for what occurs is mutual; both people work together toward achieving agreed-on objectives. At the same time, the helper must be able to communicate to clients an understanding of human behavior and have the skills to help clients change their behaviors. The helping relationship serves to increase the helpee's self-understanding and self-exploration, but it does not provide false reassurance and support. Rather, it is honest and allows for expression of the discomfort and pain that may be involved in the helping process. This honesty enables helpers to tolerate their own and the helpees' discomfort without needing to cover it up with sympathy and distancing.

The major implications of the human relations counseling model for helpers are that it

1. Defines empathic communication skills as the core of effective human relationships

2. Stresses that empathic communication skills can be taught to all helpers in all types of helping relationships

3. Provides room for diversity and flexibility so helpers can learn a variety of intervention strategies that can be effective if a successful helping relationship is developed and maintained

4. Modifies and integrates a variety of established approaches and strategies

5. Provides the versatility and flexibility necessary to meet the needs of a multicultural heterogeneous population

6. Provides for dealing with feelings, thoughts, and behaviors in a short-term, practical manner relating to the helpee's life

7. Focuses on the positive rather than negative aspects of the helpee's life (that is, on those aspects one can change rather than those over which one has no control)

8. Assists the helpee to actively assume responsibility for living and for decision making

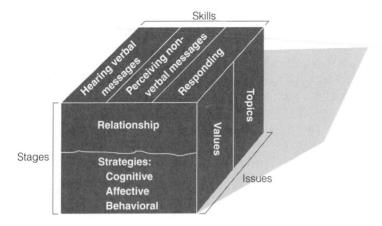

FIGURE 1.2 The counseling model in dimensional terms

Dimensions of the Model

The human relations counseling model has three integrated dimensions: stages, skills, and issues (see Figure 1.2). Outlining a counseling model in diagrammatic form necessitates some formalizing and systematizing that seems rigid and arbitrary. However, this multidimensional view is useful in conceptualizing what happens in and what constitutes effective helping. It thereby provides a useful framework for learning about counseling and developing necessary skills. Naturally, the helper will modify or redesign this conceptual model into whatever form works for him or her.

The First Dimension The first dimension comprises the two stages of the helping process described earlier. These two intertwining stages consist of the following steps:

1. Relationship (development of rapport, trust, honesty, empathy)
   a. Initiation/entry
   b. Identification and clarification of problems being presented
   c. Agreement on structure/contract for helping relationship
   d. Intensive exploration of problems
   e. Definition of possible (depending on treatment-setting policies) goals and objectives of helping relationship
2. Strategies (work)
   a. Mutual acceptance of defined goals and objectives of helping relationship
   b. Planning of strategies
   c. Use of strategies
   d. Evaluation of strategies
   e. Termination
   f. Follow-up

The thesis of this book is that the development of a warm, trustful relationship between the helper and the helpee underlies any strategy or approach to the helping process and therefore is a basic condition for the success of any helping process. Naturally, this relationship depends on one's theoretical view of people, behavior, the world, and helping. Developing a relationship is a time consuming process; however, a skilled helper can guide this development so that the relationship can aid the helpee within a short period of time. This is critical for short-term, problem-focused, managed service delivery.

Development of rapport starts with the initial contact between the helper and the helpee. A climate is provided for the helpee to explore problems and to begin to identify underlying as well as apparent concerns. Later, the client begins to understand those concerns and their implications for living and starts to clarify his or her needs and expectations of the helping relationship to facilitate self-exploration, self-understanding, and choices of action. The success of the helping relationship is crucial to the mutual determination of appropriate goals and objectives.

Once the goals and objectives have been mutually decided on, the helper reviews all available effective strategies (or courses of action for effective helping) and discusses with the helpee the rationale for choosing a particular strategy. The possible consequences and ramifications of any strategy are explored. When agreement on a course of action is reached, the helper applies the strategy, keeping his or her mind open to modifying or refining it, depending on the needs of the helpee. Evaluation of the effectiveness of the chosen strategy must be continual.

Ideally, termination (the cessation of the helping process) occurs once the outcomes agreed on by both helper and helpee have been achieved. Today, however, the helper and helpee may know from the outset how many visits they can have, and termination will be acknowledged and planned for in the first meeting. After the relationship is terminated, many helpers informally or formally check up on the progress of the helpee. This follow-up may result in closure, a decision to schedule a "booster shot" visit, or a decision to work on another set of objectives and goals. Ward (1984) conceptualizes three major functions of the termination process in situations where time allows the helper and helpee to determine the course and ending of the helping process: (1) assessing helpee readiness for the end of the helping relationship; (2) bringing about appropriate closure of the helping relationship; and (3) maximizing the helpee's self-reliance and confidence to maintain change after the helping relationship has ended. Successful termination implies that the relationship and problem-solving skills the helpee has learned during the helping process will be applied to future relationships and problems. Hence, the process of letting go and achieving closure in relationships is just as important as the process of developing a new relationship. Unfortunately, time-limit pressures sometimes cause helpers to overlook this important process.

The Second Dimension   The second dimension of the counseling model represents communication skills: hearing verbal messages, perceiving nonverbal messages, and responding to verbal and nonverbal messages. Verbal messages are the apparent and underlying cognitive and affective content of the helpee's statements. Understanding the implicit and explicit content is usually secondary in importance to understanding the feelings communicated by the helpee. Nonverbal messages are conveyed by body language (posture, gestures, eye contact), vocal tone, facial expression, and other cues that accompany verbal messages. The helper learns to recognize inconsistencies between verbal and nonverbal messages and to develop the helpee's awareness of those inconsistencies. Responding requires immediate, genuine, concrete, and empathic reaction to verbal and nonverbal messages. Both the apparent and underlying significances of messages as well as their relationships and inconsistencies determine appropriate responses.

These communication skills are required to effect the two stages of helping that constitute the first dimension. The model assumes consistency between the helper's verbal and nonverbal messages. It also relies on the helper's ability to respond to the helpee by clarifying the latter's underlying feelings and thoughts so as to increase the helpee's self-understanding.

By developing communication skills, helpers also develop their own self-awareness. As they learn to use their intuitive feelings as guidelines for hearing other people's messages, they sharpen their helping skills. Helpers are always decoding the apparent message by asking themselves, What is this person really trying to say to me? What is she or he really feeling? Then they try to communicate their understanding of the message and feeling back to the helpee.

The Third Dimension The third dimension of the counseling model represents issues, which are the values and cognitive topics that cut across the other two dimensions. These issues involve not only the ways an individual relates to others and to his or her environment, but also such subjects as sexism, racism, heterosexism, ageism, and poverty. Furthermore, this dimension includes professional matters of ethics, training, and practice, as well as the personal values and attitudes of the helper.

These significant issues affect both stages of helping. By exposing and clarifying them, helpers are able to achieve the type of helping relationship in which they do not interfere with helping. Responsive listening skills are effective techniques for clarifying and understanding these issues.

To effect values clarification, the helper and the helpee both must take responsibility for their own attitudes, beliefs, and values. For example, a counselor who tells a female client that she should not think about returning to work until her child is in school is allowing his or her sexist values to distort or interfere with counseling. If helpers are not aware of their own biases, the effects may be harmful. However, if they recognize their biases, they will be less likely to impose them on clients. Research has shown that helpers do communicate their values to helpees, regardless of whether they do so consciously. Bringing those values into the open and being constantly aware of them can keep helpers from imposing them on others.

EXERCISE 1.3 ■ With a partner or in a small group, discuss what thoughts and feelings you might experience as a helper counseling the following clients: (1) a 14-year-old pregnant girl who wants an abortion without her parents' knowing; (2) a married man who confides that he has had several homosexual extramarital affairs; (3) a 26-year-old man living at home with his parents who refuses to get a job or take responsibility for himself; (4) a recently separated mother who wants to have her drug-addicted boyfriend move in with her and her young children so that she can "help him" get better; (5) a lesbian couple who want to have a child. How do you think your true thoughts and feelings might influence the counseling process? What kinds of things would you want to say and do? What differences emerge in your group, and how do you feel about them? What have you learned about yourself and others?

Some of the current concerns affecting the helping process include how to help involuntary, reluctant, and/or at-risk clients; how to help people we really dislike; and how to deal with complex ethical issues such as informed consent, confidentiality, and abuse of power. Also, the helper's responsibility to the sponsoring institution can lead to conflicts of interest and ethical infractions such as keeping clients longer than necessary to maintain a census count and/or unrealistically trying to squeeze services into a limited time frame. The question becomes, whose needs take priority—the helper's, the helpee's, the institution's, or the insurance company's? These ethical issues will be discussed in Chapter 10.

The human relations counseling model will be discussed throughout the book. Chapter 2 defines and illustrates effective and ineffective helping relationships. Chapter 3 presents materials for developing techniques for effective communication. Chapter 4 explores the relationship stage in depth, and Chapters 5 and 6 present an overview of theoretical approaches that relate to the strategies discussed in Chapter 7. Chapter 8 explores the application of strategies, and Chapter 9 presents crisis and disaster theories and intervention. Chapter 10 gives a brief overview of issues affecting the helping process and a final postscript summarizing the entire model.

Interspersed within these chapters are case materials and exercises designed to provide you with an opportunity to use your conceptual and practical understanding of the material covered in the text. Exercises can be completed as in-class or homework assignments and discussed in supervised group settings.

SUMMARY

The intent of this book is to provide an introduction to the fundamental skills and knowledge necessary for effective helping relationships. These are needed, to varying degrees, by nonprofessional, generalist, and professional human services workers to develop and maintain satisfactory and helpful interpersonal relationships.

We began this chapter by describing the shifts that have occurred within helping professions. We then described the impact of technology and complex social change on individuals and families. The confusion and problems emanating from those changes can heighten anxiety and feelings of alienation and helplessness; hence our focus on how individuals can help themselves and others to feel less alienated and powerless by improving their own interpersonal relationships. If helpers achieve quality interpersonal relations in their own lives, they can model their skills in the helping relationship and teach others to improve the quality of relationships. Counseling, one type of helping interaction and an important part of human services, is used to demonstrate how to build an effective relationship.

The purpose of the helping relationship was defined as assisting clients to achieve greater self-acceptance and self-esteem and to gain control over their behavior and decisions. The relationship is based on the communication of empathy and application of appropriate strategies. Thus, the human relations counseling model consists of three equally important and interdependent dimensions: stages (relationship and strategies), skills, and issues. The helping process depends absolutely on the development of a trustful relationship between helper and helpee. Effective communication skills enhance that relationship and also provide a way of dealing with controversial issues. Strategies are the various approaches that helpers use to promote self-exploration, understanding, and behavior change in helpees, which in turn lead to heightened self-acceptance and responsibility. The strategies aim to increase the helpee's awareness and successful functioning in the affective (feeling), behavioral (doing), and cognitive (thinking) domains. Ideally, termination occurs when both helper and helpee feel that the helpee has resolved and worked through his or her concerns and can apply what has been learned from the helping relationship to future situations and relationships.

REFERENCES AND
FURTHER READING

Carkhuff, R. (2000a). *The art of helping* (8th ed.). Amherst, MA: Human Resource Development Press.

Carkhuff, R. (2000b). *Trainer's guide to the art of helping.* Amherst, MA: Human Resource Development Press.

Carter, R. C. (1995). *The influence of race and racial identity in psychotherapy: Toward a racially inclusive model.* New York: Wiley.

Comas-Diaz, L., & Greene, B. (Eds.). (1994). *Women of color: Integrating ethnic and gender identities in psychotherapy.* New York: Guilford Press.

Consumers value psychotherapy. (1996, January 2). *Boston Globe,* p. 4.

Convention boredom. (2000, August 7). *New York Times,* p. 2.

Corey, G. (2005). *Theory and practice of counseling and psychotherapy* (7th ed.). Belmont, CA: Brooks/Cole.

Gordon, T. (2000). *Parent effectiveness training* (3rd ed.). New York: Wyden.

Ivey, A. E., D'Andrea, M., Ivey, M. B. & Simek-Morgan, L. (2002). *Theories of counseling and psychotherapy: A multicultural perspective* (5th ed.). Boston: Allyn & Bacon.

Ivey, A. E., & Ivey, M. B. (1999). *Intentional interviewing and counseling: Facilitating client development* (4th ed.). Pacific Grove, CA: Brooks/Cole.

Kessler, R. (2005). Treating psychological problems in medical settings: Primary care as the de facto mental health system and the role of hypnosis. *International Journal of Clinical and Experimental Hypnosis, 53*(3), 290–305.

Knoff, H. (1986). Identifying and classifying children and adolescents referred for personality assessment. In H. Knoff (Ed.), *The assessment of child and adolescent personality* (pp. 1–28). New York: Guilford Press.

Kottler, J. (2004). *Introduction to therapeutic counseling: Voices from the field.* Pacific Grove, CA: Brooks/Cole.

Lakoff, G. (2004). *Edge: A talk by George Lakoff.* Retrieved February 27, 2006, from www.edge.org/3rdlakoff/lakoff/p.rhmtl

Lewis, T., Amini, F., & Lannon, R. (2000). *A general theory of love.* New York: Random House.

Mental health: Does therapy help? (1995, November). *Consumer Reports, 734*–739.

Mirkin, M., Suyemoto, K., & Okun, B. F. (Eds.). (2005). *Women and psychotherapy: Exploring identities in diverse contexts.* New York: Guilford Press.

Murphy, B. C., & Dillon, C. (2003). *Interviewing in action: Relationship, process and change.* (2nd ed.). Pacific Grove, CA: Brooks/Cole.

Okun, B. F., Fried, J., & Okun, M. L. (1999). *Understanding diversity: A learning-as-practice primer.* Pacific Grove, CA: Brooks/Cole.

Okun, B. F. (2004). Human diversity. In R. H. Coombs (Ed.), *Family therapy review: Preparing for comprehensive and licensing examinations* (pp. 122–153). Mahwah, NJ: Erlbaum.

Ratey, J. (2001). *A user's guide to the brain.* New York: Random House.

Rogers, C. (Ed.). (1967). *The therapeutic relationship and its impact.* Madison: University of Wisconsin Press.

Satcher, D. (1999). *Mental health: A report of the surgeon general.* Washington, DC: U.S. Department of Health and Human Services, National Institute of Mental Health.

Stewart, B. A., & Okun, B. F. (2005). Healthy living, healthy women. In M. P. Mirkin, K. L. Suyemoto, & B. F. Okun (Eds.), *Psychotherapy with women: Exploring diverse contexts and identities* (pp. 313–334). New York: Guilford Press.

Sue, D. W. (2002). *Counseling the culturally diverse: Theory and practice* (4th ed.). New York: Wiley.

Sue, D. W. (2005). *Multicultural social work practice.* New York: Wiley.

Sue, D. W., Ivey, A. E., & Pedersen, P. (1996). *A theory of multicultural counseling and therapy.* Pacific Grove, CA: Brooks/Cole.

Suyemoto, K. L., & Kim, G. S. (2005). Journeys through diverse terrains: Multiple identities and social contexts in individual therapy. In M. P. Mirkin, K. L. Suyemoto, & B. F. Okun (Eds.), *Psychotherapy with women: Exploring diverse contexts and identities* (pp. 9–41). New York: Guilford Press.

Ward, D. E. (1984). Termination of individual counseling: Concepts and strategies. *Journal of Counseling and Development, 63*(11), 21–26.

Visit the book companion site at www.thomsonedu.com to access tutorial quizzes.

2

The Helping
Relationship

This chapter provides a description of helping relationships, with particular emphasis on (1) the helping context, (2) empirically validated helper characteristics, and (3) the importance of communication for any helping relationship. Having an overall view of what occurs in a helping relationship will increase your understanding of subsequent chapters, in which we begin to talk about and practice helping skills and theoretical knowledge and see how they interrelate.

The purpose of a helping relationship is to meet the needs of the helpee, not those of the helper. The setting of the helping relationship may impose some constraints on this, but the relationship is meant largely to enable helpees to assume responsibility for themselves and make their own decisions based on self-awareness and expanded alternatives and approaches. Helpers neither solve helpees' problems nor reassure them merely to make them feel better.

Helpers assist and support helpees so they can come to terms with their problems by exploration, understanding, and action. For instance, if an employee comes to you in your position as a human resources worker and says he or she cannot continue working for a particular supervisor, you may, after exploration, focus on helping the employee learn to get along better in that work setting. On the other hand, helping this employee may well involve some direct form of environmental rearranging or systems change. If, in this instance, exploration determines that the supervisor is the source of the trouble and is hampering the employee's contributions to production or service, you may focus on transferring the employee to a more suitable setting, or on working directly with the supervisor to improve relations, or both. An effective helping situation does not involve doing something to someone else to make him or her better; it does involve working together to seek the best solution for that person (after considering all feasible alternatives) and, if possible, to implement that solution.

A helping relationship that benefits the helpee is a mutual learning process between the helpee and one or more other persons. The effectiveness of the relationship depends on (1) the helper's skill in communicating his or her understanding of the helpee's feelings, worldview, and behaviors; (2) the helper's ability to determine and clarify the helpee's problem; and (3) the helper's ability to apply appropriate helping strategies to facilitate the recipient's self-exploration, self-understanding, problem solving, and decision making, all of which can lead to constructive action on the part of the helpee.

KINDS OF HELPING RELATIONSHIPS

There are different kinds of helping relationships—although all are similar in concept and strategies used—corresponding to the three categories of helpers discussed in Chapter 1. There are professional relationships (doctor/patient, pastor/congregant, counselor/client, social worker/client) for which the helper has received intensive formal training in human behavior, problem solving, and communication related to helping. There are general human services relationships (employment interviewer/applicant, case aide/client, street worker/youth, teacher/student, recreation leader/youth, human resources specialist/employee, probation officer/probationer, mental health assistant/client) for which the helper has received short-term formal training such as courses or workshops in human relations. And there are nonprofessional helping relationships (receptionist/ customer, salesperson/customer, flight attendant/passenger, supervisor/employee, volunteer/client) in which the helping process may be incidental to the relationship.

Within these three categories a distinction can also be made between formal and informal relationships (see Figure 2.1). Formal situations are ones in which the helper/helpee roles are stated or implied by position or contract and the specific reason for contact is known to be for the provision of some kind of help. Informal helping occurs when the helping relationship is secondary to another relationship, whether formal or informal: principal/teacher, friend/friend. Formal relationships usually occur in an institutional setting such as an office, school, prison, or hospital; informal relationships can occur in any place—between friends, relatives, neighbors, or peers in an office, home, school, or hospital. One may see less structure, shorter time involvement, and more limited expectations for problem solving as relationships become less formal.

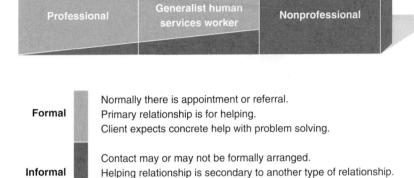

Formal	Normally there is appointment or referral. Primary relationship is for helping. Client expects concrete help with problem solving.
Informal	Contact may or may not be formally arranged. Helping relationship is secondary to another type of relationship. Client may not expect help with problem solving.

FIGURE 2.1 Kinds of helping relationships

HOW HELPING RELATIONSHIPS DEVELOP

Helping relationships begin with a helper and a helpee meeting to focus attention on the helpee's concerns. Thus, a helping relationship is distinct from other relationships in this focus on only one party's concerns and issues. However, it shares ingredients common to all satisfactory relationships—ingredients such as trust, empathy, genuineness, concern and caring, respect, tolerance and acceptance, honesty, commitment to the relationship, and dependability. These ingredients are not usually present at the beginning of a relationship but develop over time as people get to know one another. If trust does not develop, the other ingredients will dwindle and the relationship will eventually terminate. Trust is established when an individual perceives and believes that the other person in the relationship will not mislead or harm him or her in any way.

Figure 2.2 shows the helping relationship in its primary form. The helper and the helpee are always engaged in mutual communication. The principal difference between them is that the helper possesses some skills and knowledge (expertise) and the helpee possesses some concerns (problems). Put any names in the circles and put the circles in any context; the relationship will remain essentially the same. Note that helper and helpee each come to the relationship with a set of expectations, needs, values, beliefs, and skills. The degree of congruence between those two sets can affect the relationship either positively or negatively. The principals are both influenced by such variables as their gender, race, ethnicity, class, sexual orientation, geographical region from which they come, and age. However, if the helper's trustworthiness, empathy, nonjudgmentalness, and tolerance can be communicated effectively, the possibility of adverse or nonhelpful outcomes from individual differences will be lessened. The helping relationship is embedded in many contexts: sociocultural, political,

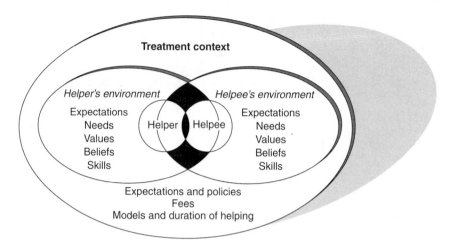

FIGURE 2.2 The helping relationship in its primary form

economic, organizational. The managed health care context, for example, requires that helpers possess expert communication skills so as to establish rapport and formulate objectives expediently. A counselor or resident aide in a dormitory may have weeks or months to develop rapport with students, whereas a counselor in a mental health agency may have only one or two sessions.

WHAT MAKES A HELPER EFFECTIVE?

The successful helper is familiar with many approaches and strategies. Having a broad range of alternatives enables helpers to select those strategies most likely to meet the needs of a particular client or client system. When the selected strategies are applied, they are filtered through the unique personality of the helper. In other words, each person's perceptions, attitudes, thoughts, and feelings affect his or her interpretation and application of the theory. In fact, it is often said that the personal attributes of helpers are more important than their strategic skills. Although some basic counseling skills and strategies seem universal in application, helpers must adapt their counseling style to achieve congruence with the value systems of culturally diverse clients. Sensitivity to the nuances and implications of cultural variables is necessary if one is to be effective with clients from a variety of backgrounds.

The helper's personal values influence significantly the effectiveness of a helping relationship. Our attitudes and feelings about kinds of people—what is "good" or "bad," what is acceptable or unacceptable, what is important for choices, and what makes people tick—lay the foundation for our value system. Thus, it is necessary for helpers to become aware of their underlying beliefs as well as their value systems in order to aid helpees in clarifying their own. And it is important to understand that our value system is shaped by the views of our culture about gender, race, ethnicity, sexual orientation, class, family system, geographical region, and so on. We cannot overemphasize the point that if you are aware of your own values you are less likely to impose them indirectly on others. Exposing clients to different value systems may be helpful; imposing values on clients is not helpful. Becoming aware of other people's value systems will help you understand, appreciate, and accept differences between your value system and others'.

A fuller treatment of the impact of cultural values on one's identity development, functioning, and lifestyle will be presented in Chapter 10, but we need to be aware of the significance of these variables from the very beginning of our discussion about effective helping. At different times of our lives, in different situations or contexts, any of these variables can have different salience with regard to our sense of who we are and who we are in relationships, as well as our views of the world in which we live.

To be comfortable applying a variety of helping strategies, the helper must be able to communicate with others in the **affective** domain (relating to feelings or emotion), the **cognitive** domain (relating to thinking or intellectual processes), and the **behavioral** domain (relating to action or deeds). By extension, the helper must teach the client to function more effectively in all three interrelated domains. Therefore, helpers must continually deepen their self-understanding in all three domains; they need to become aware of and clarify their own social, economic, and cultural values in order to recognize and separate their needs and problems from those of their clients. The strategy selected for formally helping a particular client may depend on the helper's assessment of deficits in a particular domain (affective, cognitive, or behavioral) as well as the helper's theoretical perspective. It may also be mandated by the treatment context.

EFFECTIVE COMMUNICATION
BEHAVIORS

Regardless of the setting or nature of the helping relationship, the personal values and beliefs of the people involved, the domain selected, or the theoretical orientation of the professional helper, the underlying prerequisite skill in any effective helping relationship is empathic communication. The level of trust between helper and helpee during the first stage of helping, the relationship stage, is developed using communication skills within an empathic context. **Empathy,** defined as both understanding another person's emotions and feelings from that person's frame of reference and conveying that understanding, is vital to the effectiveness of communication skills. Empathic communication skills leading to trust, then, are essential to the effectiveness of the whole helping process. Likewise, teaching empathic communication skills is an essential component of working with couples, families, organizational systems, and just about any human relations setting.

Helpers need to remember that there are cultural differences in the ways groups express empathy; in other words, what may be empathic behavior for one helpee (i.e., eye contact, touching) may *not* be so for another. Selection of strategies should be influenced by cultural factors.

How can we help people if we cannot learn their concerns and impart to them our feelings or thoughts? Both processes depend on the ability to communicate. Communication in this sense means the helper's capacity to listen, pay attention, perceive, and respond verbally and nonverbally to the helpee in such a way as to demonstrate to her or him that the helper has attended, listened, and accurately perceived. It means responding as opposed to reacting. This ability can be learned by most people, whatever their educational background or personality. It is a skill that requires continual practice, as does any other type of skill. Not surprisingly, the people considered by others to be most helpful in formal or informal settings possess good communication skills.

Research (cited in Brammer & MacDonald, 2003; Carter, 1995; Corey, 2005; Ivey, D'Andrea, Ivey, & Simek-Morgan, 2002; Sue, 2002) indicates that communication problems are the major source of interpersonal difficulties. For example, most marital, work, and family problems stem from interpersonal misunderstanding, from ineffective communication, which results in frustration and anger when implicit expectations and desires are not fulfilled. These communication problems impair problem solving. And a major problem of those who seek professional help is their inability to recognize and communicate their problems or concerns.

Many people think they know what their problem is but have difficulty in verbally communicating their concerns. Others are able to verbalize their concerns but need help in identifying the underlying problem. Still others do not even recognize that they have a problem and are what one might call "reluctant clients," in that they are required to seek help. In all cases, good verbal and nonverbal communication is essential to both stages of the helping process. Therefore, it is necessary to look closely at the process (a sequence of events that takes place over a period of time) of communication within helping relationships—at the behaviors that encourage and impede communication.

Most of us have been helpees on numerous occasions; so, based on our own experience, we should be able to recognize helpers' behaviors that have aided or hindered our receiving help. If you were asked to list those verbal and nonverbal behaviors that you, as the helpee, found supportive in any kind of helping relationship, what would your list look like? Table 2.1 lists behaviors typically cited by beginning counseling students. Most students think of more verbal behaviors than nonverbal ones. See whether you agree with these lists or can add to them.

The lists in Table 2.1 indicate that students consider helping relationships to be most effective when helpers show listening and attending behaviors that communicate empathy, encouragement, support, honesty, caring, concern,

TABLE 2.1 Helpful behaviors

Verbal	Nonverbal
Uses understandable words	Maintains good eye contact
Reflects back and clarifies helpee's statements	Occasional head nodding
Appropriately interprets	Facial animation
Summarizes for helpee	Occasional smiling
Responds to primary message	Occasional hand gesturing
Uses verbal reinforcers (for example, "Mm-hm," "I see," "Yes")	Close physical proximity to helpee
	Moderate rate of speech
Calls helpee by helpee's preferred name	Body leans toward helpee
Appropriately gives information	Occasional touching as appropriate
Answers questions about self as appropriate	Relaxed, open posture
Uses humor occasionally to reduce tension	Confident vocal tone
Is nonjudgmental and respectful	
Adds greater understanding to helpee's statement	
Phrases interpretations tentatively so as to elicit genuine feedback from helpee	

respect, sharing, affection, protection, potency, and nonjudgmental acceptance. Clients are helped because they feel worthwhile as human beings, feel accepted by another human being, and are therefore permitted to be their true selves and to explore their true concerns.

Similarly, you can undoubtedly recognize unhelpful communication behaviors.

Would you add to or change the lists presented in Table 2.2? These verbal and nonverbal behaviors involve inattentiveness, imposition of the helper's values and beliefs on the helpee, judgment, and "I-know-what's-best-for-you" or "I'm-better-than-you" attitudes. These behaviors are hindrances because they can put helpees on the defensive immediately and lead to their feeling worthless and choosing avoidance rather than approach behaviors.

EXERCISE 2.1 ■ Generate a list of helpful and unhelpful responses that you personally have experienced in specific situations—for example, when a significant relationship ended; when you received a low grade on a paper or exam; when you didn't get a desired job or were not accepted into a specific school; when someone close to you moved away, became ill, or died; when you were sick or in an accident; or when you wrecked your car. After you have identified particular responses, ask yourself why they were helpful or unhelpful. In small or large groups, share your findings and discuss why a response may be helpful to one person but not another.

TABLE 2.2 Nonhelpful behaviors

Verbal	Nonverbal
Interrupting	Looking away from helpee
Giving advice	Sitting far away or turned away from helpee
Preaching	
Placating	Sneering
Blaming	Frowning
Cajoling	Scowling
Exhorting	Tight mouth
Extensive probing and questioning, especially "why" questions	Shaking pointed finger
	Distracting gestures
Directing, demanding	Yawning
Patronizing attitude	Closing eyes
Overinterpretation	Unpleasant tone of voice
Using words or jargon helpee doesn't understand	Rate of speech too slow or too fast
Straying from topic	Acting rushed
Intellectualizing	Looking repeatedly at watch or clock
Overanalyzing	Playing with a pen or paperclip
Talking about self too much	
Minimizing or disbelieving	

EXERCISE 2.2 ■ Divide into triads of helper, helpee, and observer. The requisite materials for this exercise are crayons, large drawing sheets, and a blindfold for each triad. Each member of the triad should experience each role. The helpee is blindfolded and helped to draw a picture by the helper. It is important that each helper decide how best to help in his or her own way. The observer writes down all verbal and nonverbal behaviors and, after each member of the triad has been a helpee, the group works together to produce a list of helpful and unhelpful verbal and nonverbal behaviors. Again, discuss why a particular behavior was helpful to one person and not to another. What was comfortable and uncomfortable for you as a helper? What did you learn about your helping behaviors? What do you think you might want to change? How did you feel as a helpee? What did you find helpful and unhelpful? What was it like to be an observer?

EXERCISE 2.3 ■ To identify helpful and unhelpful nonverbal behaviors, take turns playing charades. The helpee will verbally communicate an issue or concern or describe a situation. The helper will nonverbally attempt to help. Observers will identify those nonverbal behaviors that were helpful and those that were unhelpful and discuss their observations with the helpee and helper. The helpee will also give feedback on what was experienced as helpful or unhelpful.

The purpose of Exercises 2.4 through 2.8 is to determine whether you can recognize what is effective and what is not effective communication in a helping relationship. Read each exercise and rank the helper's responses on a 0–5 scale (0 = least helpful, 5 = most helpful) before reading the text comments and discussing your fellow students' reactions. Obviously, you can respond only to the verbal content of the interactions. Comments on the exercises are found at the end of the chapter. Please remember that there are usually no right or wrong answers to the exercises in this book. They should be used as a focus for discussion of people's differences in perceptions and responses. If you want additional practice in learning communication skills, you can act out these case interactions in class.

EXERCISE 2.4 ■ Ms. James is a 26-year-old data entry clerk in the billing department of a large insurance firm. She has worked there for 16 months, and her overall annual job evaluation rating was "Fair." Specific comments that contributed to this rating were "late for work," "does not accept criticism well," and "scowls when asked to correct and reenter data." Ms. James has come into the Human Resources (HR) office to request a job change.

1. **HR counselor:** I see, Ms. James, that you haven't been doing too well in the billing department. What's going on down there?

   Ms. James: Mr. Barber is very difficult to work for. He picks on everything I do, and I just know he doesn't like me.

2. **HR counselor:** Well, Mr. Barber thinks that your attitude is poor and that you are not doing your work as quickly or as accurately as he needs it.

   Ms. James: I'm doing it as well as I can. I'm much faster than the other people in the office, and he never picks on them. Why doesn't he leave me alone? He always hovers over my desk. (*shudders*)

3. **HR counselor:** Look, Ms. James, we both know that data entry jobs are tight now and that you need to work. With such a poor reference from Mr. Barber, I couldn't possibly place you anywhere else in this company. Try real hard in the next couple of months to do better and then, after your 18-month evaluation, we'll see what we can do.

   Ms. James: (*sighing*) OK. I guess I'm stuck. I still don't think I can ever make him like me, though.

How would you rate each of the HR counselor's (helper's) statements? (Write a number from the scale in the answer blank for each statement.)

1. _____   2. _____   3. _____

What were the reasons for your ratings? What verbal behaviors from Tables 2.1 and 2.2 can you identify? What would you have said if you were the HR counselor? How do you think Ms. James was feeling during this session? What was the personnel clerk doing? What do you think the problem really was—and whose problem was it? These are the kinds of questions we continually ponder when participating in or observing helping relationships. Now look at our comments at the end of the chapter.

EXERCISE 2.5 ■ Ms. Smith is an after-school day-care worker at the local elementary school. One day, while she is supervising the children during their snack break, Tommy runs up to her and angrily accuses Steven of stealing his yogurt. In reviewing the situation, Ms. Smith discovers that Steven has indeed taken and eaten Tommy's yogurt.

1. **Ms. Smith:** Steven, why did you take Tommy's yogurt?
   Steven: I dunno.
2. **Ms. Smith:** Don't you know that it's wrong to steal?
   Steven: Uh-huh.
3. **Ms. Smith:** I'm going to have to tell Mr. Singer about this. You go sit in the corner until he comes back.
   Steven: OK.

How would you rate each of Ms. Smith's statements?

1. _____   2. _____   3. _____

Again, try to determine the reasons for your ratings. What verbal behaviors from Tables 2.1 and 2.2 can you identify? How might you have handled this situation? How do you think Steven feels? How does Ms. Smith feel? What is she doing?

EXERCISE 2.6 ■ Julie, age 22, has come to see her college counselor. She has been married for two years and is seriously contemplating divorce. (This information was given over the telephone to the counselor when the appointment was made.) The following is an excerpt from the middle part of the first session.

1. **Counselor:** Can you tell me about how things are in your marriage now?
   Julie: Pretty bad. He's always working—we never do anything together. We really have nothing to say to each other. I'm so bored I could scream!
2. **Counselor:** Things are pretty tough for you.
   Julie: (*beginning to cry*) He never wants to go anywhere or do anything. He doesn't like to be with people. We don't have any friends together at all.
3. **Counselor:** You feel angry, as if you can't go out and do what you want on your own.
   Julie: Yes. But sometimes I do go out. Like last Sunday I asked Steve if he wanted to go to the ballet with me. I asked him three times. He said no, I should go by myself. I did, too!
4. **Counselor:** Yet you felt bad about leaving him.
   Julie: I don't want to hurt him.
5. **Counselor:** You feel as if you are responsible for him.

Julie: Well, yes, of course . . . everything I do . . . I worry about what's going to happen to him.

6. **Counselor:** Wow! That's quite a burden of responsibility you're carrying around on your shoulders.

Julie: What do you mean?

7. **Counselor:** I was just thinking that it's hard enough to be responsible for oneself. You can be responsible to someone else, but if you take on the responsibility for that person's feelings, thoughts, and actions, that's quite a load! It would scare me.

Julie: Yeah, I see what you mean. But am I not responsible for my husband's feelings?

8. **Counselor:** You tell me.

Julie: Maybe that's why I always feel so hemmed in. I never seem to have any fun.

9. **Counselor:** Tell me about the last time you had fun.

Julie: Last summer I worked as a waitress in a restaurant. It was great. I loved it. I felt so alive, and I was with people all the time. I really loved it.

10. **Counselor:** You seem to miss that a lot.

Julie: I had to stop to go back to school. I didn't want to stop though.

11. **Counselor:** You think a lot about going back to that kind of job.

Julie: Yes, I wish I could. I really liked all the attention I got.

12. **Counselor:** It was exciting to have people notice you and respond to you.

Julie: Um-mm. I don't want to miss it all.

13. **Counselor:** Miss?

Julie: You know, the fun and the excitement . . .

14. **Counselor:** You feel as if you don't have any fun and excitement with Steve.

Julie: That's right. Not for a long time, probably never.

15. **Counselor:** You're really angry at Steve. You feel cheated, as if he is keeping you from having any fun and excitement.

Julie: Yes, that's it. Please, can you help me?

Although this was a rather lengthy excerpt, let's see if you can go through the same process as before and rate each response according to the scale.

1. _____	2. _____	3. _____
4. _____	5. _____	6. _____
7. _____	8. _____	9. _____
10. _____	11. _____	12. _____
13. _____	14. _____	15. _____

You will be able to identify several different verbal behaviors and feelings of both the counselor and the client in this lengthy transcript. What do you think the counselor is doing and why? See if you can trace Julie's feelings through the excerpt.

EXERCISE 2.7 ■ Joaquin, a 16-year-old high school sophomore, is called to his counselor's office. He has received three warnings in academic classes and is in danger of being removed from the school soccer team. Joaquin's mother has called the counselor several times. She wants him to talk with Joaquin and help him see how important it is for him to do well in school.

1. **Counselor:** Joaquin, your mother is very concerned about your grades, and I'm wondering what's going on with you. You know that you're a smart kid, and there really is no reason for you not to be getting at least all B's.

    Joaquin: It's OK. I'm not going to flunk or anything like that. They're just warnings. My mom just worries too much.

2. **Counselor:** Joaquin, come on now. Your parents have every reason to worry because they love you. They've worked very hard since they came to this country, and it means everything to them that you do well so you can go to college. They've been through a lot.

    Joaquin: I know that. But they're always on my back. They just don't understand. I know they love me and want me to go to college. They worry too much. I'm not doing worse than anyone else.

3. **Counselor:** For now, we need to figure out how we can get you through the term. How many hours a day are you studying after soccer practice?

    Joaquin: I dunno, uh, sometimes I forget my homework in the morning, but I always do it. I really don't know what the big deal is.

How would you rate each of the counselor's statements in this excerpt?

1. _____   2. _____   3. _____

EXERCISE 2.8 ■ Mr. Williams, age 32, is seeing his employment counselor about some forthcoming job interviews. He has been laid off for three months and has a wife and two young children to support. He has had several unsuccessful job interviews over the past two months.

Mr. Williams: I'm really uptight. And so's my wife. She gets mad when I come home from these job interviews with no job. "Who's gonna pay the bills?" she asks.

1. **Counselor:** It really is rough to be in your position. Sounds to me like you're pretty worried about the job interviews we've set up.

    Mr. Williams: (*nodding*) Well, I must be doing something wrong. None of them have even given me a chance. I must be a real dud. Why should these be any different?

2. **Counselor:** You really want to be able to do better, and you're worried that maybe you can't.

    Mr. Williams: I don't know. I never used to flub interviews. I get so nervous now.

3. **Counselor:** The tension of being out of work is really affecting everything.

    Mr. Williams: Yes. I think I come on too strong . . . too wound up. You know, it's like I'm trying to please too much. I just can't seem to help it.

4. **Counselor:** Since your next interview is tomorrow, let's take the rest of our time to practice interviewing. It might help you to feel more comfortable.

How would you rate each of the counselor's comments?

1. _____   2. _____   3. _____   4. _____

CHARACTERISTICS OF
EFFECTIVE HELPERS

Now that we've spent some time differentiating between helpful and unhelpful kinds of verbal communication, we can look more specifically at the characteristics of the effective helper. Review the lists of helpful and unhelpful behaviors shown in Tables 2.1 and 2.2, which you may have modified after working through the exercises, and then try to generalize about helpful and unhelpful traits of the effective helper. However, don't be too quick to draw conclusions.

Human relations trainers are aware that students who come into their programs with certain personal attitudes and traits seem to absorb and integrate their academic training with their lifestyle more easily than other students. Yet when we try to identify the traits that support students' progress as helpers, we—both teachers and students—become rather vague. We refer to "emotional maturity," "flexibility," "open-mindedness," "intelligence," "warmth," and "sensitivity"—yet these subjective terms tell us little that we can use directly to promote professional growth.

Professional training traditionally involves the study of the academic disciplines of psychology, sociology, anthropology, and the specialized knowledge and skill areas of counseling. Yet an increasing amount of evidence supports the idea that helpers are only as effective as they are self-aware and able to use themselves as vehicles of change. Therefore, training in academic content and theory may not be as important as training in process, communication skills, and self-knowledge (Brammer & McDonald, 2003; Corey, 2005; Kottler, 2004; Okun, 1989, 1990, 2004; Okun, Fried, & Okun, 1999; Pedersen, 2003; Rogers, 1976). Integration of personal experience with supervised field experience and academic training becomes essential for developing ability as a helper.

What Research Shows

An initial review of theory and research (Carkhuff, 2000a, 2000b; Corey, 2005; Ivey et al., 2002; Rogers, 1958, 1976; Sue, 2002) about helper characteristics can be overwhelming in that we may wonder if "self-actualized" human beings (those who have achieved self-understanding and fulfillment) really exist!

However, if we focus on the commonalities in key research studies, we can identify the characteristics of effective helpers.

The person of the therapist, his/her capacity for continuous growth and self-awareness, openness to others, respect, warmth, interest, and genuineness are considered more important than knowledge and skills. Other qualitative communication components necessary for effective helping include the ability to confront differences, mixed messages, incongruities, and discrepancies between verbal and nonverbal behaviors; the ability to clarify facts and feelings concretely; positive regard; focusing on strengths and positive assets of the helpee; and respect.

It is difficult to assess whether the knowledge base for understanding behavior or the ability to communicate that understanding has greater influence on a helping relationship. It is also important to acknowledge research findings that suggest that empirically validated strategies may not be effective outside the context of a humanistic helping relationship.

Characteristics in Context

Now let's see how the characteristics of the effective helper work in context. We believe that the following qualities, behaviors, and knowledge of helpers are most influential in affecting the behaviors, attitudes, and feelings of helpees. And those qualities, behaviors, and knowledge are the same for professional, generalist human services, and nonprofessional helpers in any context.

Self-Awareness Individuals who continually develop their own self-understanding and self-awareness are more likely to be effective as helpers than those who do not, because they are more able to separate their needs, perceptions, and feelings from those of their clients and are more able to help others develop their own self-awareness. Development of self-awareness also allows helpers to have personal experience of the process of human development, both its pleasant and painful aspects, and to know firsthand the impact of societal, cultural, and familial influences on behavior. Self-awareness can result in more effective use of the self as a vehicle to effect change in the helpee. Helpers who are self-aware continually ask themselves questions such as, What's really going on here? How come I'm feeling this way? Am I really listening to what is being said, or am I projecting my own perceptions and feelings? Whose problem is this—mine or the helpee's?

The following is one example of how self-awareness plays a role in counseling. A counseling intern in a high school is working with a 10th-grade student named Elizabeth. Elizabeth is telling the counseling intern how upset she is with her mother because her mother will not let her date an older boy from another school district.

> **Elizabeth:** I really want to see him. My mother treats me like a baby. She always has to know where I'm going, who with, and what I'm doing. She's driving me crazy! Other kids' mothers are much more trusting.

Counselor: You are angry with your mother for not letting you do what you want to do.

Elizabeth: She's always on my back, always telling me what I can and can't do, always asking a million questions about everything. I just wish she'd leave me alone.

Counselor: I don't blame you for being so angry, Elizabeth. Why don't you just tell her that you're old enough to make your own decisions, particularly about whom you date, and that you want her to leave you alone?

Elizabeth: Do you really think I can do that? Boy, she might really cream me.

Counselor: She has to learn to let you lead your own life.

Remember that this client is a 15-year-old girl! Although she may be experiencing a normal developmental desire for more independence, should she lead her own life? Instead of helping Elizabeth to explore and understand her independence/dependence conflict, the counselor is giving her permission to rebel. A discussion of this excerpt with the counselor made it apparent that the counselor was overidentifying with Elizabeth and putting words into her mouth that she, the counselor, would like to be able to say to her mother. A more self-aware counselor might say to herself, "This sounds familiar to me. I can certainly understand Elizabeth's feelings, but I must be careful not to let my own needs and feelings interfere with hers."

Gender and Cultural Awareness Helpers who are sensitive to the influence of gender and culture on their own perceptions, values, attitudes, and beliefs are likely to be open to the effects of these variables on others. For example, they can appreciate that women and other nondominant populations such as people of color and gays and lesbians have necessarily experienced life differently than have those with Eurocentric values who were born with more privileges and may never have experienced any form of oppression.

Culturally sensitive helpers are likely to be able to understand and feel comfortable with differences between themselves and others—differences of gender, race, sexual orientation, class, and ethnicity; they tend to value rather than denigrate these differences. In other words, they can think and function in what Ivey (1991) terms the "systemic cognitive dimension." They recognize the strong set of Western assumptions underlying helping theories and techniques, and realize that helpees from non-Western cultures may have altogether different perceptions of their problems and what to do about them. Western models are based on individualism, self-sufficiency, autonomy, and competition, whereas many non-Western models value family and community relations over individualism. Thus, helpers know that they may need to modify and adapt traditional views of human development and functioning as well as communication and counseling skills when working with helpees from diverse cultures.

Consider the following example. A job placement counselor describes a night-shift technical job to a recent Russian immigrant, a 34-year-old woman named Anya. The client listens politely and, through an interpreter, explains why she can't consider night work.

> **Anya:** I no can work night. My mother needs me. I must take care my mother.
>
> **Counselor:** You're feeling responsible for your mother, and as much as you need a job, you're not sure how you can do this. It must be difficult for you, being in a new country with strange ways and needing to find a job but still meet your family obligations.
>
> **Anya:** I need work, yes. I need money. I need to be good daughter.
>
> **Counselor:** I admire your sense of family loyalty, Anya. But I'm concerned about how we're going to be able to find a job for you. It's been over a month since you first came in, and this is the first time a job for which you are qualified has come up. You must realize this. I don't know if or when another opportunity will arise.
>
> **Anya:** I need work . . . I need take care mother . . . I need make life.

While the counselor is somewhat sensitive to Anya's dilemma, he is operating on the American premise that finding a job must be the first priority. He would be more helpful to Anya if he were more aware of the issues of immigration, the Russian cultural expectations that adult children will take care of their parents, and the slow process of acculturation. In other words, rather than covertly pressuring Anya to take this job, he needs to explore her confusion and conflicts with her. He needs to know what kinds of questions to ask her to facilitate her seeking resources in the Russian-speaking community to help with her mother and aid her in adjusting to her new life.

Culturally sensitive helpers also need to understand that some clients come from cultures that discourage seeking help from strangers and discourage self-disclosure. People from certain cultures might not even respond to an egalitarian helping relationship, being accustomed to more formal, directive, hierarchical helping relationships in which the helper is an expert who gives direct advice. Sensitivity to and willingness to study cultural nuances are important helper characteristics.

Honesty   One of the major variables in developing trust, honesty is a crucial ingredient for any effective interpersonal relationship. We may not always agree with what someone says, but if we believe the other person is being honest, we can respect that person. Helpers can communicate honesty by being open with clients, by answering questions within professional limits, and by admitting mistakes or lack of knowledge. Honesty is more than just being truthful; it is also being open to exploration and being fair in evaluation. One way to assess your own honesty as a helper is to invite honest feedback from clients and peers to see how they view you.

Consider the following example of honesty in a helping relationship. A registered nurse who has had specialized training in rape counseling is on call at a city hospital emergency ward that provides follow-up counseling to rape victims. She is talking with Mary, a 23-year-old woman who was assaulted three days earlier.

Counselor: You're feeling a lot of pressure from your family and the police to press charges against this guy, aren't you?

Mary: It's been just awful, and I don't know what to do. Everyone's been telling me what I should do, what the right thing is. Please tell me—you've been involved with this kind of business before. What do you think I should do?

Counselor: It's quite a dilemma, and one that only you can resolve. There really is no one right answer for everyone, you know.

Mary: What would you do if you were me?

Counselor: I honestly don't know, and I've thought about that a lot. I'd like to think I'd have the guts to testify, but after what I've seen, I'm not so sure. It's very rough going, takes a lot of time, and there's continual harassment that you really have to be tough to take. Not many people can do it, and it doesn't mean that you're not brave or good if you can't.

The counselor was then able to provide factual information about the judicial process in these types of cases and help Mary explore and understand her feelings and thoughts about the information. Because the counselor was open about her own views on the matter, she created a climate of trust and openness. At one point later in the session, Mary expressed appreciation of the counselor's "no-nonsense, honest approach."

You may be wondering how you can be honest in a situation in which you find yourself unable to like or agree with the helpee. These situations do occur, and when they do, helpers need to admit their negative reactions and to separate them from their dealings with the helpee. Occasionally, helpers will have to refer a helpee to another helper. This topic will be further explored in Chapter 10.

Congruence   Today's youth commonly accuse the adult generation of hypocrisy—that is, of incongruence or inconsistency between their words and actions. Perhaps incongruence occurs when people have not engaged themselves in a conscious process of examining, clarifying, and acknowledging their values and beliefs. Individuals who experience congruence between their values and beliefs and their lifestyle communicate more credibility and have a greater effect as models than those whose energy is used to deny incongruence. Further, people who have clarified and "own" their value systems are better able to express these values and beliefs without imposing them on others, thus allowing a more honest, nonjudgmental relationship.

If you believe that the purpose of a helping relationship is to facilitate the helpee's self-understanding and decision making and not to impose the helper's standards and values on the helpee, you'll agree that congruence, which in turn depends on the helper's self-awareness, is an important factor in effective helping relationships. This point of view does not imply that there is a "right" or "wrong" value system for helpers. Rather, it simply advocates congruence among what we believe, what we say, and what we live. Furthermore, it seems that people who are aware of and secure in their own values and beliefs are not threatened when faced with divergent or contrasting values and beliefs. Such people are better able to provide effective help to a broad spectrum of people.

An example of congruence is seen in the following exchange. A social worker is making a home visit to the Becker family. The Beckers have six children, live in a two-room apartment, and have been on welfare since Mr. Becker lost his job a year ago. One of the children requires a high-protein diet due to a metabolic disorder. They are having a very difficult time budgeting for protein-laden food.

> **Social worker:** I know how difficult it is to buy the nutritional food you need for a large family on what you get in food stamps.
>
> **Mrs. Becker:** I just can't manage, that's all. We're lucky if we have meat or anything high-protein once a week, the way things are. There just isn't enough, and pasta is about the best we can do.
>
> **Social worker:** It's frustrating and also challenging. I do believe we can all find creative ways to change our eating habits for the better.
>
> **Mrs. Becker:** It's impossible, believe me. Easy for people like you to say. You try to feed a family of eight on this kind of money. . . .
>
> **Social worker:** I'm not saying it's easy, but it is being done. There are more foods high in protein than beef. We have a nutritionist in our office now, and she is helping us put together a variety of low-cost diets for different needs. Why don't you come down to our office next week? I'll introduce you to her and see if the three of us can come up with recipes for new, low-cost dishes. I'll show you some of the ones I've found for my son; he needs a high-protein, low-carbohydrate diet for his sports practice.
>
> **Mrs. Becker:** No fooling! You people are really doing that?

This incident actually did occur and is an example of a helper implementing with action what she says (practicing what she preaches).

Ability to Communicate   As discussed earlier in this chapter, the ability to communicate verbally and nonverbally what we perceive, feel, and believe is an aid to any interpersonal relationship. Research substantiates that developing and using communication skills can have a positive effect on helping relationships. Let's carry this a step further by suggesting that we can effect positive human relations by continuously teaching (instructionally and by modeling) to our clients and others in our lives the same communication skills that we attempt to master formally or informally. (Examples of communication skills are given in Chapter 3.)

Knowledge   As you will see in Chapters 5 and 6, a knowledge of the theories on which effective helping is based is essential to the professional practitioner. Professional helpers need knowledge of psychological, anthropological, and sociological theory. Within psychological theory, they need to know about normal and abnormal development, neuropsychology, psychological assessment, learning and motivation, personality and gender development, and systems theory. Within sociological theory, they need to know about roles, organizations, and inter- and intragroup relations. Within anthropological theory, they need to know about the influence of culture on people's psychological development and behavior.

The formal study of multicultural, sexual orientation, and gender variables in psychological and sociological theory is a recent addition to academic and training institutions. As well as needing some knowledge of the different cultural backgrounds of clients, professional helpers should consider (1) the usefulness of mainstream psychological theories and practice with people of different genders and cultures, and (2) the experiences and status of helpees within their own culture in comparison with their experiences and status within a dominant culture. There will always be intracultural as well as intercultural differences.

To a lesser degree, this knowledge base is also relevant for the generalist human services worker. Likewise, knowledge of research and applied findings makes it possible for the nonprofessional helper to do a more meaningful job. In any case, the more knowledge one has about social, political, economic, cultural, and psychological issues, the more helpful one can be in aiding people to increase their self-understanding and effective decision making.

How disastrous a lack of some theoretical knowledge of development can be is illustrated in the following situation. Ms. Janssen, an older middle school social studies teacher, asked the school counselor to come in and observe two students in her class. She was concerned about two girls who were always giggling, holding hands, and kissing each other. Upon further inquiry, the school counselor learned that Ms. Janssen thought these girls were having a lesbian relationship and she did not think this was appropriate. The counselor, who knew each of the girls, agreed that this behavior was inappropriate in the classroom, but explained to Ms. Janssen that her conclusions about their sexual orientation were unfounded. He described early adolescent development as a framework for seeking intimacy and exploring all aspects of one's identity. He also talked with her about the number of "straight" students involved with the Gay and Lesbian Affiliation in the school. The counselor knew from previous dealings with Ms. Janssen that she was uncomfortable with cultural changes and earlier ages of puberty.

One further comment on counselor effectiveness: there is little doubt that experience enhances a helper's expertise. Research illustrates that increased experience leads to greater helper adaptability to clients and to the use of more eclectic strategies (Corey, 2005; Egan, 1998; Ivey et al., 2002; Kottler, 2004). With experience, helpers learn to trust their intuition, to work with a broader array of helpees, and to risk new approaches.

Ethical Integrity Overlapping the characteristics of honesty and congruence is a conscious determination on the part of the helper to behave responsibly, morally, and ethically. Deciding what helping behavior is responsible, moral, and ethical involves continued reflection; it requires awareness of potential conflicts among personal ethics, managed care and employer regulations, societal demands, and professional ethics; it requires openness to change.

Ethical dilemmas are complex and challenging; they may arise regarding confidentiality, records, and type and length of service. These issues will be discussed further in Chapter 10. Helpers need the capacity to tolerate ambiguity, uncertainty, and ambivalence. Perhaps an overriding ethical requirement is the ability to value clients' welfare over one's own needs or those of outside organizations.

Recently, a colleague of ours who worked in a counseling agency was informed by the director of the agency that she had to terminate immediately those clients who subscribed to a particular insurance plan. Although this colleague had informed her employer upon hiring that she was not yet licensed to receive third-party payments, he had unwittingly assigned her clients requiring reimbursement. When the claims for these patients were rejected, the director panicked and insisted upon sudden termination. This colleague was eager for work but disturbed by this directive. After terminating two clients and recognizing how upset they were at ending the counseling just when they were beginning to benefit from it, she began to question the ethics of this behavior. As she pondered the dilemma and consulted other professionals, she decided that sudden termination violated her personal and professional code of ethics, and she confronted her employer. As a result, she lost her job. Although she was distressed by this outcome, she felt comfortable with her ethical stand and was able to insist upon conducting her remaining terminations according to her own values over several sessions, instead of abruptly and unexpectedly.

Another colleague consulted me (BFO) about his discomfort over entering confidential client material into the computer system of the hospital where he works. He did not trust the security of the system. When a newspaper exposed some flagrant ethical violations of this particular system, he felt shame that he had gone along with the hospital policy despite his misgivings. His experience impelled both of us to study ethical guidelines and engage in invigorating discussions with colleagues about our own ethical beliefs and practices.

HELPER SELF-ASSESSMENT

To avoid a dependent or unhealthy relationship with a helpee, it's important to be aware of your own needs, feelings, and problems. As discussed previously, self-awareness enhances your ability to understand empathically the helpee's problems without adding to them by projecting your own feelings and needs.

Unfortunately, helpers are not always quick to recognize relationships in which they encourage the client's dependence or neediness. Helpees, in a vulnerable state, are often looking for someone to take over for them and tell them what to do, which may further helpers' unconscious needs to "rescue." Part of your responsibility is to refuse to do that and to encourage clients to take responsibility for themselves.

It is useful for helpers to assess continually their own needs and feelings—to think about where they are at any particular time by asking themselves the following kinds of questions and by discussing them with peers and supervisors.

1. *Am I aware when I am feeling uncomfortable with a client or with a particular subject area?* Very often helpers feel uneasy with a certain type of client who may represent something threatening or whose appearance is displeasing in some way. Helpers may also be uncomfortable with a controversial subject such as sex or drugs. It is important for helpers to recognize their discomfort, to "own" it for themselves, and to decide on an honest approach (deal with discomfort and proceed) or avoidance (refer client to another helper). "I" messages and statements can be helpful here—for example, "Look, I find I don't know enough about drugs to really discuss this with you."

2. *Am I aware of my own avoidance strategies?* Do you recognize when you avoid certain topics, allow the client to wander off, or ask too many questions to cover up your insecurities? Helpers who are aware of their avoidance behavior can say to themselves, "This really seems to be bothering me, and I'd better figure out what is going on so I can be truly facilitative with this helpee." One must, therefore, risk knowing oneself to know others.

3. *Can I really be honest with the helpee?* Is your fear of being disliked by the client making you afraid to confront or help him or her focus on something unpleasant? Do you have to be perfect and right all the time, or can you be you, a human who makes mistakes? If helpers have a strong need to be liked all the time, they will use reassuring, supportive responses to excess and diminish the possibilities for the client's development of responsibility and independence.

4. *Do I always feel as though I need to be in control of situations?* You may have some need for structure and direction in order to be accountable and achieve goals and objectives, but you should be aware of how you feel when a helpee disagrees or wants to pursue something different. For example, there may be times when you want to try a certain approach, such as a Gestalt exercise, with the helpee, and he or she refuses to participate. If you have a need to control, you may feel angry and rebuffed in this situation. If you do not have this need to control, you can accept the helpee's feelings without feeling personally attacked and can propose alternatives or delay introducing another strategy. Or you may want the client to focus on a certain topic when he or she wants to talk about something else. Can you stay with the client and not try to push this person to where you think he or she should be? Responsive listening is a safeguard against controlling the communication process.

5. *Do I become irritated when others do not see things the way I do or when helpees do not respond the way I think they should?* We need to remind ourselves continuously that there are multiple perspectives on any issue and that "good," "bad," "right," and "wrong" are relative and subjective concepts.

6. *Do I often feel as though I must be omnipotent, that I must do something to make the helpee "get better" so I can be successful?* If you often experience this feeling, you might ask whether you're in the right field! It's your relationship with clients that will facilitate their resolving their problems to their satisfaction,

not the waving of your magic wand. You can feel good about yourself when you see them gaining and acting for and taking responsibility for themselves.

7. *Am I so problem-oriented that I'm always looking for the negative, for a problem, and never responding to the positive, to the good?* This is a common concern of helpers, since they're exposed more often to negative feelings than to positive ones. However, it's important to identify and respond to positive affective and cognitive content in order to balance perspective and, more important, to reinforce positive conditions and strengths.

8. *Am I able to be as open with clients as I want them to be with me?* A common problem of people in helping professions is that they want to avoid their own feelings and problems by focusing on those of their clients. A good rule of thumb is never to ask anyone to do or talk about anything that you would not be willing to do or talk about in that or a similar situation.

Some of the preceding questions deal directly with communication, while others are more closely related to the "Issues Affecting Helping" discussed in Chapter 10. Your ability to communicate effectively is inseparable from your continuing development of sensitivity and self-awareness.

CLIENT VARIABLES

We will note when we study the various major theoretical approaches that certain approaches require certain client characteristics. For example, the client-centered and psychoanalytic approaches require a high degree of verbal ability on the part of the helpee, whereas the behavioral approaches can be used with clients who are less verbal. All approaches require some level of motivation and cooperation from the helpee to participate in the helping process. Some place more responsibility on the helper to develop that motivation, but all assume that the helping relationship will enhance the helpee's willingness to open up and accept vulnerability in order to achieve growth in the affective, cognitive, and behavioral domains.

Clients bring different sociocultural characteristics to the counseling process. Helpers need to understand cultural influences on such variables as emotional expressiveness; verbal and nonverbal language; attitudes toward family, friends, and work; attitudes toward space, time, and the pace of life; and attitudes toward seeking help, control, responsibility, decision making, sex roles, parenting, and identity.

SUMMARY

A helping relationship involves verbal and nonverbal communication between helper and helpee. Communication facilitates the development of rapport between them, which in turn allows for exploration of the helpee's beliefs, values, attitudes, feelings, and behaviors. The aim is to increase the helpee's self-understanding and understanding of others. The self-aware helpee will possess higher self-esteem, resulting in greater tolerance and acceptance of others. He or she will be better able to decide on and adopt a course of action to attain agreed-upon objectives, and to assume responsibility for the consequences.

There are many different kinds and levels of helping relationships and many different approaches to helping people, but clear communication is the basis of all helping. Informal helping relationships are characterized by a reciprocity—helpers and helpees can switch roles—that does not exist in formal helping relationships. Experience and research both indicate that certain traits and characteristics of helpers appear to have positive effects on helping relationships. The more in touch people are with their own gender and culture biases, beliefs, behaviors, and feelings, and the more able they are to communicate genuinely, clearly, and empathically their understanding of themselves and others, the more likely they are to be effective helpers. Self-awareness, honesty, congruence, the ability to communicate, and knowledge of human behaviors and the impact of gender, culture, and social factors on behavior all enhance the helping relationship.

Certain communication behaviors—verbal and nonverbal—also affect the process and outcome of helping relationships. The exercises in this chapter were designed to help you recognize verbal and nonverbal behaviors that are consistent with your personal style and beliefs and to become aware of which behaviors different helpees find helpful.

COMMENTS ON EXERCISES

Exercise 2.4 We can't tell from the excerpt who has the problem, Ms. James or Mr. Barber. The HR counselor assumed that the problem was Ms. James's and made no attempt to verify that assumption by gathering new data from her. By learning more about Ms. James's thoughts, feelings, and behaviors, and exploring the work atmosphere within her department, the HR counselor might have begun to help her clarify the nature of the problem, what part of it she was responsible for, and what her options and alternatives were for coping with the problem.

The HR counselor should have helped Ms. James to feel that she was worthwhile as a human being, regardless of what she was or was not doing, so that she could retain her dignity; at the same time he or she might have encouraged Ms. James to explore more fully and understand what was happening to her, to take responsibility for herself.

The HR counselor's three statements were not helpful; no clarification or change occurred. Behaviors included judging, blaming, and telling the client what to do. Ms. James felt defensive, as one is likely to feel when attacked. She had come to the HR department to see about a job change, and she never really got the chance to do so; she was immediately pushed into a corner.

Exercise 2.5 This short excerpt is all too typical of the interactions between adults who see themselves as being helpful and youngsters who have been "caught in the act" of doing something wrong. Ms. Smith was not helpful, because she did not help Steven to retain his feelings of self-worth and dignity or to understand his own behavior. Nor was Steven helped even to begin to verbalize what the problem really was all about, much less to understand what he could do about such problems in the future. Ms. Smith was apparently not concerned with

Steven's feelings, nor was she concerned with trying to understand him. Behaviors that she used are judging, punishing, threatening, and blaming.

She also asked a "why" question, which typically elicits defensiveness. Questions such as those of Ms. Smith cut off communication and encourage denial and withdrawal. Exploration and understanding cannot occur if communication is cut off. Like Ms. James, Ms. Smith most likely felt angry and frustrated at not being able to control a situation. A more appropriate response for Ms. Smith would have been, "Steven, it's very difficult when somebody else has something that you really want." This response would have allowed Steven the opportunity to tell his side of the story to an empathic listener.

Exercise 2.6 Julie's counselor demonstrated effective responsive listening skills and succeeded in eliciting much affect (feeling) and content (information) from her. Some of the responses were more helpful than others, but overall this was a productive first session in what subsequently became a short-term helping relationship. (At the end of this helping relationship, Julie was able to decide for herself and take responsibility for her decision and action regarding her marriage.) This is a lengthy excerpt, so let's examine each of the counselor's statements.

1.   This is a good opener, eliciting more information on an open-ended level.
2.   This is a reflective, empathic statement in that it conveys the counselor's understanding of Julie's intense feeling.
3.   Again, this statement clarifies the problem by focusing on Julie's feelings.
4.   Some interpretation is involved here in that the counselor interprets the nonverbal behavior that accompanied this statement (nonverbal behavior was apparent from the tape of this case).
5.   Again, there is some interpretation. The client's response indicates that the counselor was on target.
6–7. Counselor focuses on the issue of responsibility, adding some possible materials for client to consider.
8.   Counselor backs away from imposing own values here and succeeds in putting the issue back in the client's hands.
9.   Another exploratory statement—open-ended.
10. There is some interpretation of the underlying message here.
11. This is a probing statement. The counselor is not quite sure if this is the right track.
12. Again, probing.
13. Strictly reflection.
14. This response reflects the client's statement but brings the conversation back to her relationship with her husband.
15. The counselor is responding to the intense underlying feeling and focusing this feeling on the husband.

In this excerpt, the counselor had to make some decisions about what she would focus on with the client; there were many different directions she could have followed, and no one direction was necessarily correct. Julie was helped to begin to explore what was bothering her and to begin to understand some of her feelings. From this beginning the counselor could continue to develop the relationship and help Julie assume responsibility for herself and make her own decisions.

Exercise 2.7 Joaquin's counselor did not even recognize Joaquin's feelings, much less show concern for them. He totally ignored the possibility of Joaquin's underlying yearnings for assimilation and assumed that Joaquin's mother's concern was stereotypical immigrant upward-mobility anxiety. Thus, he was not helpful to Joaquin at all, because he did not explore Joaquin's feelings and he imposed his own needs on Joaquin by focusing exclusively on "getting through the term." If Joaquin had been allowed to explore his feelings and his desire to become more independent of his parents, he might have decided to put more effort into his schoolwork.

The first statement was moderately helpful in that it allowed Joaquin the open-ended opportunity to pursue what was on his mind and communicated positive regard for Joaquin's academic capabilities. However, the counselor's second and third statements were not helpful in that they conveyed judgment and a desire for expedience. Thus, Joaquin did not have the opportunity to learn about himself and his real concerns so as to decide for himself how to function in school.

Exercise 2.8 Mr. Williams's counselor demonstrated helpful communication skills. He took his time in drawing out his client so that it was the client, not the counselor, who clarified the problem by elaborating on his "coming on too strong" in job interviews. A less patient counselor might have simply accompanied the client in bemoaning his misfortune rather than clarifying what might be done about it. Each of the counselor's three responses demonstrated an empathic understanding, reflection of feelings, and congruence. The counselor's last statement was action-oriented, taking into consideration the nature of the problem and the available time for intervention.

REFERENCES AND FURTHER READING

Atkinson, E. R., Morten, G., & Sue, D. W. (Eds.). (1998). *Counseling American minorities: A cross-cultural perspective* (5th ed.). New York: McGraw-Hill.

Brammer, L. M., & MacDonald, G. (2003). *The helping relationship: Process and skills* (8th ed.). Boston: Allyn & Bacon.

Carkhuff, R. (2000a). *The art of helping* (8th ed.). Amherst, MA: Human Resource Development Press.

Carkhuff, R. (2000b). *Trainer's guide to the art of helping.* Amherst, MA: Human Resource Development Press.

Carter, B., & Peters, J. K. (1996). *Love, honor, and negotiate.* New York: Pocket Books.

Carter, R. C. (1995). *The influence of race and racial identity in psychotherapy: Toward a racially inclusive model.* New York: Wiley.

Combs, A. (1989). *A theory of therapy: Guidelines for counseling practice.* Newbury Park, CA: Sage.

Corey, G. (2005). *Theory and practice of counseling and psychotherapy* (7th ed.). Belmont, CA: Brooks/Cole.

Egan, G. (1998). *The skilled helper: A problem management approach to helping* (6th ed.). Pacific Grove, CA: Brooks/Cole.

Gladding, S. T. (2004). *Counseling: A comprehensive profession* (5th ed.). Englewood Cliffs, NJ: Prentice Hall.

Gottman, J. M., & Silver, N. (1999). *The seven principles for making marriage work.* New York: Crown.

Hackney, H. I., & Cormier, L. S. (2004). *The professional counselor: A process guide to helping* (3rd ed). Boston: Allyn & Bacon.

Ivey, A. E. (1991). *Developmental strategies for helpers: Individual, family, and network interventions.* Pacific Grove, CA: Brooks/Cole.

Ivey, A. E., D'Andrea, M., Ivey, M. B., & Simek-Morgan, L. (2002). *Theories of counseling and psychotherapy: A multicultural perspective* (5th ed.). Boston: Allyn & Bacon.

Ivey, A. E., & Ivey, M. B. (1999). *Intentional interviewing and counseling* (4th ed.). Pacific Grove, CA: Brooks/Cole.

Kottler, J. (2004). *Introduction to therapeutic counseling: Voices from the field.* Pacific Grove, CA: Brooks/Cole.

Okun, B. F. (1989). Therapists' blind spots related to gender socialization. In D. Kantor & B. F. Okun (Eds.), *Intimate environments: Sex, intimacy, and gender in families* (pp. 129–163). New York: Guilford Press.

Okun, B. F. (1990). *Seeking connections in psychotherapy.* San Francisco: Jossey-Bass.

Okun, B. F. (2004). Human diversity. In R. Combs (Ed.), *Family therapy review: Preparing for comprehensive and licensing examinations* (pp. 122–153). Mahwah, NJ: Erlbaum.

Okun, B. F., Fried, J., & Okun, M. L. (1999). *Understanding diversity: A learning-as-practice primer.* Pacific Grove, CA: Brooks/Cole.

Pedersen, P. B. (2000). *A handbook for developing multicultural awareness* (3rd ed.). Alexandria, VA: American Counseling Association.

Pedersen, P. B. (2003). Increasing the cultural awareness, knowledge, and skills of culture-centered counselors. In F. D. Harper & J. McFadden (Eds.), *Culture and counseling: New approaches* (pp. 33–46). Needham Heights, MA: Allyn & Bacon.

Rogers, C. (1958). The characteristics of a helping relationship. *Personnel and Guidance Journal, 37,* 6–16.

Rogers, C. (1975). Empathy: An unappreciated way of being. *The Counseling Psychologist, 5*(2), 2–10.

Rogers, C. (1976). *The therapeutic relationship and its impact.* Madison: University of Wisconsin Press.

Sue, D. W. (2002). *Counseling the culturally diverse: Theory and practice* (4th ed.). New York: Wiley.

Sue, D. W. (2005). *Multicultural social work practice.* New York: Wiley.

Sue, D. W., Ivey, A. E., & Pedersen, P. (1996). *A theory of multicultural counseling and therapy.* Pacific Grove, CA: Brooks/Cole.

Visit the book companion site at www.thomsonedu.com to access tutorial quizzes.

3

Communication Skills

To be effective, helpers must use communication skills that enable them to hear verbal messages (cognitive and affective content), perceive nonverbal messages (affective and behavioral content), and respond verbally and nonverbally to both kinds of messages. To ensure that these communication skills become an integral part of your helping techniques, you must practice them frequently. Because you, like most people, have probably taken your communication behaviors for granted, you may not have had the opportunity to focus on and develop an awareness of them. When you start concentrating on your communication behaviors (these behaviors were briefly reviewed in Chapter 2), at first you may feel uncomfortable and tired. It's relatively easy to talk about communication skills and theoretically understand their importance to effective helping relationships; however, it's much more difficult to put this understanding into practice. Indeed, practicing communication skills is more difficult than completing written exercises about them!

Because the practice of communication skills is so important, incorporating the exercises in this chapter into your group discussion will make this practice more fun. Sharing what you have experienced during the exercises, your feelings, and your recognition of what you are willing to do and what you tend to shy away from (**approach** and **avoidance reactions**) is the most beneficial aspect of the exercises. More understanding comes from the discussion after an exercise than from the exercise itself. In this kind of discussion, called processing, one talks about one's feelings and reactions rather than about the actual content of the exercise. The ability to process feelings and reactions will also be useful in your work with clients.

PERCEIVING NONVERBAL MESSAGES

The reason it is so important to understand nonverbal communication is that it is the foundation on which human relationships are built. Some anthropologists believe that more than two-thirds of any communication is transmitted on a nonverbal level. We must interpret patterns of gestures, posture, facial expressions, spatial relations, personal appearance, and cultural characteristics. Thus we, as helpers, should try to develop a conscious awareness of nonverbal manifestations and their various meanings.

Because the perception of nonverbal messages has not been emphasized in our culture, some of the exercises in this chapter may lead to frustration and tension as we become aware of our dependence on nonverbal cues for understanding verbal messages. Remember, your brain is constantly absorbing information below your level of consciousness. This makes nonverbal communication even more important than you may have realized (Lewis, Amini, & Lannon, 2000). Chapter 2 listed various facilitative and nonfacilitative nonverbal behaviors in helping relationships. The kinds of nonverbal cues that we attend to in a communicative relationship are listed in Table 3.1. We, as helpers, look to see whether the nonverbal behavior is consistent with the verbal behavior and if we can pick up any clues that will help us identify the affective messages (underlying feelings) we hear. Nonverbal behavior provides us with clues to, not conclusive proof of, underlying feelings. However, research has shown that nonverbal clues tend to be more reliable than verbal clues! We also need to pay attention to culture-specific expression and meaning of nonverbal behaviors.

TABLE 3.1 Nonverbal cues in a communicative relationship

Feature	Examples
Body position	Tense, relaxed, leaning toward or away from
Eyes	Teary, open, closed, excessive blinking, twitching
Eye contact	Steady, avoiding, shifty
Body movement	Knee jerks, taps, hand and leg gestures, fidgeting, head nodding, pointing fingers, dependence on arms and hands for expressing message, touching
Body posture	Stooped shoulders, slouching, legs crossed, rigid, relaxed
Mouth	Smiling, lip biting, licking lips, tight, loose
Facial expression	Animated, bland, distracting, frowning, puckers, grimaces
Skin	Blushing, rashes, perspiration, paleness
General appearance	Clean, neat, sloppy, well groomed
Voice	Fast, slow, jerky, high pitched, whispers, mumbles

EXERCISE 3.1 ▪ What do the following gestures mean to you? When you have completed this exercise, compare your answers with those of your classmates and those suggested at the end of the chapter.

1. A man walks into your office, takes off his coat, loosens his tie, sits down, and puts his feet up on a chair.

2. A man walks into your office, sits erect, and clasps his arms across his chest before saying a word.

3. A client rests her cheek on her hand, strokes her chin, cocks her head slightly to one side, and nods deeply.

4. A woman walks into your office, sits as far away as she can, folds her arms, crosses her legs, tilts the chair backward, and looks over your head.

5. A client walks into your office and avoids eye contact with you.

6. A client gazes at you and stretches out her hands with the palms up.

7. A client quickly covers his mouth with his hand after revealing some sensitive material.

8. While talking with you, a client holds both arms behind her back and clenches one fist tightly while using her other hand to grip her wrist or arm.

9. A woman in your office crosses her legs and moves her foot in a slight kicking motion; at the same time, she is drumming her fingers on the arm of her chair.

10. A person sits forward in his chair, tilting his head and nodding at intervals.

EXERCISE 3.2 ▪ Cut out some pictures of people from a magazine. Try to select people of different genders, ages, ethnic groups, cultures, and races. Remove the captions and ask a partner what he or she believes is being communicated. Then, in groups of four to six, ask other people to respond to the same pictures. Talk about the various responses, and see if it is possible to reach a consensus. After you have identified the feelings that are being communicated in several pictures, see if you can establish some patterns in your group's identifications. The purpose of this exercise is to examine different responses to the same nonverbal stimulus. What were the reasons given for a particular identification? In cases of disagreement, what were the major areas of difference? How do people project their own attitudes, values, and beliefs onto their perceptions of subjects' feelings? How can you explain the variety of perceptions? What kinds of stereotypes did you uncover in your group discussion?

EXERCISE 3.3 ▪ The purpose of this exercise is to give you the opportunity to identify the feelings underlying another person's nonverbal behavior. This is an important skill because effective helpers must learn to identify feelings and emotions using many different cues, including nonverbal behaviors. In triads or small groups, have one person identify a specific feeling, tell it to an observer, and then try to communicate it nonverbally to his or her partner or to the other members of the group. After the feeling has been properly identified, have someone else choose a feeling and attempt to communicate it to the group. Process your experiences as you did in Exercise 3.2.

EXERCISE 3.4 ■ Another way to become adept at giving and identifying nonverbal messages is to play a nonverbal form of "telephone." A group sits in a circle and one person selects a feeling to start the game. Everyone closes his or her eyes, and the starter taps the person on the right, who opens his or her eyes, tries to understand the nonverbal communication, and then repeats the communication process by tapping the person on the right, who opens his or her eyes and receives and sends the nonverbal message. This entire exercise is nonverbal until the last person in the circle receives the message and verbally identifies the feeling. The group then processes what happened, where and how the message became distorted, if it did, and what the members felt about the nonverbal communication.

EXERCISE 3.5 ■ This exercise helps participants identify complex nonverbal messages by having them observe a scene rather than the acting out of an isolated feeling. A pair leaves the room and plans a 10-minute role-play scene of a couple talking at the dinner table, a teacher and principal conferring, or whatever seems appropriate (and fun!). They come back into the room and, using nonsense syllables, carry on a dialogue that has no verbal meaning for the observers. The role players strive to convey their intentions and feelings. The observers are to identify and reconstruct what is occurring strictly by observing nonverbal behavior. The observers usually find that they can understand the meaning of the scene without verbal information. A variation of this exercise is to watch (either individually or in a small group) a videotape or DVD without sound, sharing interpretations within the group.

EXERCISE 3.6 ■ The purpose of this exercise is to become more aware of the nonverbal behaviors associated with feelings. Develop a list of emotions, and describe the nonverbal behaviors you associate with each emotion. For example, "When I'm mad, I frown, clench my fists, tighten my body, sit back away from people, and feel knots in my stomach." Share your list in small groups, and note similarities and differences. Again, see if you can elicit a variety of influences, including gender, age, race, and ethnicity.

EXERCISE 3.7 ■ In pairs (or triads), take turns being helper and helpee (and observer). The helpee describes a real or imagined concern and uses facial expressions, vocal tones, postures, and gestures that are opposite to the feelings he or she is expressing in the verbal message. For example, I (BFO) may tell you how excited I am about a trip I'm going to make this weekend and slump, frown, and slur my words. What feelings do you perceive? The helper states what he or she perceives the major expressed feeling to be. Then group members discuss their experiences with verbal and nonverbal incongruence. Which cues did you find most powerful and important? What did you make of this?

EXERCISE 3.8 ■ The purpose of this exercise is to explore gender- and ethnicity-related characteristics of nonverbal behaviors. As each member of the group acts out a concern or event nonverbally, jot down what you think may be gender or ethnically linked. During the next week, observe nonverbal behaviors of as many different people as possible: on buses, in restaurants, in waiting rooms, and so on. If you live in a homogeneous area, you may focus on differences related to age or religious affiliation. Pay particular attention to the use of space/distance, body movements, gestures, and displays of affection. At your next group meeting, share your findings, and see if your group can agree on differences in nonverbal behaviors related to gender, ethnicity, or other factors you selected.

HEARING VERBAL MESSAGES

We are all aware of the need to listen to verbal messages, and we sometimes can accurately restate another person's simple verbal messages if we are in a one-to-one situation. But if we think back to the "telephone" game that we played at childhood parties, we can remember how simple verbal messages became distorted as they were passed along by several different people.

As difficult as it sometimes is to understand apparently clear-cut verbal messages, it is much more difficult to understand the underlying affective content of verbal messages. One reason is that we tend to respond more to the cognitive content than to the affective content. Cognitive content comprises the actual facts and words of the message. Affective content may be verbal or nonverbal and comprises feelings, attitudes, and behaviors.

Receiving verbal messages really involves understanding both cognitive and affective content and being able to discriminate between them. The cognitive content is usually easier to understand; it is stated. The affective content sometimes differs from the cognitive content and is often less apparent. The difference between hearing only the apparent cognitive content of a verbal message and hearing both the cognitive and underlying affective messages is the difference between being an ineffective and an effective listener.

Your response to a client's statement will depend on your ability to hear and understand what is being said and to uncover the underlying message. Your response will, in turn, influence the direction of the client's next statement. Thus, before you can learn to respond appropriately to a client's statement, you must learn to hear and discriminate between his or her apparent and underlying cognitive and affective messages.

Verbal Cognitive Messages

As previously stated, cognitive messages are easier for us to recognize than affective messages, for our schooling stresses cognitive knowledge. Cognitive messages usually involve talking about things, people, or events and may involve one or several simple or complex themes. The client is often more comfortable talking *about* thoughts or behaviors than actually feeling them.

If we find ourselves responding only to the client's cognitive concerns, we never really get down to his or her underlying feelings or see the inconsistencies between cognitive and affective content. For example, a client may come in and talk about trouble with a supervisor. If the helper asks only "What happened?" "What did your supervisor say?" and "What did you say then?" the entire session can pass without uncovering the client's underlying concerns and feelings. The only possible outcome of this type of helper response would be the helper's suggestion that the client make different verbal responses or offer different behaviors to the supervisor. The helper's suggestions may work out, but they really don't contribute to the client's understanding and choice of his or her own course of action. The solution of one obvious problem may not touch on the helpee's underlying concerns.

The theme (problem or concern) that the helper focuses on affects the direction of the ensuing discussion. A helper hopes to choose a theme that will be the most productive in developing the helping relationship. It is difficult to determine which cognitive theme is most important, and there could be several of equal importance, but it is necessary to respond to and focus on one major theme at a time in order to clarify and explore all aspects of the situation.

The objective of the following exercises is to help you identify cognitive themes in communication.

EXERCISE 3.9 ■ Read the following client statements, and pick out as many different cognitive topics as you can. Then check your answers with ours at the end of the chapter. Remember, list only cognitive content, not affective content (feelings).

1. "I'm really up a tree at this point as I have so many bills to pay and Tom isn't working and I don't know what to do. This job doesn't pay enough, and I guess I should see if I can get an extra evening job, like waitressing or telephone soliciting. I wanted to go back to school at night this term, but that doesn't seem possible now."

2. "Why should I stay in school when there are so many people with degrees who can't get jobs? I don't feel as if I'm learning anything here anyway, nobody seems to care what happens to anybody, and the classes are so large and impersonal. It's a waste of money."

3. "I couldn't find a parking place today, so I missed this morning's briefing session. Somebody ought to do something about this situation. I can't find that memorandum, and I'm not sure what to say to Mr. Jones when he calls this afternoon."

4. "Look, I've got a sick kid, and we just moved here and don't know anyone. The landlord won't turn on the heat, and I need to find a job to pay the bills. I don't know where to turn first, and I also need to get the rest of my furniture delivered!"

5. "Wow, what a time we had! We went swimming every day, bicycling at night, fishing several times, and just had a great time. Oh yes, we sailed the Meyers's boat—did you know they were down there?"

Now go over your list of topics and see whether you can rank them in order of importance or immediacy of concern for each statement. If you had to respond to only one of the themes in each case, which would it be?

Because this exercise provides the client statements only in written form, it is obviously difficult to rank the cognitive topics objectively in terms of their importance to the client. However, once you have learned to hear the verbal cognitive content, you will be able to use affective content as a clue for establishing priorities. In verbal communication, we tend to respond more often to the most recent verbal theme rather than to the most important one. We need to train ourselves to hear the whole message and discriminate among themes.

A variation of this exercise would be to read the statements aloud to a partner and have him or her verbally recall the cognitive themes.

EXERCISE 3.10 ■ This exercise has many different forms and names. Its purpose is to develop students' attending skills by having them repeat verbal cognitive messages. It is effective in groups that divide either into pairs (helper, helpee roles) or into triads (helper, helpee, observer roles). One person, the helpee, communicates to the helper statements that last no longer than three minutes and that involve a real or imagined concern. The helper must then restate the helpee's verbal message to the latter's satisfaction. The helpee and the observer (if there is a triad) then process this interaction by evaluating the effectiveness of the helper's restatement of the helpee's verbal cognitive content. Everyone in the pair or triad should have the chance to be the helpee and the helper. The observer can jot down what he or she has heard and compare it to what the helper restates.

After the pairs or triads have completed this exercise, they should recombine into a group and process their experiences by sharing their difficulties and concerns. Group members should then make suggestions for dealing with those difficulties and concerns. Observers should share their observations about the helper's verbal and nonverbal behaviors, such as posture, eye contact, and gestures.

This exercise helps us realize that we often spend more energy preparing our responses than listening to what is actually being said to us. It is also a good exercise to show us how we often hear another person's verbal message through our own "filters" (selective perception). We often hear and see what we need or want to hear and see, rather than what is actuall1y being communicated.

EXERCISE 3.11 ■ In this exercise, choose the helper response that best reflects the cognitive content of the helpee's statement. Remember that you are trying to paraphrase the main idea of each statement without changing it. Check your answers at the end of the chapter.

The following situation occurred in a professional accounting firm. The helpee is a recent college graduate who was hired six months ago and has been absent and tardy more and more frequently. The helper is the partner in the firm responsible for personnel and office management.

1. **Helpee:** I'm not so sure what it is you people are so uptight about here.
   Helper:
   a. You think we make too much of things here.
   b. You're concerned about how we feel about your absences and tardiness.
   c. How do you feel you're doing here?

2. **Helpee:** I graduated at the top of my class, and I know this stuff cold.
   Helper:
   a. Sounds like you think you're better than the rest of us.
   b. You have a lot to teach us.
   c. You seem concerned about how well you're doing here and how you're fitting in.

3. **Helpee:** In the past six months, I've moved to a strange city and had a devil of a time finding an apartment and a roommate and trying to make ends meet.
   Helper:
   a. You've had a lot of change in your life recently.
   b. Your personal life is really not related to what's happening here.
   c. Being out in the real world is very different from college life, isn't it?

4. **Helpee:** Well, I'm really getting bored doing what I'm doing. My education seems wasted. How soon can I move on to something more in line with my qualifications?
   Helper:
   a. Sounds like you really need to move on quickly.
   b. You're eager to make more money.
   c. It's frustrating for you to feel that you're not working up to your potential.

5. **Helpee:** I look at some of the guys who've been here for years and really haven't gotten very far. I won't let that happen to me.
   Helper:
   a. It's important for you to get ahead quickly.
   b. Young people today have a hard time working their way up. They want everything to happen so quickly.
   c. You're afraid that you may get stuck and not get where you want to go.

6. **Helpee:** There's just too much junk work to do around here and too much politicking. I want to get on with it.

   Helper:

   a. It's hard for you to do the scut work that needs to get done.

   b. You're angry that this job didn't turn out the way you wanted it to.

   c. It's hard for you to get yourself to do what you don't want to do.

7. **Helpee:** Sometimes I wonder what I'm doing here. I'm sure I could make more money someplace else.

   Helper:

   a. You're confused about whether or not to stick it out here.

   b. You're very worried about your financial affairs.

   c. You're unsure whether money is more important than the job training you're receiving.

8. **Helpee:** Being on time and sticking in the office is hard for me. I'm used to being able to do what I want when I want.

   Helper:

   a. The structure here really gets to you.

   b. You get angry at us for making demands on you, so you just don't bother to come in.

   c. Sounds as though you're having a conflict—you really want to work, but you're having trouble getting used to the routine and structure here.

EXERCISE 3.12 ■ This exercise demonstrates the incongruities that can exist between verbal and nonverbal communication in cognitive messages. Divide into your pairs or triads and repeat Exercise 3.10 with one difference: the helper should deliberately attempt to use facial expressions, vocal tones, posture, and gestures that are *opposite* in meaning to the cognitive messages being sent. For example, if you talked about your concern about finding a legitimate parking place in time to get to a downtown meeting and at the same time smiled, seemed relaxed, and nonverbally expressed casualness, your actions and your words would be incongruent. The point of this exercise is for the helper to experience how such incongruities between verbal and nonverbal behaviors can affect perception of cognitive messages. Helpees will experience the discomfort involved in communicating incongruous messages on a conscious level.

Verbal Affective Messages

Affective messages are communicated to us both verbally and nonverbally. Affective messages involve feelings: emotions that may be directly or indirectly expressed. They are much more difficult to communicate than cognitive messages and much more difficult to perceive and hear. Clients are often so much more aware of thoughts than feelings that the helper's responses, clarifying and identifying feelings, come as a surprise to them and uncover a whole new area for exploration and experiencing. By understanding affective messages and in turn responding to them, the helper is communicating not only acceptance of the helpee's emotions but also permission for the helpee to experience and "own" those feelings. We have already practiced nonverbal communication of emotions in several exercises; for the present we will restrict ourselves to verbal communication.

Some helpers find it useful to group feelings into four major categories: anger, sadness, fear, and happiness. Very often a feeling from one category covers up one from another (for example, sadness sometimes masks anger or vice versa, or anger may mask fear). We can use many different words to identify feelings in these four categories, and it is helpful to select vocabulary that is comfortable for the client. For example, if a teenager is using the current slang of his peer group, instead of using the word "angry" when identifying his feelings, you may say "pissed off," as long as you feel comfortable doing this (and do not come across as phony). You will also want to select feeling words that convey the same intensity as the client's statement. For example, if the client says she feels "irritated," it would be more appropriate to reply that she seems to feel "annoyed" than that she seems to feel "enraged." Identifying underlying feelings in verbal messages is difficult at first and is related to how comfortable and proficient you are in recognizing and expressing your own feelings. It is crucial that you listen to the client's messages and identify his or her feelings rather than project your own onto the client. Again, this requires continual, repeated practice.

EXERCISE 3.13 ■ The purpose of this exercise is to clarify your own ways of expressing feelings and emotions. Write down all the words you can think of that express each of the four major categories of emotion: happiness, anger, fear, and sadness. What words do you use to express those feelings? For example, under "happiness" you might write "glad," carefree," "tip-top," and so forth. When you have completed your list, share it with two others and see if there are many differences. All groups can then compile a master list, which you may want to keep and refer to as you complete these exercises and begin your work with helpees.

EXERCISE 3.14 ■ Now take each of the four major categories of emotion (happiness, anger, fear, and sadness) and list as many verbal behaviors as possible that you are aware of enacting when you feel each emotion. For example, when you're mad, you may swear, use short, clipped sentences or monosyllables, or yell. Share your lists in small groups, and learn how different people express the same emotion. Again, pay particular attention to gender, generational, racial, and ethnic differences within your group.

EXERCISE 3.15 ▪ This exercise is called listening for feelings. For each of the following statements, write what you think the person is really feeling. Ask yourself, what is the underlying feeling here?

1. "Two big boys were picking on me when I was coming home from Boy Scouts today."

2. "The doctor told me to come over here and have all these tests. I'll sit over there and wait until you're ready for me."

3. "Poor Lenny! He works so hard, and he never gets home for dinner anymore."

4. "I can't wait until final exams are over."

5. "I'm really too busy to take a coffee break now, though I'd love to talk to you."

6. "I can't work on that report today. Professor Ramirez gave me four rush letters to get out by three o'clock, and I still have to get the exams ready for tomorrow."

7. "Please put down that newspaper. You never talk to me anymore!"

8. "I think people are out to get what they can for themselves."

9. "If Jim hadn't been transferred, this project would have gotten off the ground in plenty of time."

10. "Have you heard anything about the new social worker? I'm supposed to see her at three o'clock."

11. "I hear the new office manager is a real clock watcher."

12. "Only two more weeks until vacation!"

13. "Look, Ms. Jones, if you can't get this material entered, I'll have to see if someone else can do it."

14. "My husband is out of work, and I don't know how we're going to pay the rent next month."

15. "All children steal at that age, don't you think?"

16. "Young people today really have a lot more sexual freedom than we did in my day!"

17. "Javaid, I want to tell you that, after much careful consideration, I'm stepping down as chairperson so as to have more time for my family and to do my research."

18. "Ms. Green is a lousy teacher. She doesn't know how to explain things."

19. "Please bring the car home by eight o'clock. I don't want you driving in the dark."

20. "Why should I stay in school? I don't know what I want to do. What do you think?"

21. "I hate staff meetings. No one ever gives me a chance to talk."

22. "Coming to see you just doesn't seem to be helping me. We talk about the same stuff over and over, and I still don't know what to do."

23. "No one ever picks me to be on his team at school."

24. "Are you going to see me again this week, doctor?"

25. "I'd like to talk to you when you have a minute. Be sure and see me before you leave the office tonight."

After you have completed this exercise, discuss your answers either in small groups or as a large group. Then look at the answers at the end of the chapter.

You will note that people may identify different underlying feelings for the same statement and that, in discussing these statements, various projections begin to emerge. For example, one group of students told me (BFO) that some members felt so threatened by statement 25 that they identified the underlying feeling as anger, whereas other members perceived it as eagerness, hypothesizing a situation in which one person wants to invite another person over but doesn't want others in the office to know about it and feel excluded. For the statements on which the group disagrees, try reading them aloud with varying affect and intonation, and see what different kinds of reactions you get.

EXERCISE 3.16 ■ Read the following client statements (they are the same as in Exercise 3.9) and list the major feelings in each situation.

1. "I'm really up a tree at this point as I have so many bills to pay and Tom isn't working and I don't know what to do. This job doesn't pay enough, and I guess I should see if I can get an extra evening job, like waitressing or telephone soliciting. I wanted to go back to school at night this term, but that doesn't seem possible now."

2. "Why should I stay in school when there are so many people with degrees who can't get jobs? I don't feel as if I'm learning anything here anyway, nobody seems to care what happens to anybody, and the classes are so large and impersonal. It's a waste of money."

3. "I couldn't find a parking place today, so I missed this morning's briefing session. Somebody ought to do something about this situation. I can't find that memorandum, and I'm not sure what to say to Mr. Jones when he calls this afternoon."

4. "Look, I've got a sick kid, and we just moved here and don't know anyone. The landlord won't turn on the heat, and I need to find a job to pay the bills. I don't know where to turn first, and I also need to get the rest of my furniture delivered!"

5. "Wow, what a time we had! We went swimming every day, bicycling at night, fishing several times, and just had a great time. Oh yes, we sailed the Meyers's boat—did you know they were down there?"

As you go over your answers, see if you listed your own feelings or what you believe the subject is feeling. How can you tell? How did you decide? Discuss your list in small groups.

EXERCISE 3.17 ■ This exercise is similar to Exercise 3.10 (verbal cognitive messages), but in this case you'll identify the feelings rather than the cognitive content.

In pairs, with people's backs to each other to block out nonverbal cues, have the helpee talk for up to three minutes, and have the helper identify the feelings that are being communicated. The helpees should not verbally identify their own feelings for the helpers but should make the same types of comments they did in Exercise 3.10 and allow the helper to identify the underlying feelings. The results of this exercise should be processed in the same manner as those in Exercise 3.10.

EXERCISE 3.18 ▪ Have two pairs (or triads) work with each other, with two people identified as helpers and two as helpees (and two as observers). The purpose of this exercise is to show each helper how two different people may express the same feeling with different verbal messages and different nonverbal cues. The two helpees are to separate themselves from the rest of the group, select one feeling (for example, elation, frustration, or boredom), and tell the two observers secretly which feeling they have selected. Then each helpee is to make verbal statements expressing, but not verbally identifying, that feeling to each of the two helpers separately. After listening to both helpees, each helper is to identify the feeling. The observer will let the helper know when he or she is correct, and the helpee is encouraged to continue making statements until this identification occurs.

Hearing and discriminating among affective and cognitive verbal messages without body language cues is extremely difficult. The process is naturally hampered by the artificiality of out-of-context role playing. Nevertheless, as you become used to role playing, you will become less artificial and more comfortable.

After you have practiced identifying cognitive and affective contents separately, try Exercise 3.19.

EXERCISE 3.19 ▪ In pairs (or triads), assign helpee and helper (and observer) roles. The helpee is to talk for five minutes (it will seem like a very long time!) about a real or imagined concern. The helper is not to ask any questions, but can make exploratory statements such as "Tell me more about that" and "I'm wondering if" to probe for more data. At the end of the agreed-on time, the helpee is to stop and the helper is to identify both the cognitive and affective messages to the helpee's satisfaction. A suggested format is "You feel _____ when _____ because _____." Allow each person the opportunity to be helpee, and then process the results of the exercise in small or large groups.

The purpose of this exercise is to sharpen helpers' discrimination skills and to focus their attention on the helpee's message and the development of messages. It encourages client-centered listening in that it does not allow questions. If the role of observer is assigned in this exercise, the person playing that role should assist the helper to identify messages.

RESPONDING VERBALLY
AND NONVERBALLY

Developing an awareness of one's own verbal and nonverbal cognitive and affective messages, as well as those of helpees, is an important first step in learning how to be an effective helper. Helpers must be skilled in responsive listening as a basis for responding to helpees both nonverbally and verbally. **Responsive listening** is defined as attending (paying careful attention) and responding to the verbal and nonverbal messages and the apparent and underlying thoughts and feelings of the client. This is easier said than done and involves developing awareness of oneself as a communicator as well as refining hearing and perceiving skills.

Responsive listening implies that the helper is able to communicate his or her genuine understanding (empathy), acceptance, and concern for the helpee and, at the same time, increase understanding of the issue by clarifying the helpee's statement. Thus, helpers must be able to communicate to the client their caring, as well as identification and understanding of the primary cognitive concern and the underlying feeling. It's essential that the helper be congruent in his or her own verbal and nonverbal communication, or the helpee will be just as confused by double messages from the helper as the helper is when he or she receives double messages from the helpee.

The following is an example of responsive listening:

Helpee: I know I'm too fat. That's why nobody ever asks me out.
Helper: You really feel sad when you see everyone around you having a
    good time, and you're scared, wondering what will happen to you if
    you don't improve your appearance.

Saying "Don't worry" or "You should go on a diet" is not helpful. Those kinds of responses do not help clients increase their self-understanding. What makes the preceding excerpt an example of interpretive responsive listening is that in it the helper identifies an underlying feeling, relates it to the major cognitive concern, and adds clarity and understanding to the helpee's statement.

We'll develop more examples of responsive listening skills as we proceed through this chapter. Let's focus first on developing our awareness of our own nonverbal communication behaviors.

Nonverbal Responding

Nonverbal behaviors communicate warmth, understanding, attentiveness, and efficacy, apart from and in congruence with verbal behavior. Desirable nonverbal behaviors for effective helping include occasional nodding, smiling, and hand gesturing; maintaining good eye contact; using facial animation; leaning toward the helpee (sitting near, with no desk as a barrier); speaking at a moderate rate; and talking with a firm, supportive tone of voice.

We must adapt our nonverbal behaviors to our client's level of comfort. For example, one person may want you to sit close and lean toward her, whereas another may feel more comfortable with greater distance. In addition to cultural influences, there are individual differences.

EXERCISE 3.20 ▪ This is an important Gestalt exercise that helps us get in touch with our own comfort or discomfort with nonverbal behavior. (We'll discuss the Gestalt approach more in Chapters 5, 7, and 8.) Pairs sit facing each other and communicate for three to five minutes by eye contact only. No other body language or verbal language is permitted. After the time is up, the partners can continue their eye contact, but they can also communicate with their hands for three to five minutes. Then they are allowed to communicate nonverbally any way they choose for five more minutes. At the end of this exercise, the pairs are to process verbally, by sharing their feelings, thoughts, intentions, and reactions. Then, in small or large groups, everyone can share his or her experience.

Many people find themselves very uncomfortable maintaining eye contact at first, but this form of communication becomes more comfortable and meaningful with practice and experience.

EXERCISE 3.21 ▪ Another significant Gestalt exercise is mirroring. In this exercise the group divides into pairs who sit facing each other. One person is the communicator; the other is the nonverbal "mirror." The communicators talk about anything they want to for five minutes. The mirrors nonverbally mirror each gesture, movement, and expression of the communicators. (They do not verbally mirror what they think the other is saying, because they are concentrating on nonverbal behavior.) At the end of five minutes, the mirrors express their feelings, the communicators share their feelings, and they both share what they have learned from participating in this exercise. (If you do not have a partner, you can do this exercise alone by talking to yourself in front of a mirror.)

Because we rarely see ourselves communicating, we are generally unaware of our nonverbal behaviors. However, the mirror exercise allows us to observe and discuss whether our nonverbal behaviors are facilitative or nonfacilitative. For example, one student discovered that by sitting back and rocking in his chair, he was distancing himself from others and not being facilitative.

EXERCISE 3.22 ▪ In triads, the helpee communicates a real or imagined stress or crisis. The helper attempts to respond to these messages, and the helpee and the observer give direct feedback to the helper about his or her nonverbal behavior. Observers can refer to "Nonverbal Behaviors" in Appendix A as a guide to evaluating and developing helpers' awareness of nonverbal behaviors.

Verbal Responding

When we respond verbally, we attempt (1) to communicate to helpees that we are truly hearing and understanding them and their perspective; (2) to communicate our ability to help, our warmth, acceptance, respect, and caring; and (3) to increase the client's self-understanding and self-exploration as well as his or her understanding of others by focusing on major themes, clarifying inconsistencies, reflecting back the underlying feelings, and synthesizing the major apparent and underlying concerns and feelings. To be more effective in our responses, we need to learn about language and nuances that are culture specific. Sue (2005) and Sue and Sue (2002) suggest we consider vocal cues, volume of speech, and when it is and is not appropriate to speak. Okun, Fried, and Okun (1999) emphasize the importance of tone of voice and rate of speech, as well as the value and meaning given to language.

We have already begun to focus on verbal responding by identifying the major affective and cognitive contents of helpee statements. We are also developing the ability to generate **additive** (facilitative) **responses,** which help the client understand his or her thoughts and feelings and add some understanding of what the client is trying to communicate. This form of responsive listening is particularly helpful during the relationship stage of helping because it facilitates the objectives mentioned above. Responses that are simply reflections or paraphrases of the client's verbalized and nonverbal thoughts and behaviors are considered interchangeable, and responses that do not pertain at all to the client's message are subtractive, or nonfacilitative.

Following these guidelines will help you reach the goals of verbal responding just listed:

1. Listen to the helpee's basic message.
2. Respond to the most important part of the helpee's statement that coincides with the basic apparent or underlying verbal and nonverbal messages.
3. Reflect the helpee's feelings at a matching intensity.
4. Reflect both implicit and explicit feelings of the helpee, and help him or her differentiate between thoughts and feelings.
5. Respond to the helpee's nonverbal behaviors.
6. When the helpee changes topics, respond to the primary cognitive or affective theme of the topics by verbal tracking.
7. Always allow the helpee to modify or reject your perceptions.
8. Use your own feelings as the basis for clarifying, confronting, **leading,** and so on (see "Advanced Verbal Response Skills," later in this chapter).
9. If you are unable to rephrase your questions as statements, ask only open-ended questions (see below) that clarify issues for the helpee or that elicit feelings.
10. If the helpee doesn't pause to give you a chance to respond, and you feel lost or confused, break in with a statement such as "I feel confused . . ." in

order to focus on major themes. But don't feel you have to respond to every single helpee statement.

The next exercise will give you an opportunity to identify responses that are interchangeable, subtractive, or additive in terms of communicating your goals to the helpee.

EXERCISE 3.23 ■ Rate each of the following statements as either − (subtractive: does not increase the client's understanding), = (interchangeable: neither increases nor decreases the client's understanding), or + (additive: increases the client's understanding). Each rating may appear more than once in each numbered set. (See answers at the end of the chapter.)

1. **Client:** I need to find a job quickly. I've got a family to support.
   Helper:
   ____ a. Why did you leave your last job?
   ____ b. You really are scared about how you're going to make ends meet.
   ____ c. You want to find a job right away so you can take care of your family.

In this situation, the first response would be rated − because it asks a "why" question and puts the client on the defensive, not adding to his or her understanding of the problem. Response b is rated + because it identifies the underlying feeling and communicates empathy. Response c is rated = because it neither increases nor decreases understanding but merely paraphrases the message. Now finish rating the statements and then check the answers at the end of the chapter.

2. **Client:** Put the flowers over there and the newspaper there, and bring me my slippers and robe, please.
   Helper:
   ____ a. You really want me to be able to give you more attention.
   ____ b. You want me to put down your flowers and newspaper so I can bring you your slippers and robe.
   ____ c. Here you go again. I have other patients to care for, too!

3. **Client:** I'm not going to be able to come back to school next year.
   Helper:
   ____ a. Why not?
   ____ b. People who graduate have a better chance of getting jobs.
   ____ c. You're not coming back for your junior year.

4. **Client:** Yeah, well, you gotta be tough if you're gonna make it on the outside. Nobody gives an ex-con a chance anyway, so you gotta take what you can get and see that you get it.
   Helper:
   ____ a. You really feel that no one's going to give you a break.
   ____ b. You're wondering if you're tough and smart enough to make it. It's scary.
   ____ c. Ex-cons don't have a very good track record, you know.

5. **Client:** When I'm at home, my mom lets me eat whatever I want.

Helper:

___ a. Wow! Your mom sure spoils you!

___ b. You don't want to have to eat what you don't like.

___ c. You're unhappy that you can't always do what you want to here.

6. **Client:** I'm so angry at my mother that I'd like to kill her! She never says a nice thing to or about me. I wish I never had to see her again.

    Helper:

    ___ a. You're really angry that you seem to need her approval.

    ___ b. It's wrong to even think about your mother like that.

    ___ c. You're really angry with your mother. Tell me more.

7. **Client:** This is an awful place to work. No one is ever where they should be, and I do more work than anyone else.

    Helper:

    ___ a. You don't like working here.

    ___ b. All offices are like that in this kind of business.

    ___ c. It seems to you that nobody cares about you here and that nobody values your work.

8. **Client:** It's unfair that you can't find more money for me. How am I supposed to manage? I've got a wife and four kids.

    Helper:

    ___ a. You're concerned about making ends meet.

    ___ b. You're getting as much as you're entitled to under the law.

    ___ c. Why do you think you should get more than anyone else?

9. **Client:** People today care more about money than they do about one another.

    Helper:

    ___ a. You feel lonely and scared that people don't seem to care about you.

    ___ b. You're angry that people are so materialistic.

    ___ c. Yes, that's the world we live in today.

10. **Client:** It's a lousy course. I've had all that stuff before, and it's a waste of my time and money. Most of the courses around here are pretty bad.

    Helper:

    ___ a. You're not sure you should be in that course.

    ___ b. It's a required course for this program.

    ___ c. You seem to have ambivalent feelings about being in this program. Can we talk about that?

11. **Client:** I'd love to go back to work, but my husband feels I should be home when the kids get back from school.

    Helper:

    ___ a. I can see why he feels that way. It's much better for the children when their mom is home.

    ___ b. You're not sure whether to work or stay home.

    ___ c. Sounds like you feel some anger toward your husband because he imposes his expectations on you.

12. **Client:** I've really had a rough year.
    Helper:
    ____ a. You've had a tough time this year.
    ____ b. Everyone has a bad year at some time or another.
    ____ c. You seem very tense about how you've handled things this year.

13. **Client:** Well, he's got a hell of a nerve telling me what to do in that tone of voice. Who does he think he is?
    Helper:
    ____ a. Bosses are known to do that. Don't take it to heart. I'm sure his bark is worse than his bite.
    ____ b. You get angry when someone pushes you around!
    ____ c. You're really angry that he doesn't treat you with respect and accept you as a person who has feelings.

14. **Client:** Look, I'm only here because Mr. Smith sent me. I've got nothing to talk about.
    Helper:
    ____ a. Mr. Smith wanted you to come see me.
    ____ b. You don't want to be here, and you're angry that you got yourself into this.
    ____ c. He must have had some reason for sending you here.

15. **Client:** Every night my wife complains about everything that's happened during the day. It's getting so I don't want to go home anymore. I'd much rather stay in town and drink with the boys.
    Helper:
    ____ a. All wives are like that. After all, what else have they got to do?
    ____ b. You find it so intolerable at home that it's easier for you to stay away. Sounds as if you're pretty angry at your wife.
    ____ c. Your wife really rides roughshod on you when you get home every night.

Note that the subtractive, nonfacilitative responses in Exercise 3.23 neither increase the client's understanding of the problem nor focus on the underlying feelings. Rather, they tend to moralize or preach and avoid the affective parts of the client statements. The interchangeable responses do not close the door for further development, but they do not add to what has already been stated. Helpers who continually make interchangeable responses need to examine carefully their own avoidance behavior. Are they afraid to risk testing their understanding? Facilitative responses communicate the helper's listening, understanding, and caring; they help focus on the implicit and explicit affective and cognitive content; and they may encourage further exploration. A helper's response that incorrectly identifies the client's underlying feeling would still be considered facilitative. As long as the client has the opportunity and encouragement to say something like "No, not that, but . . . ," further exploration is facilitated. So it is not so much a question of a right or wrong response as of how facilitative the response is in terms of empathy, honesty, and open-endedness.

At this point, you may be thinking, "But isn't this kind of verbal responding putting ideas and thoughts into the client's head?" The answer to that question is that genuine, client-centered, empathic responses are your best insurance *against* putting words, ideas, or your values or needs into your client's head, because making those kinds of responses means that you are hearing and understanding client messages and, at the same time, continually allowing for feedback and reactions to your responses. By your manner and responses, you can communicate to clients your respect and confidence in their ability to think, feel, and act for themselves. You neither want nor need to do that for them. If the client doesn't like or agree with what you say, that's fine; it doesn't mean that you are no good or that the client is resisting you. It does mean, however, that you can both continue to explore what is going on until you can agree on what the problem is all about. It is a good idea to remember that timeliness and individual variables will influence your choice of responses. For example, some clients may become defensive if they receive an additive response too early in the relationship.

The next exercise asks you to write a facilitative response to each client statement. Check your responses against ours at the end of the chapter to see if you're in the ballpark. There is no one right response to any statement. Discuss your responses with others in your group.

EXERCISE 3.24 ■ For each helpee statement, write the best verbal response you can think of to meet the communication goals discussed in this chapter. Remember that these statements are presented out of context, and therefore you can respond only to verbal cues.

1. **Client:** I had a great time last night. I didn't think about Dave one minute!
    Helper: *(possible answer)* You're relieved that you were able to have fun and not think about Dave.

2. **Client:** John was snorting coke at the party, and he wanted Tom and me to do it, too. But I was scared we'd get into trouble.
    Helper:

3. **Client:** We'd like to get married, but we know we have many problems. What do you think we should do?
    Helper:

4. **Client:** You know, I wrote that financial report, but because I'm only an assistant, I can't even get credit for it.
    Helper:

5. **Client:** We don't need his folks' help. We can do it ourselves, and I wish Jack would realize that his mother is always butting into our affairs.

Helper:

6. **Client:** I refuse to let my kid be sent to that school with all those kinds of kids. She's gonna stay right here where she belongs.
    Helper:

7. **Client:** I'm not so sure that I can handle this job. It may be too much for me. The others are so much faster and don't make as many mistakes as I do.
    Helper:

8. **Client:** Listen, mister, you better believe that once I get outta here, there's no way you're gonna get me back. I'll die first, and I'll take some of your kind with me, you wait and see.
    Helper:

9. **Client:** The boys won't let me play ball with them. They're always teasing me and calling me names. I hate them!
    Helper:

10. **Client:** I think people are two-faced.
    Helper:

11. **Client:** You're always late. I've got more important things to do than sit around your office waiting for you, you know.
    Helper:

12. **Client:** I can't take that test. I have a splitting headache. Will you talk to Ms. Goldstein for me?
    Helper:

13. **Client:** I didn't do nothin'. You're always picking on me.
    Helper:

14. **Client:** I made it through school on my own. Why should I pay his tuition? Let him work like I did.
    Helper:

15. **Client:** I'm always telling Jim not to argue with his father. His father has a terrible temper.
    Helper:

16. **Client:** I'm so mad at my boss! I'd like to wring his neck. I do all the work around here, and he doesn't even recognize that.

Helper:

17. **Client:** How can he expect me to work full-time, take care of the house, and raise the children? He better find work pretty soon so we can afford some help.
Helper:

18. **Client:** I managed just fine until the accident. I'm blind now, and I just have to face the fact that I can't do what I used to do.
Helper:

19. **Client:** Other people have no idea how expensive it is to care for a handicapped child. We have to keep borrowing from my family.
Helper:

20. **Client:** I now have a job, Yuichi is in day care, and I just can't believe how wonderful everything is. For the first time in 44 years, I feel like a whole person!
Helper:

Now that you have had an opportunity to respond in writing to client statements, it is time to try out verbal responses. The next few small-group exercises allow you to verbalize responses that demonstrate responsive listening. A useful adjunct to these exercises is to tape-record sessions with actual helpees or with a friend or member of your family and then analyze your tape. Remember that this is a learning process, that putting concepts into practice is very difficult, and that it will take continual practice and time to achieve effective responsive listening skills.

EXERCISE 3.25 ■ In this exercise, you should divide into triads. (It is a good idea for these triads to remain the same for the duration of the course so that, as trust develops within the group, you will feel freer to voice real concerns rather than role-play.) Each triad meets for at least one hour per week, in or out of class. Each member of a triad should have the opportunity to be helper, helpee, and observer for at least 15 minutes at each meeting. The helpee may present a real personal issue or concern (it does not have to be a crisis or even a negative issue) or role-play a concern.

The helper demonstrates effective responsive listening skills. Problem solving and solution giving are to be avoided. The purpose of these interactions is for helpees to express their concerns and for helpers to convey understanding and to facilitate further exploration. The observers are free to break in if they feel the helper is getting off track or getting into problem solving. At the end of about 15 minutes, the triad processes the practice counseling session. It is as important for observers to give honest feedback to helpers as it is for helpees to share their reactions and feelings. You may find that you learn most about the significance of effective and noneffective listening when you play the role of helpee. Helper and helpee should discuss whether they felt they were on the same wavelength at the same time.

With regard to observer ratings, Kagan (1980) has found "interpersonal process recall" to be helpful in processing counselor interactions. When processing the triad sessions, the observer asks the following questions of the helper:

1. What do you think the helpee was trying to say?
2. What do you think the helpee was feeling at this point?
3. Can you pick up any clues from the helpee's nonverbal behavior?
4. What was running through your mind when the helpee said that?
5. Can you recall some of the feelings you were having then?
6. Was there anything that prevented you from sharing some of your feelings and concerns about the person?
7. If you had another chance, would you like to say something different?
8. What kind of risk would there have been if you had said what you really wanted to say?
9. What kind of person do you want the client to see you as being?
10. What do you think the client's perceptions of you are?

The observer can also use a rating scale (see Appendix A) to aid in providing feedback to the helper, or he or she can make audio- or videotapes of the session and then analyze them. The rating scale focuses on the verbal and nonverbal behaviors desired in helping situations and aids in assessing the level of communication the helper uses. In general, appropriate participation occurs when the energy levels of the helper and helpee are about equal and the helper feels comfortable with occasional silences and pauses. Overparticipation occurs when helpers feel very anxious, think they must say something at every pause, and put much of their energy into filling gaps. Underparticipation occurs when helpers are so insecure about their verbal responses that they allow helpees to go on and on and rarely intervene. They may even convince themselves that it is rude to interrupt the client, not realizing that nonstop talking by the client is not counseling. Once you become aware of your own patterns and style of communication, you will be able to modify your responses in the best interests of the helpee.

EXERCISE 3.26 ■ This is a variation on Exercise 3.25. In this exercise, small groups of six to ten people sit in a circle. One person volunteers to be the helpee and begins to communicate a personal concern. Each time the helpee makes a statement, a different person in the circle makes a facilitative response. For example, the helpee makes an opening statement, and person A responds to that statement. The helpee then replies to person A, and person B responds to that reply. When the helpee replies to person B, person C responds, and so on around the circle. This exercise is processed in a manner similar to Exercise 3.25. It has the advantage of involving more people in the processing and producing various levels of responses to the same person. Thus, the helpee is able to provide valuable feedback: whose responses were most helpful, why, and whose were not helpful. Actually, the most important benefit of this exercise is for the helpee, in that he or she is able to feel the effects of "connected" and "unconnected" responses.

EXERCISE 3.27 ▪ Read the following statements. Try to imagine that the person is speaking directly to you, the helper. Then write a response that (1) includes your understanding of both feelings and content and (2) will encourage the helpee to continue talking.

1. **30-year-old woman:** I'm really upset. My parents keep needling us about having a baby. Joe and I aren't sure that we want to have children. They can really disrupt your life. Most of our friends who did have kids really got bummed out. Anyway, my parents keep wanting us to come home for the holidays, but every time we do, it gets really tense. I wish they'd leave us alone.
   Helper: (*possible answer*) You really are concerned about how you and Joe can lead your own lives and make your own decisions without hurting your parents.

2. **Asian male graduate student:** My adviser says I have to talk more in seminar. All they do is argue in there. I get very nervous.
   Helper:

3. **Female college student:** I don't understand why grades are so important. College should be a place to have fun, but my folks are always on my back about my grades. They say if I ever want to go to graduate school, I need to focus on work, study hard, and all that stuff. They really get annoyed if I'm having a good time.
   Helper:

4. **14-year-old boy:** I'm really worried about my older sister [age 16]. She thinks I don't know what's going on, but I know she's into drugs and that she's screwing her boyfriend. And the folks act like nothing's going on. She's moody and rotten to everyone at home.
   Helper:

5. **Nurse:** It's impossible to spend any time talking to patients. The head nurse is always on us about wasting time with patients when we're so understaffed and there's so much paperwork. If I'd known that nursing would turn into this, I'd never have done it.

Helper:

6. **Secretary:** I was supposed to meet my brother for dinner tonight. But Ms. Palkovic asked me to work late tonight to get this report finished, and she's been so good to me I don't see how I can let her down.
   Helper:

7. **39-year-old business executive:** There's never enough time to get everything done. Business is slow and everyone is on edge around here. There are rumors that maybe payroll can't be met. And I just found out my kid needs braces and my wife wants the kids to go away to camp next summer. I don't know how I'll pay my heating bills this winter.
   Helper:

8. **22-year-old college graduate:** I have been on umpteen interviews. I know exactly what kind of job I want, and I can't seem to get it. Someone else will have already gotten there, or there just isn't anything open now. I don't know where else to look or what to do, and I'm going stir crazy sitting around the house waiting for people to call me back.
   Helper:

9. **63-year-old woman:** My children never come to see me. They're always too busy. When I call to talk to them, they always seem rushed. I don't understand it I was always good to my mother. I spent the best years of my life being a mother, and this is what I get for it.
   Helper:

10. **38-year-old African American worker:** Look, I try to get here on time. But I have to come across town from my other job, and sometimes I run into traffic. Yes, this job is important, but I have to work two jobs in order to feed my kids.
    Helper:

ADVANCED VERBAL
RESPONSE SKILLS

After you have learned to recognize facilitative and nonfacilitative responses, you can begin to develop patterns of verbal responding that are congruent with the types of issues involved and the stage of the helping relationship. Ten of the most commonly used kinds of verbal response are the microskills of (1) making a minimal verbal response, (2) paraphrasing, (3) reflecting, (4) using questions

(5) **clarifying,** (6) **interpreting,** (7) **confronting,** (8) informing, (9) summarizing, and (10) processing the relationship.

Making a Minimal Verbal Response Minimal responses are the verbal counterpart of occasional head nodding. These are verbal cues such as "mmmm," "I see," "uh-huh," which indicate that the helper is listening and following what the client is saying. Be careful when you use such minimal verbal responses as "yes," "right," or "okay," because clients may sense you are agreeing with the content of what they are saying, rather than just encouraging them to continue talking. Also, remember that you do not need to say something after every client statement. It is OK to say nothing!

Paraphrasing A paraphrase is a verbal statement that restates the content of what the client has said. It is similar to the client's statement, although the words may be synonyms of words the client has used. These are typically considered interchangeable rather than additive responses, so you don't want to rely exclusively on these types of responses. For example:

> **Client:** I had a lousy day today.
> **Helper:** Things didn't go well for you today.

Reflecting Reflecting refers to communicating to the helpee our understanding of his or her concerns and perspectives. We can reflect stated or implied feelings, what we have observed nonverbally, or what we feel has been omitted or emphasized. Examples of reflecting are "You're feeling uncomfortable about seeing him," "You really resent being treated like a child," and "It sounds as if you're really angry at your mother."

Using Questions The kinds of questions you can ask a client vary. Questions may be open-ended, leading to a fuller discussion of an issue, thoughts or feelings ("What can you tell me about this?"), or closed-ended, often eliciting just a "yes" or "no" response or brief information ("Did you give him an answer?" or "How old are you?"). Questions may also be reflective, a way to communicate your understanding of cognitive content or feelings in a nonthreatening way ("Are you saying that you're afraid she'll be angry at you if you disagree?"). You can repeat a word or two in a questioning voice (the client says "I'm just tired of everything," and the helper asks "tired?" or "everything?"), or you can respond with "and" or "but" in a questioning tone after a phrase (the client says "I was planning to exercise," and the helper responds "But?"). You may ask questions when you feel they will augment the communication flow, but unless you need specific information, such as in an interview setting, it is best to make them indirect and open-ended.

However, one glaring form of an often unhelpful open-ended question is a "why" question. This kind of question suggests that there is a "right answer" and that the person should know that answer. Often a client will respond "I don't know." "Why" questions can be perceived as judgmental and threatening, and the helpee may become defensive. If you cannot reframe the question, such as "Tell me what you think is behind this . . . ," asking a "how" question is more open-ended and allows clients to discover the "why" on their own at their own pace.

Please note that questions must be used sparingly. They usually hinder the development of the helping relationship more than they help it. Asking questions is often a way for the helper to avoid responding and can be distancing. The counselor may be directing what the client discusses, and the client may learn to rely too much on the helper to structure the session. Thus, it is highly preferable to rephrase questions into statements until you have mastered communication skills and learned when and how to ask questions. For example, instead of asking "What did you do next?" say "Tell me what happened then."

Clarifying Clarifying is an attempt to focus on or understand the basic nature of a helpee statement. It can be expressed as a question or a statement. Examples are "I'm having trouble understanding what you are saying. Is it that . . . ?" "I'm confused about. . . . Could you go over that again, please?" and "Sounds to me like you're saying. . . ."

Interpreting Interpreting occurs when the helper adds something to the client's statement or tries to help the client understand his or her underlying feelings, their relation to the verbal message, and the relation of both to the current situation. For example:

> **Client:** I just can't bring myself to write that report. I always put it off, and it's hanging me up right now.
> **Helper:** You seem to resent having to do something you don't want to do.

If the interpretation is useful, it will add to the client's understanding, and you will receive a reaction reflecting "Yes, that's it." If it's not useful, the client may say "No, not that but . . . ."

Confronting Confronting involves providing the helpee with honest feedback about what is really going on. The confrontation may focus on genuineness, reflected in statements such as "I feel you really don't want to talk about this," "It seems to me you're playing games here," and "I'm noticing that you always take the blame. What do you get out of that?" Or the confrontation may focus on discrepancy, reflected in statements such as "You say you're angry, yet you're smiling," and "On the one hand you seem to be hurt by not getting that job, but on the other hand you seem sort of relieved, too." An effective way of using confrontation is to send "I" messages, to "own" your responsibility for the confrontation by openly sharing your own genuine responses to the helpee or by focusing on the helpee's avoidance or resistance.

A 21-year-old client was discussing a pattern of hooking up with many different sexual partners. When asked about contraceptive use and "safe sex" practices, the client responded that she was not doing anything to protect herself.

It was clear from prior conversations that the client was well educated in this area. The therapist told the client that she was putting herself at great risk, which the client acknowledged that she already knew. The therapist then said that the client was behaving irresponsibly, and it was important for her to understand her actions. The client was taken aback that the therapist confronted her in such a direct way, but then began to discuss how she hated herself and just did not care what she did.

Informing   Informing occurs when you share objective and factual information, such as what you know about a particular college in terms of student enrollment, types of programs, and so on. It can also be a way of validating a client's experience: "The bad dreams and withdrawal you are experiencing are very typical after someone is mugged." It's important for the helper to separate informing from advising, which is subjective and verges on telling the helpee what to do. (Advice may be all right as long as it is tentative, with no strings attached, and as long as it's clearly advice, not a demand. Its success as an intervention depends on timing and on your relationship.)

Summarizing   By summarizing, the helper synthesizes what has been communicated during a helping session and highlights the major affective and cognitive themes. Thus, a summary is a type of clarification. This response is important at the end of a session or during the first part of a subsequent session. Summarizing is beneficial when both the helper and the helpee participate and agree with the summary. It also provides an opportunity for the helper to encourage the helpee to share his or her feelings about the helper and the session.

Processing the Relationship   By commenting on what is happening in the here and now, within the helping relationship, the counselor may help the client gain awareness of particular patterns of behaviors, thoughts, or feelings. "I noticed that you become angry at me every time I ask you about your visit with your mother." This skill can facilitate the development of an empathic, effective helping relationship.

The following are general guidelines when using the 10 major kinds of verbal responses:

1. Phrase your response in the same vocabulary that the helpee uses.
2. Speak slowly enough that the helpee understands each word.
3. Use concise rather than rambling statements.
4. Help the client stay focused on relevant issues or themes, rather than going off on tangents.
5. Talk directly to the client, not about him or her.
6. Send "I" statements to "own" your feelings, and allow the client to reject, accept, or modify your messages.
7. Encourage the client to talk about his or her feelings.

TABLE 3.2 Role behaviors and verbal responses appropriate to stages of counseling

	Stages	Role Behaviors	Verbal Responses
Responsive Listening	Relationship	Attending	Minimal verbal response
		Clarifying	Paraphrasing
		Informing/describing	Using questions
		Probing/inquiring	Reflecting
		Supporting/reassuring	Clarifying
			Processing
			Informing
	Strategies (working)	Attending	Using questions
		Informing/describing	Processing
		Probing/inquiring	Interpreting
		Supporting/reassuring	Confronting
		Motivating/prescribing	Informing
		Evaluating/analyzing	Summarizing
		Problem solving	Terminating

8. Time your responses to facilitate, not block, communication.

9. Be aware of cultural differences in helpee preference for and response to helper interventions.

The 10 major kinds of verbal responses may be applicable throughout the helping relationship and/or during particular stages. For example, minimal verbal response and paraphrasing may facilitate beginning relationship sessions or interviews, whereas interpreting, confronting, and informing may be more appropriate during the strategies (working) stage. Table 3.2 lists the verbal responses that apply to the first and second dimensions of the human relations counseling model.

SILENCE

Another powerful intervention, one that beginning helpers often find quite difficult and scary, is not listed as one of the verbal responses above because it does not use words at all. Silence—saying nothing in response to helpee statements— is a necessary and important technique for helpers. Yet most beginning helpers feel uncomfortable with it.

Here are some important points to keep in mind when using silence:

1. Remind yourself that what seems like hours is probably just a few seconds. Be aware of, and reduce, your own anxiety in response to the silence so that you can focus on your client and not feel inner pressure to break the silence.

2. Remind yourself that important therapeutic work can be done during silences. In fact, silence can help your client slow down and spend more time on an issue. If you talk too much, you may interrupt the client's progress.

3. Don't stare at your client during the silence.

4. Try to understand what your client is experiencing. Is the client thinking about what you just said? Is she feeling her emotions? Is he anxious or angry about the silence? Is she waiting for you to break the silence and take charge of the session? Is there a cultural meaning to the silence? Is your client someone who is particularly at ease with long silences during conversations? Your response to the silence will depend on what you observe and understand about your client. You might respond, "What are you feeling right now?" or "You'd like me to bring up the next topic."

EXERCISE 3.28 ■ Silence is necessary in a helping relationship, but helpers but often feel uncomfortable with it. Work through the following series of Gestalt-type exercises in triads, rotating the roles of helper, helpee, and observer each time you've completed the series.

1. The helpee talks about a real or imagined concern, and the helper is not allowed to respond in any way, either verbally or nonverbally. After five minutes, share reactions and feelings.

2. Maintaining the same roles, repeat the first sequence; now the helper is allowed to make two nonverbal responses within a five-minute period. Again, process.

3. Now the helper can make one verbal and two nonverbal responses within a five-minute period. Process after completion.

4. The helper can make four responses, either verbally or nonverbally, within a five-minute period.

5. The helper can respond in any way and as often as he or she chooses in the last five-minute period.

Discuss your reactions to the entire series of exercises; then change roles and start over again.

EXERCISE 3.29 ■ The purpose of this exercise is to see whether you can recognize and identify the major types of verbal responses. The exercise will help you become aware of your own verbal responses and perhaps encourage you to expand your repertoire. Read the following client and counselor statements, and identify the counselor's response in each case as making a minimal verbal response, paraphrasing, reflecting, using questions, clarifying, interpreting, confronting, informing, summarizing, or processing the relationship.

1. **Client:** That's why I'm here. Ingrid said you were a good one to talk to.
    Helper: You're hoping that I can help you with your problem.

2. **Client:** Do you think they have a good benefits package there?
   Helper: The National Conference Board reports that that particular company ranks in the top third for employee benefits.

3. **Client:** Eddie made me get kicked out of class today.
   Helper: How did you feel about that?

4. **Client:** I have to get the house cleaned before we can have company over.
   Helper: I see.

5. **Client:** In my family, my dad and brother don't do any of the work around the house.
   Helper: The men in your family don't do any housework.

6. **Client:** I can't decide what to do. Nothing seems right.
   Helper: You're feeling pretty frustrated.

7. **Client:** I don't want to talk about it.
   Helper: You always seem to back away when things get personal. It seems to me that it's much easier for you to talk about the situation than feel it.

8. **Client:** Anyway, I'm unable to do it because it's too expensive, and besides they won't help me anyway.
   Helper: Let me get this straight. You feel the tests will cost too much and the results won't be worth the cost. Is that it?

9. **Client:** Nobody in this world cares about anyone else.
   Helper: It's scary to feel that nobody at all cares about you.

10. **Client:** I guess that about covers it.
    Helper: Let's see if we can review what we've talked about today. . . . Does this seem right to you?

SUMMARY

In this chapter, we have discussed the cognitive and affective components of verbal and nonverbal messages, identified and elaborated the elements of responsive listening, and outlined 10 major kinds of verbal responses. A progressive series of individual and group exercises was presented, first to develop awareness of your own style of nonverbal and verbal communication behaviors, then to test your understanding of the concept of responsive listening—the differences among subtractive, interchangeable, and additive responses—and finally to allow you to practice and develop more effective communication skills. The exercises also help you to attend to cultural influences on verbal and nonverbal communication behaviors.

We are focusing our exercises and work on responsive listening as the core communication skill. It is also the most difficult to learn and master, in that it is the least commonly used form of communication in our society. Not only is responsive listening essential to establishing rapport and attending to the helpee's verbal and nonverbal messages, but it is also helpful in identifying and clarifying the helpee's underlying concerns. We have also described 10 commonly used forms of verbal responses that can be used in connection with overall responsive listening in the two stages of the helping relationship.

Guidelines are given in this chapter for developing communication skills. The effectiveness of the exercises will depend largely on the supervisory and modeling capabilities of your supervising trainer, but an instructor cannot spend a great deal of time supervising any one individual. Members of a group, however, can learn to be effective observers and provide one another with beneficial instruction in the form of honest feedback. Communication skills are the fundamental basis of the helping relationship and can be learned and practiced in many different formats, so you will have further opportunities to develop them in the chapters to come.

EXERCISE ANSWERS

Exercise 3.1 Possible answers might be (1) openness or trying to demonstrate control, (2) defensiveness, (3) evaluation or thoughtfulness, (4) rejection, (5) rejection or shyness or respect, (6) helplessness, (7) embarrassment, (8) self-control, (9) boredom, (10) acceptance.

Exercise 3.9

1. a. I don't have enough money.
    b. I have bills to pay.
    c. Should I take another job?
    d. Should I go back to school?

2. a. Is school worth the money it costs?
    b. I'm not learning anything here.
    c. People who go to school don't get jobs later.
    d. People get lost in such a big, impersonal place.

3. a. I don't know what to say to Mr. Jones when he calls later.
    b. Somebody ought to fix the parking situation.
    c. I need to be able to park in order to get here on time.
    d. I lost a memorandum.
    e. There aren't enough parking places here.

4. a. My apartment is not satisfactory because there is no heat.
    b. My kid is sick.
    c. I don't know what to do or where to start.
    d. I need money to pay the bills.
    e. I need a job.
    f. I am alone here.
    g. I just moved here.

h. I have not received all my furniture.

i. I have a disagreeable landlord.

5. a. We had a great time.

b. The Meyers were down there.

c. Swimming

d. Bicycling

e. Fishing

f. Sailing

(c through f could be interchangeable)

Exercise 3.11 1. a; 2. c; 3. a; 4. a or c; 5. c; 6. a or c; 7. c; 8. c

Exercise 3.15

1. Fear of bullies

2. Fear of illness or pleasure at attention from doctor

3. Sympathy for Lenny or anger at Lenny for never getting home

4. Anxiety about coming exams or anticipation of vacation after exams

5. Feeling pressured and rushed or bitter and angry about not being able to take a coffee break

6. Anger at being overworked by Professor Ramirez or distressed at being too busy to type report

7. Frustration and anger or loneliness

8. Fear of being hurt or anger at others' selfishness

9. Exasperation and frustration about delay or anger at dependence on Jim

10. Anxiety about new social worker or excitement about meeting her

11. Fear

12. Anticipation

13. Anger at Ms. Jones or concern for Ms. Jones

14. Desperation

15. Fear that something is wrong with child

16. Anger at young people for having more sexual freedom, or jealousy

17. Relief at stepping down or bitterness about pressures

18. Frustration at inability to learn

19. Concern

20. Confusion, fear

21. Anger at being ignored

22. Discouragement about not getting anywhere or anger at helper for not being better helper

23. Anger at rejection, or loneliness
24. Fear of rejection, or loneliness
25. Anger or concern

Exercise 3.23

2. a. +	3. a. −	4. a. =	5. a. −	6. a. +
b. =	b. −	b. +	b. =	b. −
c. −	c. =	c. −	c. +	c. =
7. a. =	8. a. +	9. a. +	10. a. =	11. a. −
b. −	b. −	b. =	b. −	b. =
c. +	c. −	c. −	c. +	c. +
12. a. =	13. a. −	14. a. =	15. a. −	
b. −	b. =	b. +	b. +	
c. +	c. +	c. −	c. =	

Exercise 3.24 Possible helper responses might be the following:

2. "Sounds to me as though you were annoyed at them for tempting you."
3. "You're confused about whether your marriage will work if you haven't worked through your problems."
4. "You feel angry and inadequate when you're not given credit for your work."
5. "You're pretty angry at Jack for not being able to wean himself away from his folks."
6. "You're afraid something will happen to her, and you care so much."
7. "You're afraid that you may be inadequate and may fail on this job."
8. "You're furious at the thought of returning to a place where you've been so unhappy."
9. "You feel sad and lonely when they won't let you play with them."
10. "You've been hurt often, and you're afraid to trust people."
11. "You feel like I don't care enough about you if I keep you waiting."
12. "You're so afraid you won't do well on that test."
13. "It seems to you that I don't like you, that I'm unfair to you."
14. "You're angry that he wants your help when you were strong enough to do it on your own."
15. "You're afraid of anger."
16. "You don't feel appreciated."
17. "You're really scared and overwhelmed with responsibilities."
18. "You're very independent, and you seem determined and proud."

19. "You're very angry that you have to be dependent on your family."

20. "Things are finally going well for you, and you don't want anything to happen."

Exercise 3.28

1. Processing the relationship

2. Informing

3. Using questions

4. Making a minimal verbal response

5. Paraphrasing

6. Reflecting

7. Confronting

8. Clarifying

9. Interpreting

10. Summarizing

REFERENCES AND
FURTHER READING

Brammer, L. M., Abrego, P. J., & Shostrom, E. L. (1993). *Therapeutic counseling and psychotherapy* (6th ed.). Englewood Cliffs, NJ: Prentice-Hall.

Brammer, L. M., & McDonald, G. (2003). *The helping relationship: Process and skills* (8th ed.). Englewood Cliffs, NJ: Prentice-Hall.

Cormier, L. S. & Nurius, P. S. (2003). *Interviewing and change strategies for helpers: Fundamental skills and cognitive behavioral interventions* (5th ed.). Pacific Grove, CA: Brooks/Cole.

Gordon, T. (2000). *Parent effectiveness training* (3rd ed.) New York: Wyden.

Hill, C. E. (2001). *Helping skills: The empirical foundation.* Washington, DC: American Psychological Association.

Ivey, A. E., & Ivey, M. B. (2003). *Intentional interviewing and counseling: Facilitating client development in a multicultural society* (5th ed.). Pacific Grove, CA: Brooks/Cole.

Kagan, N. I. (1980). Affect simulation in interpersonal process recall. *Journal of Counseling Psychology, 16,* 309–313.

Kagan, N. I., & Kagan, H. (1992). IPR—A research/theory/training model. In P. W. Dowrick (Ed.), *A practical guide to video in behavior sciences.* New York: Wiley.

Lewis, T., Amini, F., & Lannon, R. (2000). *A general theory of love.* New York: Random House.

Long, V. O. (1996). *Communication skills in helping relationships.* Pacific Grove, CA: Brooks/Cole.

Murphy, B. C., & Dillon, C. (2003). *Interviewing in action: Relationship, process and change* (2nd ed.). Pacific Grove, CA: Brooks/Cole.

Okun, B. F., Fried, J., & Okun, M. L. (1999). *Understanding diversity: A learning-as-practice primer.* Pacific Grove, CA: Brooks/Cole.

Sue, D. W. (2005). *Multicultural social work practice*. New York: Wiley

Sue, D. W., & Sue, D. (2002). *Counseling the culturally diverse: Theory and practice* (4th ed.). New York: Wiley.

Westra, M. (1996). *Active communication*. Pacific Grove, CA: Brooks/Cole.

Visit the book companion site at www.thomsonedu.com to access tutorial quizzes.

4

Stage 1: Building Relationships and Establishing Goals

In Chapter 1, we posited the development of the helping relationship as crucial to the effectiveness of any helping strategy. We then turned to a discussion of successful helper characteristics and communication skills. We move
on now to examine the conditions and steps necessary for creating the type of
empathic climate in which the helpee can begin to explore his or her world
and gain self-awareness.

CONDITIONS AFFECTING
THE RELATIONSHIP STAGE

Before discussing the five steps of the relationship stage, let's look at the important conditions affecting this stage. These conditions may appear obvious to
you, but unless they are taken into account consciously, they may hinder the
helping relationship.

Initial Contact

The term *interview* (or *intake interview*) is often used to describe the first one or
two helping meetings, because these sessions are usually for information gathering. For some people, the word has threateningly formal connotations: we can all
think of job and school interviews we've endured that have been more like

inquisitions. Whether the interview is initiated by the helper, the helpee, or a third party, the helpee often feels anxiety about being accepted and fears saying the "wrong" things and being judged. Nonetheless, we'll use the term *interview* for those initial encounters when the participants first meet and collect information. If the helping relationship proceeds, subsequent meetings can be called *sessions.*

The purpose of interviewing is for both interviewer and interviewee to share pertinent information during these initial stages of establishing the helping relationship, setting boundaries, and establishing goals. It is important for interviewees to learn the "rules" of the helping context to determine whether the helper/helpee "fit" is comfortable and to gain awareness of what can and cannot be provided.

The tone of an interview is set at the first moment of initial contact, whether that be when the appointment is made or when the interview begins. First the helper and the helpee must establish a mutually convenient meeting time. Right away, the helper should be frank. If unable to devote adequate time to the helpee at that particular moment, rather than trying to rush through a few frantic exchanges on the phone or in a corridor, the helper is better off saying, "I see you really need to talk to me about that. I'm tied up now. Could you come (call) back at three o'clock?"

The helper must quickly determine the realities and priorities of any given situation: Is this a crisis? Can I rearrange my schedule? Can this person wait until later to see me? Sometimes the only way to determine the nature of a situation is to ask helpees whether they can wait. In any case, at this critical moment of initial contact, the helper can communicate genuine concern and willingness to be available to the helpee. The following are some points to remember when arranging an appointment.

1. Schedule a specific time for an appointment; avoid saying "later," "next week," or "soon," and suggest specific alternative times.

2. Tell the helpee that you want to be available to him or her when you both can give full time and attention to the helpee's concerns.

3. Communicate support (reinforcement) to the helpee for initiating contact (for example, "I'm so glad you've come to see me about this"). People often feel a bit foolish and unsure about asking for help, and giving support helps them feel more secure about talking to you.

If you work in a setting where appointments are made for you, you must assume responsibility for seeing that whoever makes appointments communicates the same kind of concern and helpfulness to the client. There is nothing more deflating to a person seeking help than to be put off rudely by an appointment maker who refers to how busy you (the helper) are, seems reluctant to schedule a meeting, or is too inquisitive and asks too many personal questions.

If at all possible, arrange to have a corner where people waiting to see you cannot be observed by others in your setting. Many people feel uncomfortable if a peer knows they are talking to a supervisor, a counselor, or some other helping person.

If you are initiating the first interview, tell the helpee why you are arranging this meeting, preferably at the appointment-making time or at the beginning of the first contact. It is necessary that the helpee understand why you've arranged the contact so that he or she can learn to trust you, and to offset his or her resistances and defenses.

Duration

A helping relationship can last one, a few, or many sessions. The number depends on the following three points:

1. The nature of the relationship—whether it is formal or informal, voluntary or involuntary

2. The nature of the problem—whether it is short-term or long-term; how easily it is defined, clarified, and accepted; whether it is a crisis situation or one that is preventive or developmental; whether it relates only to the individual seeking help, involves others, or is a matter of poor fit between the person and the environment (for example, racism, layoffs, sexism)

3. The setting in which the relationship occurs—whether it is a counseling center, a human services institution, a business, an education system, a military setting, or some other situation—and the fee policies that pertain to that setting

In some cases, the nature and duration of the helping relationship cannot be determined until the problem is clarified. Thus, most initial sessions begin in a similar fashion, with the dual purpose of having the involved parties establish rapport and identify the problem. Increasingly, however, the helper and the helpee know from agency or third-party payer policies that a fixed number of sessions (typically 4–8) is allotted and that the helper will have to make a strong case for further sessions.

Applications and Forms

If applications or forms are required, it is usually better to ask the helpee to complete them before you begin the interview so that the meeting time can be used to establish a positive relationship. However, if your time allows, assisting the helpee in filling out the forms can be useful in establishing the helping relationship. Just remember not to become so involved in the content of the forms that you miss what the helpee is really communicating.

Employment and vocational counselors have traditionally collected informational forms and sometimes test battery results prior to an initial session. Increasingly, mental health counselors are requesting written information forms (see Appendix C) in advance so that the first meeting can focus on rapport building, rather than on information gathering. The kinds of information usually elicited include name, address, phone, e-mail, date of birth, insurance information, prior experiences with counseling or therapy or treatment for medical conditions (including current medications), history of alcoholism and drug abuse, brief family history including a history of violence or abuse, current family profile, legal history, helpee's definition of presenting problems and description of symptoms and complaints, helpee's perceptions of causes and contributing factors to these problems, other agencies or helpers currently involved, and expectations about the helping relationship.

Record Keeping

Record keeping is becoming increasingly important in today's treatment context. It is important and often legally required for helpers to maintain some basic written information. In addition to the written information forms already mentioned, mental health helpers today are required to record their diagnosis of the helpee's condition in accordance with the American Psychiatric Association's *Diagnostic and Statistical Manual TR*, 4th edition (2000). Furthermore, most third-party payers require helpers to record specific behavioral goals and objectives for the overall helping process as well as the strategies that will be utilized to achieve these objectives and criteria—all of which will be used for evaluation. In addition, helpers are required to maintain brief records of each meeting: date, time, duration, and specific objectives and outcomes of each meeting. Not only is this information required by third-party payers, employing clinics, and organizations, but in many states it must be available to subsequent helpers and to other agencies involved with the client.

The ethical and legal implications of record keeping will be discussed in Chapter 10. We (BFO and REK) usually share with helpees from the outset just what information we record, any disposition of that information, and regulations regarding confidentiality. We also discuss with a client our ideas about the implications of the diagnosis code submitted to a third-party payer, and together we reach a conclusion as to the appropriate diagnosis to submit to the payer for the client's particular circumstances. Some clients prefer to pay out of pocket to avoid submission of the personal details required by many third parties; some states require submission of personal records only for additional sessions.

If you intend to take written notes or use a video- or audiotape recorder during the interview, you can begin by explaining your rationale for this procedure and by clarifying who will and will not have access to the recorded data. Do not assume that a helpee who says nothing about the record keeping doesn't have any questions or feelings about it. You should bring it up and frankly discuss what it is all about. Both helper and helpee usually become oblivious to recording devices after the first few moments. Very often, helpees ask to review video- and audiotapes, which can prove to be an excellent strategy for developing both the helpee's and the helper's self-awareness. Taking notes during sessions or interviews can be distracting and can impair helper and helpee attentiveness; on the other hand, note taking may convey to clients that what they are saying is important—so important that "I must write it down" in front of clients so they can see that the helper is not making any judgments via note taking. Legal and ethical issues regarding note taking that will be elaborated in Chapter 10.

This is a good time to provide the helpee with a written statement of your professional policies (regarding matters such as cancellation and confidentiality) along with a copy of the federal HIPAA compliance requirements (see Appendix D). When multiple helpers or organizations are involved, you may need a Release of Information Form (see Appendix B) to carefully share information and coordinate services. In this situation, accurate written records can be invaluable.

Facilities

To establish trust and support, it is necessary that the helper provide a meeting place where client confidentiality can be ensured. Conferences in open offices with thin partitions or in the corner of an occupied room can be difficult situations in which to uncover a client's real concerns. If a private room is not available, try to find an out-of-the-way section in a stairwell or corridor, or go out of the building.

If you do have a private office, try to arrange the furniture so that you can sit facing the helpee without any barriers between you. For example, you can sit on one side of your desk close to the helpee, rather than across from him or her. Some people prefer to work away from their desks and arrange chairs facing each other in another part of the room.

Timing

Except in unusual circumstances, try to keep appointments as scheduled. It is terribly frustrating for someone to come to see you and find you unavailable. You can let the helpee know just how much time you have at the outset, if this is not already understood. During all interviews and sessions, it is important that you demonstrate your involvement with the helpee by refusing to accept telephone calls and by not allowing interruptions of any kind. A common complaint voiced by people seeking help is that they had just begun to get down to their real concerns when the mood was interrupted by a call or a knock on the door.

Another aspect of timing is a consideration of the time of day or evening when both helper and helpee function best. Some people are aware of being more alert during certain periods of the day. One client described a former therapist who ate dinner during his session with her. When she asked him about this, he told her he had diabetes and could not skip a meal. She questioned why he did not schedule a nonworking dinner hour for himself and decided to end therapy.

Other People

Sometimes a helpee will bring someone such as a friend, relative, or interpreter to the interview. According to the nature of the situation and setting, you will have to decide whether the presence of another person will help or hinder the helping relationship, and act accordingly. When an interpreter is necessary, remember that the communication process between you and the helpee is filtered through another layer and that the relationship between the interpreter and helpee and between you and the interpreter is never neutral. Having a friend or relative present gives you the opportunity to observe and hear differing or new perspectives about the helpee; it also has the potential benefit of strengthening support resources for the helpee.

Often, people from other cultures expect to bring in friends or family members as a matter of course. Recently, when one of us (BFO) was counseling a female student from Kenya about her homesickness, she brought in her African American roommate and assumed that was OK, which indeed it was. Our personal belief is that anyone within the helpee's social network who is willing to participate should be included for at least some sessions.

Some of the preceding points fall under the heading of obvious common courtesy. Yet we can all think of situations when we, as helpees, have been stymied by a helper's failure to consider one or more of the conditions affecting the relationship stage. Think back to interviews you have participated in. What conditions did you find threatening and what helpful? Try to relate them to what we will now discuss. We are going to cover the five critical steps in the relationship stage: (1) initiation/entry, (2) clarification of presenting problem, (3) structure/ contract for the helping relationship, (4) intensive exploration of problems, and (5) establishment of possible goals and objectives of the helping relationship.

STEP 1: INITIATION/ENTRY

A warm, smiling welcome is the best way to begin any interview or session. The obvious purpose is to help put the helpee at ease and hence get down to the business of identifying issues and concerns as quickly as possible. And, of course, you want to let clients know that you are genuinely glad to see them. Often some informal conversation about the weather, parking, and so forth is necessary to help the client relax. Ice-breaking remarks such as "Tell me what I can do for you" or "I'm interested in what's going on with you now" can help focus on the reason for the meeting. Your manner—relaxed, pressured, genuine, distant—will often provide the climate for how this initial meeting proceeds.

Drawing Out the Helpee

At the beginning of most interviews or sessions, you can better draw out the helpee and get more information by making responsive listening statements than by asking questions. Some examples of drawing out the helpee follow.

> **Client:** My husband has never been out of work so long before. It's having a terrible effect on the kids. That's why I'm here, I guess.
> **Helper:** That's a scary situation for all of you, I know. Let's talk more about what it's doing to you and your family.

In the preceding example the helper is communicating support and understanding while at the same time steering the conversation toward specific effects of the husband's unemployment on his family.

> **Client:** My friend Joan Astin said you helped her decide if she should stay with her boyfriend. I thought I'd come and see if you can help me decide what to do about my boyfriend. He just doesn't seem to want to make any decisions, and I think he should know by now if he wants us to get married.
>
> **Helper:** You seem to be confused about what you want to do. Can you tell me more about your relationship with your boyfriend?

In this example, the helper is seeking clarification of the nature of the situation.

> **Client:** (*fidgeting and avoiding eye contact*) I dunno why you sent for me. I ain't done nothin' wrong.
>
> **Helper:** You're concerned that I've asked you here because you're in some kind of trouble. I've asked you to come in so that I can get to know you better and find out more about how you're doing in shop. Mr. Jones seems to feel you're having some difficulties there.

Here the helper responds to the request for an explanation of the interview in a nonthreatening, honest manner.

> **Client:** I don't know whether I should come to you with this. I hate to complain. My daughter is awfully unhappy with Keisha [her camp counselor].
>
> **Helper:** I'm glad you've come to see me, Mrs. Woo. Tell me what you think is troubling Mikage about Keisha.

In this case, the helper is assuring the helpee that it's OK to deal with this issue, while asking for some further information.

> **Friend:** Hi! Got time for a cup of coffee?
>
> **Friend:** Just a sec. I've been wondering how things are going with you.

In this informal setting the helping friend responds promptly to the cue for a visit and starts right in expressing concern.

Statements or **leads** such as those in the preceding examples, which draw out information in a nonthreatening, open, indirect manner, are door openers or ice breakers. Their purpose is to keep the communication flowing without any judging, confronting, or manipulating. Other such leads are "Tell me more about that," "I'm wondering about . . . ," "Seems to me that . . . ," and "That sounds really interesting." Minimal verbal statements can also keep the communication flowing, as can head nodding, smiling, and encouraging gestures, such as raised eyebrows or a hand signaling "more, more."

Helpers need to be supportive and encouraging in order to establish an effective helping relationship. However, if you as a helper confuse reassurance with support and encouragement, you may help people avoid rather than approach their true concerns. If you are too reassuring, you are denying the legitimacy of the helpee's concerns and, by doing so, imposing your values and judgments, even though you think you are being nice and making someone else "feel better."

EXERCISE 4.1 ■ In triads, rotate role-playing helper, helpee, and observer. The helpee should imagine having an anxiety-producing secret that must be revealed if he or she is to benefit from a helping relationship. The helper should seek to establish a safe, empathic environment that will enable the helpee to self-disclose. After 20 minutes, the members of the triad should process what verbal and nonverbal behaviors of the helper were helpful and what were less helpful.

Working With Reluctant and Resistant Clients

The ambivalence of reluctant clients to engage in the helping relationship can negatively affect the counseling process and outcome. The first step for the helper is to explore the reasons for reluctance. It may be a "healthy cultural paranoia" (Boyd-Franklin, 2003) that African American and other marginalized groups may feel toward a European American psychotherapist. Many people from marginalized groups have an ingrained self-protective mistrust of white-controlled institutions and their white staff based on their history of and current experiences of racism. Other clients may be reluctant because of past experiences with counselors and agencies. These experiences may have been positive, and now the client is hesitant about starting over, negative, or even damaging.

Reluctance may also emanate from shame, embarrassment, or fear of exposure of secrets (such as substance abuse or physical abuse). Many people fear the counselor's indirect or direct judgment. For example, a gay or lesbian couple may be uncomfortable sharing with a heterosexual helper their concerns about having a child together. Some people may be reluctant to seek and engage in a helping process because a court, employer, or family member is requiring their participation or because their family or ethnic group does not approve of counseling.

Exhibiting a great deal of patience and empathy and allowing sufficient time for the counseling process can help to diminish the ambivalence and defensiveness of reluctant clients. Your genuineness, which includes discussing alternatives and their consequences, enables the reluctant client to decide whether it will be in his or her best interest to cooperate with you. The client will not be able to make this decision, however, unless you can spell out just who you are, what you are doing there, and what you see as the nature and objectives of your prospective helping relationship.

Helpers often become enmeshed in a game with reluctant clients that does little more than pass the time. It is the "I'm only here to help you" kind of game. One way of combating this game is to encourage the reluctant client to take the initiative for structuring the relationship. An example of this occurred in a halfway house, where the youth worker stayed in close physical proximity to a reluctant client, shrugged off verbal abuse, and communicated caring and genuineness more by nonverbal presence than by words. After four days of testing the youth worker in every conceivable fashion, the 14-year-old boy began to shed his bravado and share some of his underlying feelings and thoughts. It was almost a test of endurance: who could outlast whom.

Larrabee (1982) suggests the use of affirmation techniques with reluctant clients. Based on responsive listening, these techniques help the client face the reality of his or her problematic situation and understand the reasons that maintain the situation. Reluctant helpees may not perceive the negative aspects of their situation and may resist help out of misguided loyalty to peers or others. For example, the helper might suggest to the client some of the possible outcomes of helping and propose meeting for a limited number of sessions to explore possibilities before the helpee makes a final decision. The use of interchangeable and additive responses enables the helper to paraphrase or reflect the helpee's feelings and thoughts without communicating devaluation, sarcasm, or impatience—and at the same time allows the communication of genuine caring and respect for the helpee's different views. Larrabee also suggests that open-ended leads can help reluctant clients focus on self-examination. There are times when it may be necessary to use silence as the only way of responsibly attending to a reluctant client.

Try not to feel guilty about or hurt by rejection from a reluctant client. Instead, try to become aware of possible aspects of your approach to this helpee, as well as aspects of your setting and situation, that may be contributing to that rejection. You may find that your style of helping is not working for a particular client in a particular setting. In that case, you can either modify your style or arrange for a referral. You might also reflect the helpee's reluctance, clarify the consequences of not working together, and/or wonder out loud if there is anything at all you can do to help, even if the focus is not what the referral source had in mind.

Resistance can occur initially, as with the reluctant clients described above, or at any time in the helping relationship, and can vary in intensity and duration. Resistance is often the helpee's response when a trustful relationship has not yet been established and the helpee is feeling threatened, whether by the relationship, the material being explored, or the helper's probing or interpreting of sensitive issues before the client is ready to talk about them. It typically can be identified when the client does not appear to collaborate in developing the helping relationship or in establishing and/or striving toward goals.

Resistance can range from subtle forms of inattention, failure to keep appointments, or other indications of ambivalent attitudes, to outright rejection of the helper. Otani (1989) describes four categories for classifying aspects of client resistance: (1) amount of verbalization, (2) content of message, (3) style of communication, and (4) attitude toward helper and helping sessions. For example, clients can show resistance by verbalizing too little, limiting their verbalizing to safe topics, chattering irrelevantly or giving monosyllabic answers, missing sessions, being late, or not paying attention.

The sensitive helper uses the helpee's resistance to focus more closely on the characteristics of their relationship. In other words, the helper can be alert to the helpee's resistance without reacting directly to it, and by recognizing the resistance, the helper can gain an understanding of the helpee's unique defensive style. The effective helper will try to reduce defensiveness, perhaps by changing the pace, topic, or level of the discussion, and by communicating as much support and acceptance as possible. If the relationship has already been well established when resistance occurs, the helper may perhaps reflect back the feelings of resistance and decide with the helpee how to deal with them. A helper can often reduce resistance by sharing an awareness of the resistance with the helpee; changing strategies; modifying his/her style, such as by judicious use of humor or self-disclosure; or using some temporary diversion, such as changing the subject or referring the helpee to a different source of help.

It is usually futile to get into a win/lose power struggle with a resistant client, as the helper can only lose. Remember, you can lead a horse to water but you cannot make it drink! Helpers often experience anxiety, frustration, and anger by struggling against the resistance. The more a helper pursues a resistant helpee, the stronger and more manipulative the resistance may become. It is more useful to "go with" or follow the helpee's resistance in a supportive, non-threatening manner. If all else fails and the helpee refuses to cooperate at all or attempt to deal with the resistance, a "sabbatical leave" from helping may be appropriate. Many helpees need time on their own to work through their resistances and, if a period of time is allowed between sessions, may feel more in control of the situation.

Although resistance is often an indication of the client's inner conflict, sometimes it results from inappropriate helper behavior, such as empathic failure leading to unhelpful responses. It is important that you stay aware of the part you might play in the helpee's resistance. Remember, blaming yourself or the helpee is not the issue; what is important is understanding and recognizing the value and inevitability of resistance as part of the change process.

EXERCISE 4.2 ■ After each of the following helpee statements, pick the response(s) that you think would best address the helpee's reluctance or resistance. Our answers are given at the end of the chapter. An alternative exercise is to have students form small groups. One person reads the helpee statement, and each other member provides a helper response.

1. **Helpee:** I've never told anyone before, and I am just not comfortable telling you.
   Helper:
   a. That seems like a waste of my time and yours.
   b. Talking about it is the only way you will ever feel better.

    c. Have you been abused? Is that what you don't want to talk about?

    d. It's important for you to go at the pace you are comfortable with.

    e. Perhaps you would like a referral to another therapist.

2. **Helpee:** (an adolescent boy) You can't make me talk.
   Helper:

    a. You're right. I know you don't want to be here, but I'm wondering if there is anything I can help you with as long as you are here.

    b. We might as well end the session now.

    c. Now I understand why you've been referred here.

    d. I'll need to tell your parents that you are not cooperating.

    e. You have some real anger problems.

3. **Helpee:** I just don't want to talk about my abuse today. I'm not ready.
   Helper:

    a. You're in counseling now, so it is important to talk.

    b. OK, what else would you like to talk about today?

    c. I've also been abused, so you don't have to worry about telling me.

    d. Tell me about not being ready.

    e. How old were you when the abuse started?

4. **Helpee:** (looking repeatedly at the clock) When is this session ever going to be over?
   Helper:

    a. In ten minutes.

    b. You don't wear a watch?

    c. Are you angry at me?

    d. The session seems like it is going on forever.

    e. You've been sent by the court and it is important for you to participate for the full session.

5. **Helper:** Would you tell me about your relationship with your mother?
   Helpee: (irritated tone) Why? There's nothing to tell.
   Helper:

    a. You seem irritated by my question.

    b. Seems like this may be a difficult topic for you.

    c. OK, tell me about your relationship with your father.

    d. So your relationship with your mother is quite problematic.

    e. Running away from a topic does not make it go away.

6. **Helpee:** How do I know I can trust you?
   Helper:

    a. Because I am telling you that you can trust me.

    b. No wonder you have had difficulty in relationships.

    c. Trust is something that will, hopefully, develop over time.

    d. How has lack of trust been an issue in your life?

    e. Tell me more about what you mean by trust.

7. **Helpee:** How old are you? How much experience have you had doing this? You look like my granddaughter.

Helper:

a. I'm 25, but I just finished my master's degree in counseling.

b. How old is your granddaughter?

c. You're wondering whether I can be helpful to you.

d. I look a lot younger than I really am.

e. It's difficult to tell your concerns to someone who is much younger than you are.

8. Client has come to the session today after missing two of the last four appointments. Until this point, the client had never missed a session.
   Helpee: I forgot our sessions.
   Helper:

   a. You need to stop being so irresponsible.

   b. I wonder if there's anything that we've been discussing lately that's been difficult for you.

   c. No problem. Where would you like to begin today?

   d. When did you start having memory problems?

   e. My time is just as important as yours.

9. **Helpee:** I don't know why you keep focusing on me. As I've told you, my husband is the one with the problem.
   Helper:

   a. Bring him in. I'll fix his ass.

   b. It's often frustrating when the person with whom you're upset isn't in the room. We can certainly talk about whether a couple referral makes sense, but I'm wondering if we could also look at your personal goals for interaction with him.

   c. I really think you need to divorce him. He's clearly scum.

   d. Well, you say that about everyone. Maybe you're the real problem.

   e. I'm wondering if we might look at how you'd like to respond to situations with your husband.

EXERCISE 4.3 ■ After each of the following helpee statements, circle the letter of the helper response that you believe would best facilitate the development of an empathic relationship and lead to clarification of the presenting problem. Our answers are given at the end of this chapter.

1. **Helpee:** Ms. Alvarez said you wanted to see me.
   Helper:

   a. Yes, Elena. She tells me you're not getting on very well in that group.

   b. Oh? That's right, I did. Can you tell me what's going on in your group? I understand production is way off and there are a lot of personality conflicts.

   c. I have been wanting to talk to you, Elena. How do you feel about the way things are going in the group?

    d. Yes. I want to see if there's any way we can help you feel good here. Can we talk about how things are going in the group?

    e. Ummmm. I want to hear your version of what's going on in the group.

2. **Helpee:** I'm not going to be able to get through that interview. I know I'll mess it up like all the other times!

  Helper:

    a. No, you won't—not if you make up your mind not to.

    b. Come on! Have some faith in yourself. Of course you'll do OK.

    c. You're worried that you'll fall apart once you get in there?

    d. Why don't you talk to some people who've already had their interviews and see if they can clue you in as to what it'll be like.

    e. You feel that because you've had some bad experiences interviewing, this one will be bad, too.

3. **Helpee:** I don't understand why we're always fighting. We just can't seem to talk about anything anymore.

  Helper:

    a. Tell me about it.

    b. All married people fight sometimes.

    c. It's frightening to be so angry with your husband most of the time. Makes you worry about what's happened to change your relationship.

    d. What do you fight about?

    e. You probably need a change. How about changing your routine a bit—maybe go out to dinner or to a movie or do something different.

4. **Helpee:** I've come to see you because I need help. What do you think I should do about this?

  Helper:

    a. You seem to want me to tell you what to do.

    b. The first thing is to check out some information. Have you looked into financial aid?

    c. I can't solve your problems for you, you know.

    d. What do you want to do?

    e. I don't know. Let's talk some more about it.

5. **Helpee:** Business has really fallen off. They're talking about laying people off.

  Helper:

    a. You're worried that you may be laid off if things don't start to get better.

    b. I know. I'm worried too. Don't know what will happen.

    c. Yeah, times are rough. Every day the papers report more layoffs.

    d. Don't worry. I'm sure things are just exaggerated right now.

    e. Don't you think we're all in the same boat?

6. **Helpee:** I want to take Laurel home for Thanksgiving. But I know my mom will be upset about our religious differences, and I just don't feel like getting into all that.

  Helper:

    a. Sounds as though you've been thinking a lot about it.

b. You're sort of caught between not wanting to upset your mother and sharing your real life with your family.

c. Have you talked to your dad or brothers about this?

d. Are you afraid you'll have to choose between Laurel and your mother?

e. I can see you're unhappy about having to make a decision. What could be done to help you?

7. **Helpee:** My coming to see you really won't help. You can't change anything.

Helper:

a. You wish I could make things easier for you.

b. You're pretty discouraged. You wish there were some way I could change things for you.

c. Sounds to me as though you're not even willing to try.

d. Maybe there are some things you could change!

e. I'm wondering if you really want to change.

8. **Helpee:** If only I had listened to my dad. He told me this wouldn't work.

Helper:

a. Well, you live and learn. It's not so terrible to make a mistake.

b. Crying over spilt milk won't help.

c. It's rough. Tell me why you think it didn't work.

d. It's sort of scary to think your dad might be right about things. What else might he be right about?

e. It makes you nervous to find out you're not always right.

9. **Helpee:** I don't want to go back to school, ever. I'm not learning anything, and the teachers are terrible. I want to get a job now.

Helper:

a. You know, Misha, if you don't finish school, you'll be sorry later on, and it will be too late.

b. I know how you feel, but it's pretty difficult getting a job these days.

c. You really are feeling down about that school. Sounds as though you really want to get away from there.

d. You're not sure what you're getting out of being in school. Seems like a waste of time for you.

e. I'm wondering what you're doing to help yourself out over there.

10. **Helpee:** My parents are always on my back. They always want to know where I am, what I'm doing, and who I'm with. They never leave me alone.

Helper:

a. It does seem as if parents worry too much, doesn't it?

b. You're really upset because it seems to you that your parents don't trust you.

c. I'm sure they really love you and are just worried. It's so hard these days with teenagers.

d. Have you ever done anything to give them cause for worry?

e. It's nice to know they care so much, isn't it?

After you have completed this exercise, look at the suggested answers at the end of the chapter, then discuss your answers in small groups and see whether you can determine why some are more appropriate than others.

STEP 2: CLARIFICATION
OF PRESENTING PROBLEM

It may take some time and patience to uncover the problem that is of concern to the helpee. Understandably, most people test helpers with superficial concerns before they trust them enough to reveal more basic ones. Some clients might not even be aware of their real concerns. For example, a woman came in to see me (BFO) and told me she had come because she was worried about one of her children. However, as we proceeded to develop a relationship, it became apparent that she was angry at her husband and concerned about her marriage. In this case, it had been less painful for the woman to focus on her child than on her troubled marital relationship. You must actively listen and carefully respond to the helpee in order to avoid being sidetracked by superficial concerns.

It is possible that a helpee will present several different concerns. By using responsive listening techniques, you can aid the helpee in sorting out and ranking the different problems.

The following examples show two different approaches to the same client statement expressing many concerns.

Client: I'm really having family problems. My fiancée and I have a mutual uncle, and he is close to my parents and me. Her parents have not seen or spoken to him in 15 years. They have forbidden her to visit him or come to my house if he is there.

Helper: That's rough. You seem to feel guilty about your relations with your uncle.

Client: Yes. The problem is the wedding. My mother insists he come, and my fiancée says it's impossible.

Helper: You're really in a bind, and you don't know how to get around this.

Client: I'm beginning to think we should elope. You know large Italian family weddings; I don't know how we can make everyone happy.

Helper: Let's talk about the different ways you can deal with the wedding invitations.

■ ■ ■

Client: I'm really having family problems. My fiancée and I have a mutual uncle, and he is close to my parents and me. Her parents have not seen or spoken to him in 15 years. They have forbidden her to visit him or come to my house if he is there.

Helper: You seem to be upset that your fiancée's parents have such control over her.

Client: Yes, I guess they really do.

Helper: It's uncomfortable for you to be in the middle of the two families, and for her not to be taking a stand with you.

Client: I think her first loyalty should be to me! After all, I'm going to be her husband!

Helper: Sounds to me like you're wondering how she'll react to her parents' pressures after you're married.

Client: That's really it.

The helper in the second example was able to clarify the real issue, rather than be sidetracked by an apparent problem. You can see how important it is to take the time to get to the real problem and not rush too quickly into problem solving. It has been our experience, both as counselors and with colleagues at meetings, that unless the time is taken to clearly identify the problem and its "ownership," a large amount of problem-solving activity is futile. What we mean by *problem ownership* is identifying which person has the problem. A person must feel that he or she "owns" at least part of the problem before that individual will invest much energy in the problem solving process.

Another example illustrating the problem-clarification step is the following:

Client: I'm not going to be able to come in for work tomorrow. I know you need me for the inventory, but I just can't make it.

Helper: Sounds like something is bothering you.

Client: No, not really. I'm going to have to start looking for a place of my own to live.

Helper: Your present living situation isn't working out.

Client: I'll say! My roommate is really bitchy and giving me a hard time. I need an apartment of my own, even though I don't know how I'll manage.

Helper: You seem scared about the financial responsibilities and torn between getting a place of your own and putting up with a bad situation.

Client: That's right. I've never been on my own before. I don't know if I can do it. Everything seems to cost so much.

Helper: Let's see if I can help you plot out what it will cost.

Again, by taking the time to listen to what the helpee was really saying, the helper was able to identify the helpee's underlying fear and insecurity, rather than be sidetracked by the helpee's relationship with the roommate.

In many cases, presenting problems cover up more pervasive underlying problems, and many sessions may be required before those problems emerge. This may be because some people take longer than others to develop trusting rapport or because the client does not understand or acknowledge to himself or herself what the real issues are. The steps of the relationship stage may be completed with the presenting problem and then begun again for newer, emerging problems.

Exercise 4.4 In small groups, discuss the following situations. Then, if possible, role-play the courses of action listed with the goal of clarifying the problem. Share with the other members of your group your feelings about and reactions to these scenarios, and see if they help you to clarify the problem(s). Give your rationale for accepting or rejecting each alternative, and then supply some of your own.

1. Tanya, age 10, comes to you, her Girl Scout leader, to tell you that two other Scouts in your troop stole some candy from a local store yesterday. She's been with them when they've done that before, too. What would you do, and why?
    a. Call in the other two girls and confront them with Tanya's report.
    b. Discuss with Tanya the morality of shoplifting, tattling, and one's association with wrongdoers even if one doesn't misbehave.
    c. Explore with Tanya her own concerns about this problem and what her options are.

2. Mr. Domingo comes into your public employment office to insist that he did, in fact, show up for a scheduled job interview, even though the employer claims that he did not. What would you do, and why?
    a. Tell Mr. Domingo that you know he has lied and that you can no longer refer him for job interviews.
    b. Ask him to tell you what happened, and explain what you can and cannot do for him and what options are available to him.
    c. Suggest that he join a vocational counseling group for practice in interviewing.

3. Tom, age 14, comes to your gymnastics class at the local recreation center "stoned." Despite his steady attendance, you've been concerned about Tom's erratic participation in this class for a few weeks. Every time you've asked him what's wrong, he tells you, "Nothing. Don't bug me." What would you do, and why?
    a. Tell Tom that you want to have him in your class but he really can't come when he is stoned, because that is not fair to you and the others in the group.
    b. Tell him that you're concerned about him and will be available to talk to him about whatever is bothering him whenever he's ready.
    c. Ask him if you can take him home and talk to his parents with him.

4. You are a store manager in a fashionable suburban shopping center, and you have noticed for several weeks that your senior salesperson has been making errors during the nightly audit. You also have noticed that she is irritable and snapping at coworkers over every little thing. What would you do, and why?
    a. Tell her you've noticed she seems upset and that you're concerned. Can she tell you what's going on?
    b. Explain to her that your regional manager is on your back about these errors and you need to know if she needs help at night.

    c. Suggest to her that she seems to be troubled and perhaps needs to talk to someone. You know someone at a local agency that you would be happy to refer her to.

5. You are a volunteer for a local crafts program for the elderly. One gentleman, Mr. Roberts, appears to be withdrawn and cranky. When you talk to him, he tells you that his daughter-in-law is being nasty to him, and he is unhappy living with her. What would you do, and why?

    a. Discuss with him how unsympathetic in-laws often are and sympathize with his position.

    b. Discuss with him the different capabilities he has and the options he has for various activities within the community.

    c. Empathize with his loneliness, and discuss what you and others can offer him in the way of companionship and activities.

Again, act out as many of the previous responses as you can, and see how effective they are. Get in touch with your own feelings and values as you identify with both helper and helpee.

STEP 3: DEFINITION
OF STRUCTURE/CONTRACT

Once the problem has been clarified and acknowledged by the helpee as one needing resolution, you can decide whether you are able to provide help in solving that kind of problem. Your decision will most likely be influenced by your assessment of the helpee's motivation to collaborate actively in the process. If you feel that you are unable to provide help, you can aid the helpee in obtaining assistance elsewhere by means of **referral.**

    Referrals are arrangements for clients to see a designated individual or agency for a specific purpose. In helping relationships, early referrals are especially important because they can take some time to effect. There may be a waiting period before a referral appointment can take place, and during that period you may want to maintain a supporting, encouraging relationship. The helpee may be reluctant to accept a referral, and acceptance (readiness) may become the goal for your helping relationship. If you serve in a helping role in a setting where personal or long-term counseling is not available, you can maintain a list of available community resources so that you can quickly make contacts for helpees.

    An example of a referral is the following:
    Ms. White, age 42, has been employed as a supervisor in the packing unit for eight years. She has recently lost a lot of weight and has displayed irritable, irrational behavior with her workers. Her behavior is unusual; for eight years she has been regarded as one of the most easygoing supervisors in the company.

The following excerpt occurs at the end of her second session with the human resources manager, someone with whom Ms. White has talked before. Ms. White requested these sessions because she felt the need "to talk to someone."

> **Ms. White:** And so it seems as if my whole world is falling apart. I can't eat, I can't sleep, I can't think.
>
> **Human Resources Manager:** I'm concerned about you. You're really having a difficult time.
>
> **Ms. White:** I went to the doctor a couple of days ago. He says except for the weight loss and nerves, it's all in my head and I just have to stop worrying. I don't even know what I'm worrying about.
>
> **Human Resources Manager:** Thelma, I'd like to be able to help you, but I really think you need a different kind of help than I can give.
>
> **Ms. White:** What do you mean? I'm not mental or anything like that.
>
> **Human Resources Manager:** No, I know that. But you are having problems that lots of people have at one time or another in their life. And there are people around who are trained to help you. They can help you find out what's worrying you.
>
> **Ms. White:** I don't know. I don't think I could talk to anyone the way I can to you. And I can't afford much.
>
> **Human Resources Manager:** You can still talk to me. Let me try and find out who in your town can be of help, and the cost. Then we can talk some more about it.
>
> **Ms. White:** If you really think that's what we should do.
>
> **Human Resources Manager:** Can you come see me tomorrow morning? Around 9:45—just before coffee break? We can talk some more about it then.

Ms. White is frightened of a referral, and the HR manager is sensitive to her fear. In a case such as this, the helper should take the time necessary to allow the trustful relationship with the helpee to serve as a vehicle for helping him or her accept a referral. Because the HR manager knows that Ms. White has already had a medical examination, she can take the time to be supportive and effect what she believes will be a satisfactory referral for Ms. White.

To feel good about making a referral, you must learn what you can and cannot deal with and learn who around you can handle what kinds of situations. However, if the nature and extent of the problem are such that you feel you can provide help, you must state clearly to the helpee just what you can and cannot do, what you expect from the helpee, how you perceive his or her expectations of you, and how much time you can devote to this helping relationship. These directions apply to both formal and informal helping relationships, whatever the setting. Unfortunately these guidelines are often neglected, and unhappiness and frustration result on both sides when (unclarified) expectations are unmet.

Knowledge of a variety of resources is particularly important today, when so many people do not have access to traditional helping services. It is often advantageous to make use of as many different approaches and services as are available for a particular situation. We often refer clients to such available resources as Alcoholics Anonymous, marriage encounter groups, parenting groups, groups for parents of learning-disabled children, and groups designed for patients with a specific illness. Support groups are also available for military families, divorced or widowed families, and trauma survivors (such as those impacted directly or indirectly by 9/11 and the Iraq War). Also available are many informal and formal illness groups, as well as stress-reduction, mindfulness, meditation, and yoga classes. A recent client, upon release from a psychiatric hospital, returned to her home state and began a group for women with manic-depressive disorder. This proved to be enormously helpful in providing the same kind of peer support and understanding that she had benefited from when in the hospital.

EXERCISE 4.5 ■ Each member of the class can select a particular problem (such as alcoholism, marital problems, parenting a sick child, dealing with a rebellious adolescent, or coping with being laid off) that a helpee might present. During the week, contact community agencies (clinics, hospitals, schools, churches, and other organizations) and peruse local newspapers and bulletins in order to identify all possible helping resources. Share your findings with classmates, and begin to develop a referral pool.

When the nature of the problem remains uncertain or other factors seem to be involved, you may want time to seek a consultant's advice about your own options as a helper, or you may suggest that the helpee seek consultation with another helper. If a medical condition, such as headaches or poor digestion, might possibly be contributing to a client's distress, you will want to refer the helpee to a physician before you proceed further. Or if a client is having problems with an ex-spouse, you may want to suggest legal consultation.

If you and the helpee agree to it, one way to clarify expectations is to make a contract. A contract can be written or spoken; it is clear, understood by all parties, and always open to revision. For example, if you tell a helpee you would like to meet five times and then see how things are, you can always decide to lengthen or shorten that time as long as you both agree. Agreement is the key factor. The terms of the contract can include time of sessions, length of sessions, site of sessions, fees (if applicable), an estimate of number of sessions needed, who may or will attend sessions, procedures for changing any of these terms, and identification of helper and helpee expectations.

The following example demonstrates the making of a contract.

Marianne, an 18-year-old college freshman, has been referred to the counselor by her residence adviser because of continuing homesickness. The following excerpt occurs at the end of the first session, during which the counselor has identified the problem as one of low self-concept with resulting feelings of inferiority and inadequacy.

Counselor: Our time is almost up, Marianne. I'm wondering how you feel about our talk today.

Marianne: It's been OK.

Counselor: Would you like to come in again?

Marianne: Yes, I think so. Do you think I should?

Counselor: It's up to you. I do think we can talk some more about what you're doing and feeling.

Marianne: Uh-huh.

Counselor: Why don't we plan on having three more sessions—one hour per week—and then we can see where to go from there. You may want to think about joining a group then, or you may want to continue coming in. We can leave that open for now.

Marianne: That sounds OK. Do I make the appointments with you or with your secretary?

In this case, the counselor suggests that there is more material to gather and that, in a few weeks, they may have some other options to consider. This kind of structuring provides a frame of reference so that the helpee does not feel caught up in an endless process.

Another example involves a reluctant client on probation after conviction on drug and truancy charges.

Liam, a 17-year-old high school junior, has been referred to a counselor by his probation officer. During the first session, he informs the counselor that his problems are due to his mother's homosexuality and that unless his mother is willing to change her sexual orientation, he cannot work through his issues. He is reluctant to return to the counselor and furious that the terms of his probation require weekly counseling sessions.

Counselor: I can understand that you don't want to come to see me.

Liam: I hate shrinks. I don't see why I have to come here.

Counselor: It's upsetting that you can't choose for yourself what you can do . . . it must be hard to have someone else have control over you.

Liam: Yeah.

Counselor: I'm wondering what will happen if we decide not to meet again.

Liam: Make an appointment for me for next week.

Counselor: What? I'm surprised and confused . . . thought you didn't want to.

Liam: Make the appointment. Mr. C. said I have to come for the rest of the school year, so I'll come six more times.

Counselor: Sounds like you want to finish school. I appreciate your frustration, and we'll see what we can do to arrange for meetings the next six weeks. Perhaps we'll even find some topics that are of interest to you.

In this case, the immediate problem was meeting the probation terms so that Liam could finish school. During the next six weeks, further clarification and exploration of presenting and underlying problems occurred. Note that the counselor did not fight the helpee's reluctance.

STEP 4: INTENSIVE EXPLORATION
OF PROBLEMS

Using the responsive listening model of communication, you can begin to aid the helpee to look at the aspects, implications, and ramifications of his or her problems. Of course, many new problems will emerge throughout the helping process. Again, it is important to know just what the problem is, who has responsibility for the problem, and to what extent the helpee is able to effect some problem solving.

A helpee's problem is often part of the system in which he or she lives. In such a case, the helpee is likely to feel very frustrated, hopeless, and help-less. However, the same principles apply in such cases as in other problem situations: you try to learn as much as you can about the helpee, the system, the possibilities for change, and the choices that exist. Throughout this period, you are learning more about the thinking processes, feelings, and behaviors of the helpee as well as his or her strengths and difficulties in prob-lem solving, both in and out of the helping relationship. You are discovering the client's values, beliefs, attitudes, defense and coping strategies, relation-ships with others, hopes, ambitions, and aspirations. This is a time when you encourage the helpee to express whatever thoughts or feelings he or she is experiencing, without fear of being judged or instructed. All the while, you are promoting the development of trust, genuineness, and empathy, so that you can create a safe climate in which the helpee feels free to explore his or her own self-awareness.

The following excerpt is from the third counseling session with Marianne and demon-strates intensive exploration of her problem.

Counselor: So you've felt for a long time that you couldn't do much on your own.

Marianne: My mom and Pat [older sister] always did everything for me.

Counselor: And so you feel sort of . . .

Marianne: Dopey. They even would check over my homework every night. You see, Pat got married right after high school and never went on to college. She had been an honor student, and now here she is widowed and back home with a baby.

Counselor: Seems like you're supposed to make up to your mom and Pat for what they didn't have.

Marianne: They always say they want me to have what they didn't have. That's why it was so important for me to come to college.

Counselor: It was important to you, too?

Marianne: I don't know. I never thought about what was important to me. I never want to upset my mom; she cries so easily.

Counselor: And your dad . . .

Marianne: Oh, he wants whatever my mom wants. He never interferes or anything.

Counselor: I hear some anger in your voice.

Marianne: I was just thinking that there have been times when I wished my dad would stick up for me.

In this example, the counselor is learning as much as possible about Marianne's background and all the aspects of her feelings of inadequacy. This takes much time and skill, but some exploration is necessary before goals and objectives can be established. Intensive exploration is a continuing process that occurs throughout the helping relationship. For many helpers, it is one of the most challenging and exciting steps of the helping relationship. In fact, many relationships end at this step, because the act of mutual exploration is in itself therapeutic as it engenders new perspectives that can result in new feelings, thoughts, and behaviors.

STEP 5: ESTABLISHMENT OF POSSIBLE GOALS AND OBJECTIVES

After the problem has been thoroughly explored, the helper and helpee can more specifically develop goals and objectives for the relationship. This step can be accomplished in a systematic or casual fashion, depending on the style of the parties in the helping relationship, the theoretical orientation of the helper, and the requirements of the helping context.

The important point is that both parties agree to whatever the goals and objectives are and that they are in line with what the treatment organization allows. It certainly would not be helpful for the client if the goals represented only the helper's needs. If there is conflict between the established goals and what is allowed within the treatment context, both helper and helpee need to discuss how to deal with this conflict.

Helpers and helpees may establish immediate and long-range goals, specific and diffuse goals. Goals may be either outcome, focusing on problem resolution, or process, focusing on the relationship between helper and helpee. A student who is referred to a counselor because he or she faces possible failure in a course may also have family problems. The counselor and the student may choose to work on the more specific, immediate goal—passing the course and staying in school—rather than the long-range, more diffuse goal of solving family problems. These goals may not be equally valid or important, so it is up to the helper and the helpee to determine mutually which goals are feasible, given the nature and conditions of the particular helping relationship.

It is important not only to prioritize goals but to consider what Murphy and Dillon (2003) term "partializing goals"—taking a larger goal and break-ing it down into smaller (partialized) objectives. For example, a person who wants to find a job can partialize that goal into smaller, measurable behavioral steps, such as getting a newspaper, circling ads for jobs one is qualified for, preparing an appropriate resume and cover letter, practicing interviewing skills in the helping session, and going for interviews. Each of these is a par-tialized goal.

The process goal of the helping relationship may simply be to develop the relationship further, so that the helpee's self-concept is enhanced, or to provide a vehicle for self-understanding. That could very well become the goal in the case of Marianne. Or it may be that the goal is to make a decision or seek alter-native forms of behavior, which are specific outcome goals. The point is that both the helper and the helpee need to know why their relationship exists and what their goals are. When I (BFO) ask students what distinguishes a particular session in a counseling center from a friendly talk over coffee, they usually reply that a helping relationship involves goals and objectives that one does not con-sider in a friendly conversation.

When a helper and a helpee formulate several different goals, they should decide which goal has priority and how long that priority should last. Sometimes the ranking of goals falls into a logical sequence; other times helper and helpee arbitrarily decide on the order.

The following example illustrates goal setting at the end of a first session.

Mr. Winsor, age 32, has come to see the adult adviser at the local commu-nity college. He wants to take some courses that will give him upward job mobility. He is feeling trapped in a job that will not take him anywhere, and he worries about impending layoffs.

Counselor: It's really important for you to see some possibilities of moving ahead.

Mr. Winsor: Yes. I have a growing family, we're having a hard time making ends meet, and we do want to be out of the city by the time the oldest starts school.

Counselor: But you're not really sure just what courses you might want to take or what kinds of jobs to aim for.

Mr. Winsor: At this point, I just want to move . . . up.

Counselor: It seems to me we ought to find out more about what kinds of work you'd really like and are suited for, rather than just sign you up for some courses.

Mr. Winsor: What do you mean?

Counselor: Why don't you take our battery of vocational interest and aptitude tests, and then we can go over the results and try to decide together what would be the best path for you to follow?

Mr. Winsor: I guess so. Will it take long?

Counselor: I can set you up for a testing session next week, and we can talk before registration.

Mr. Winsor: I've heard about those tests . . . can't do any harm. I'm game.

The objectives of the relationship have become focused on vocational testing and exploration.

All outcome goals should be specific, behavioral, and measurable. They are formulated over several sessions and are always open to modification. As they are made, it is a good idea for helper and helpee to decide how they will evaluate the achievement of these goals—how they will know when the problem is resolved. For example, a vague goal such as an increase in self-esteem can be measured by an increased number of positive self-statements or social activities.

Goal setting is also important with children. Like adults, children increase their motivation—which usually results in better performance—by participating in goal setting.

EXERCISE 4.6 ■ In the following situations, what would you consider to be the primary helping goal? How would you measure achievement of this goal? Remember, you need to be specific. Discuss your answers with others in your group.

1. Mr. O'Leary was laid off three months ago along with 4,500 other technical workers from a major corporation. He had been pretty confident about finding a new job, but he is finding that the competition is fierce for the few available positions in his community. He has lost weight, is irritable, has low energy, and bickers more with his wife and kids. He is particularly concerned because his daughter may have to leave college in the middle of the year due to financial strains.

   Primary goal:

2. Ms. Gonzalez has been referred by the battered women's shelter. She came to this country four years ago from Central America, and her husband, stressed by his inability to get work and provide for his family, has become increasingly violent. The children do not want to go to school, and Mrs. Gonzalez feels threatened by school personnel who are insisting they attend.

   Primary goal:

3. Johnny, aged 16, is a high school football star. Recently, since his dad left the city and his mother had to go on welfare, his grades have been sliding to the point that he may be removed from the football team. He is angry and scared, and feels trapped in doing his schoolwork, playing football, working a part-time job, and being "the man of the family."

Primary goal:

4. Ms. Robinson, a mail order clerk for a large publishing house, has been threatened with dismissal if she does not improve her attendance. Ms. Robinson suffers from chronic major depression along with panic and agoraphobia disorders. Periodically, she has episodes when she cannot leave her house. She has used up her medical leave and now she is feeling panicky about how she will meet her monthly bills. Her parents want her to apply for social service disability, and her psychopharmacologist wants her to work as much as possible in order to achieve some independence and well-being. She is referred to you by a friend.

   Primary goal:

5. Amy, a 23-year-old Asian American, is distraught. Her family will not allow her to go out with her boyfriend without one of them accompanying her. Her American boyfriend is beginning to run out of patience, and Amy says that she "is caught between a rock and a hard place."

   Primary goal:

The following exercises will give you the opportunity to become familiar with the different steps of the relationship stage. The more you actively participate in and process exercises and discuss your feelings and reactions to them with others, the more meaningful the concepts discussed in each chapter will become.

EXERCISE 4.7 ■ Which of the five steps of the relationship stage (initiation/entry, clarification, definition of structure/contract, exploration, establishment of possible goals/objectives) is evident in the following example?

1. **Client:** If I am pregnant, my folks will murder me.
   Helper: You're scared of what your parents will do to you.
   Client: You don't know them! They're always yapping at me and telling me I'm gonna end up just like my sister.
   Helper: You don't want to be like your sister.
   Client: You bet your sweet ass I don't! She had to marry Ron when she was in high school, and now she's really stuck with two brats and a husband who beats her up.
   Helper: That's scary. You seem afraid that you may have gotten yourself into a situation where you can end up the same way.

In this excerpt, the counselor is in step 2: clarification of the problem. She is trying to determine whether possible pregnancy (the presenting symptom), relationship with parents, or fear of being "trapped" is the major issue.

Now decide which step each of the following examples illustrates, and discuss in pairs or small groups what you've decided. Then see the comments at the end of the chapter.

2. **Helper:** There are only two more weeks of school left. Would you like to spend that time working on your shyness in class, so that you can start off next year in high school feeling more comfortable?

   Client: Do you think I'll ever be able to answer out loud in class without getting all messed up?

   Helper: There are exercises we can practice that will help you become less nervous.

   Client: That would really help. If I could learn that, my marks would go up.

3. **Client:** Am I too early?

   Helper: No, right on time. Come in and sit down.

   Client: Over here?

   Helper: Fine. Now, tell me about how your father-in-law's illness is affecting you.

   Client: Yes, I'm so worried about him. You see . . .

4. **Client:** Do you think you can help me find a job?

   Helper: We can work together on preparing a resume and choosing leads to follow.

   Client: I don't really know where to start. What do you charge for this?

   Helper: Let's set up three sessions to get things rolling. Here's a copy of my fee schedule. There are also some forms for you to fill out.

5. **Client:** I just don't know whether it's best for me and the kids to stay with Joe or to leave.

   Helper: You feel a lot of ambivalence about your marriage.

   Client: Well, I don't want the children to grow up without a father, and he says we can't afford financially to split up. But then, I'm 37, and I hate to think of spending the rest of my life this way. There must be something better for me.

   Helper: Let's focus on this ambivalence for a while. What do you gain for yourself by staying in this marriage?

EXERCISE 4.8 ■ In this exercise, if possible, you should form triads with people with whom you have not worked or formed relationships. Rotate the roles of helper, helpee, and observer, and select one or more of the following 10 situations (or choose one of your own) as a presenting problem. Choose whatever setting feels comfortable to you. The helper is to work with the helpee for about half an hour; the observer uses the rating scales in Appendix A and makes notes about the behaviors of the helper and the steps he or she follows. At the end of the session, take as much time as necessary to fully process the exercise so that both the helpee and the observer can provide as much specific feedback as possible to the helper. What steps were you able to accomplish as the helper? How did you feel? What do you feel you need to work on? This exercise is one that can be used for weeks of training, in or out of class.

1. You've had a blowup with your husband.
2. You're never able to get assignments in on time.
3. You want to lose weight.
4. You're afraid you'll be laid off at work.
5. Your car is in the shop for repairs, and you don't know how you'll manage because you need a car for work.
6. You're afraid of flying and you have an upcoming trip to make.
7. You're shy and have difficulty meeting new people.
8. You're not sure why you're here.
9. You have trouble saying no to people when they ask you for something.
10. You're worried about a friend who might have AIDS.

This exercise allows you to experience the power of the helper–helpee interaction. Helping relationships can vary in intensity, depending on the situation. Factors that affect the intensity are the helpee's expectations and feelings of insecurity and anxiety at the beginning of a session, as well as the expectations, feelings, competencies, and skills of the helper. Try to pinpoint these as you work through the exercises.

SUMMARY

In this chapter, we have discussed conditions affecting the relationship stage. These conditions can be grouped under the categories of initial contact, duration, applications and forms, record keeping, facilities, timing, and other people. An important distinction was made between interviews, initial meetings to establish rapport and determine whether or not the relationship is to proceed, and sessions, subsequent meetings that begin with the structure/contract step and last through termination of the strategies stage.

The five major steps of the relationship stage—initiation/entry, clarification of presenting problem, definition of structure/contract, intensive exploration of problems, and establishment of possible goals and objectives—were discussed, with illustrative case examples. An important point to remember is that each of these steps takes varying amounts of time and contact. In some cases, the first four steps occur in one or two meetings; in others, it takes many meetings before intensive exploration can occur. The amount of time spent in helping relationships is determined not only by the nature of the relationship and the issues addressed, but also by context. Some institutions and agencies have delineated the number of sessions possible; others are more flexible.

The issues of reluctance and resistance were also presented in this chapter, with the viewpoint that supporting and understanding reluctance and resistance are more effective than struggling against them. Resistance is a necessary part of the change and growth process, one that can be worked with rather than feared and avoided.

Research has been unable to prove that one helping strategy is more effective than another, but studies do show that the effect of any given helping relationship depends as much on the quality of the relationship as on the techniques and strategies used. With this knowledge, and with practice of the exercises in this chapter to help you gain proficiency in enhancing helping relationships, we can proceed to the next stage of the helping relationship: the strategy stage.

EXERCISE ANSWERS

Exercise 4.2 Possible answers: 1. d; 2. a; 3. b or d; 4. d; 5. a or b; 6. c or e; 7. c or e; 8. b.; 9. b or e

Exercise 4.3 Possible answers: 1. d; 2. e; 3. c; 4. a; 5. a; 6. b or d; 7. b; 8. d or e; 9. c or d; 10. b

Exercise 4.7 Example 2 represents the fifth step, setting possible goals and objectives. There is a time limitation here, and helper and helpee choose to use the time to focus on assertive behaviors. Example 3 represents the initiation/entry step. Example 4 represents the structure/contract step, when fees, time, and specific commitments are discussed. Example 5 is a brief sample of intensive exploration, when helper and helpee are covering all the aspects and consequences of the helpee's concerns.

REFERENCES AND
FURTHER READING

American Psychiatric Association. (2000). *Diagnostic and statistical manual of mental disorders TR* (4th ed.). Washington, DC: Author.

Boyd-Franklin, N. (2003). *Black families in therapy: Understanding the African American experience* (2nd ed.). New York: Guilford Press.

Brammer, L. M., & MacDonald, G. (2003). *The helping relationship: Process and skills* (8th ed.). Englewood Cliffs, NJ: Prentice-Hall.

Corey, G. (2005). *Theory and practice of counseling and psychotherapy* (7th ed.). Belmont, CA: Brooks/Cole.

Egan, G. (1998). *The skilled helper: A problem management approach to helping* (6th ed.). Pacific Grove, CA: Brooks/Cole.

Ivey, A. E., & Ivey, M. B. (2002). *Intentional interviewing and counseling: Facilitating client development in a multicultural society* (5th ed.). Pacific Grove, CA: Brooks/Cole.

Larrabee, M. J. (1982). Working with reluctant clients through affirmation techniques. *Personnel and Guidance Journal, 61,* 105–109.

Murphy, B. C., & Dillon, C. (2003). *Interviewing in action: Relationship, processing, and change* (2nd ed.). Pacific Grove, CA: Brooks/Cole.

Otani, A. (1989). Client resistance in counseling: Its theoretical rationale and taxonomic classification. *Journal of Counseling and Development, 67,* 458–462.

Visit the book companion site at www.thomsonedu.com to access tutorial quizzes.

5

Helping Theory

Now that we have covered the steps of the relationship stage, we can proceed to the second stage of the helping relationship, the application of strategies. To provide a framework for understanding how to apply counseling skills and strategies, however, we must first review the major formal theories of helping. Chapter 5 discusses the major traditional theories. Chapter 6 will present the theoretical perspectives of the late 20th and early 21st centuries that cut across these major formal theories. In Chapters 7 and 8, we'll explore the strategic application of the major theories of helping.

This chapter's review of foundational theories will cover their basic principles, their views of the helping relationship, their significant techniques, and their implications for helpers. Suggestions for further reading on each of the major theoretical viewpoints appear at the end of the chapter.

Before studying these major theories, we will explore the values and needs that make up your "personal" theory. Understanding your personal theory of human behavior and how people change is important, because it will undoubtedly affect your understanding of, and your acceptance or rejection of, the formal, scientific theories of helping.

PERSONAL THEORIES
OF HUMAN BEHAVIOR

You may now be asking yourself why we should bother exploring abstract theories when we are learning about practical skills to apply in the context of
unique helping situations. Perhaps you are asking this question because you are
uncomfortable with what may seem to be an ivory tower approach to a down-
to-earth situation. Furthermore, the term *theory* is somewhat threatening to
many of us, possibly because it implies rigidity or the need to choose and justify our positions.

However, each of us already has views or assumptions that form our personal theory. These personal theories have been influenced by many factors,
including biology, gender, past experiences, exposure to different schools of
thought, the people with whom we work and study, opportunities in our lives,
our personalities and temperaments, our degree of self-awareness, and our
ethnic, socioeconomic, and familial backgrounds. Regardless of whether we are
able to express them or are even aware of them, these theories affect our behavior, especially in interpersonal relationships. Unless we acknowledge our personal theoretical base, we may "help" people more in order to apply our theory
than to satisfy their needs.

EXERCISE 5.1 ■ To start thinking about some of your theoretical assumptions, ask
yourself the following questions:

1. What are human beings? Are they good or bad? Are they born that way? Are they
   controlled or controlling?

2. What motivates human beings? How can we motivate people?

3. What is my explanation of maleness and femaleness? Are differences due to
   biology? To socialization? Are racial and ethnic differences inherent or
   learned?

4. How do human beings learn? Are there different kinds of learning? What affects
   how people think?

5. How do personality traits develop? Are they inherent or learned? Are certain personality types distinguishable by behavior?

6. Can people change? How do they change? Does something external cause them
   to change, or does it come from within?

7. What is social deviance? Who decides what it is? What can or should be done
   about deviance? What behaviors (in myself and others) do I find acceptable and
   unacceptable? Are these behaviors deviant?

8. What impact do group memberships have on our behavior? What is the impact of
   various sociocultural factors?

Try answering these questions in your own words, from your own frame of reference.
You may be surprised to find that you do have answers to these questions! Compare

them to others' answers. Your answers are neither right nor wrong, and today's answers could—and probably will—change as you continue to learn and become more aware of your own views and feelings.

How open are you to different viewpoints? Open-mindedness will affect your flexibility and adaptability, which in turn will affect the range of people with whom you're able to work and the settings in which you feel comfortable. Helpers who are aware of their beliefs and have consciously grappled with these questions are aware of the influence of their own theoretical views on their perceptions, attitudes, and behaviors toward helpees and develop helper styles that are consistent with their own personal theories. If we believe that by changing behavior we can change attitudes and feelings, we are more likely to adopt action-oriented counseling strategies focusing on behavioral changes than if we believe that behavior will change only through the development of self-awareness. In the latter case, we are more likely to adopt an approach using verbal techniques to develop insight. Likewise, an understanding of basic learning theory will enable us as helpers to be aware of and consciously use our potential as role models in helping relationships.

Unfortunately, there is often little congruence between what people involved in human behavior fields say they believe (espoused theory) and what they actually practice (theory in action). Many advocate for empathic, supportive orientations, for example, but reports of their actual behaviors reflect different orientations. In other words, one's actions do not always match one's words. If we can become more aware of our own personal theory, we will be able to see how it relates to formal theory and to our own helping practices.

Now examine the following, necessarily brief overview of the major theoretical views of helping, and see what parts of them you accept and reject. Remember, if you want to learn more about a theory, there are suggestions at the end of the chapter. You may see some of your present assumptions reflected in these theories; however, your assumptions may change by the time you finish this book.

PSYCHODYNAMIC THEORY

The psychodynamic approach to helping, which is based on psychoanalytic theory, was introduced by Sigmund Freud and has the longest history of all the current theories. Freud is recognized for his great insight in developing procedures for treating disturbed or unhappy persons based on his concepts and observations of mental and emotional processes. The development of many later theories of helping can ultimately be traced back to Freud's theory. Freudian theory has been modified and developed by later psychoanalytic theorists, including Alfred Adler, Erik Erikson, Erich Fromm, Karen Horney, Carl Jung, Wilhelm Reich, Harry Stack Sullivan, the object relations school, and ego and self psychologists.

We'll now briefly review the Freudian contributions to psychodynamic theory. We want to stress that there is no one psychodynamic therapy; today's psychodynamic approaches range from orthodox Freudian to humanistic ego psychology and object relations, from long-term psychoanalytic treatment to brief psychodynamic psychotherapy. We'll also review key concepts of Carl Jung, Alfred Adler, ego psychology, and object relations and self psychology theorists, whose thinking was influenced by Freud's but developed into separate, major schools of psychodynamic theory.

Freudian Theory

Psychoanalysis and derivative psychoanalytic treatments make up the strategies of Freudian theory. Freud's view of human beings, based on his clinical observations, was negative and pessimistic in that he perceived them as being inherently selfish, impulsive, and irrational. His view of human behavior was **deterministic**—that is, he saw behavior as predetermined by biological instincts and drives along with previous life experiences. This is a comprehensive view, encompassing people's inner experience, external behavior, biological nature, social roles, and individual and group functioning. Freud emphasized the goal of health as effective functioning in love, work, and play.

Freudian theory, based on a psychology of internal, **intrapsychic** conflict between competing internal drives or instincts, hypothesizes the existence of the following personality structures:

1. The **id,** an instinctually derived structure that represents the primitive, selfish aspects of humans. The unconscious (unaware) id demands immediate gratification by increasing pleasure and reducing tensions.

2. The **ego,** a structure that rationally attempts reality orientation by consciously mediating (thinking, perceiving, and deciding) among the aggressive id, the moralistic superego, and the external world.

3. The **superego,** a structure that represents the internalization of parental, societal, and cultural moral and ethical injunctions (the conscience).

Behavior is considered to be the product of conflictual interaction among these three structures, which can occur consciously (with awareness) and/or unconsciously (without awareness). Freud's concept of the unconscious as a repository of all experiences and memories underlies his theory of motivation. According to Freudian theory, all psychological distress stems from the unconscious. **Anxiety,** the major symptom of distress, is caused by repressed emotions arising from basic conflicts among the id, the ego, and the superego over control of **libido.**

Libido is one of two motivational instincts postulated by Freud. The basic driving force of the personality, libido is stored in the id. It comprises survival or life instincts such as hunger and sex. Aggression, the second motivational instinct, comprises death instincts such as hostility and self-destruction. Thus, libido is the drive energy directed at objects needed to fulfill instincts and biological needs. Libido must be either diverted or discharged.

When conflict between impulses and wishes is suppressed, the resulting anxiety triggers the ego **defense mechanisms,** including **repression, isolation, regression, rationalization, reaction formation, sublimation, projection, denial, displacement, compensation,** and **intellectualization** (remember that all boldface terms are defined in the glossary). The purpose of the defense mechanisms is to reduce anxiety. While successfully reducing anxiety, defense mechanisms can obscure the true nature of the intrapsychic conflict and, therefore, can result in **neuroses.** Neuroses are derived from childhood conflicts and can emerge in childhood, adolescence, or adulthood when the balance between the libidinal drives and the ego defense mechanisms is upset and anxiety is heightened. This lack of balance can occur during normal developmental transitions or through disappointment, loss of love, physical illness, or other crises or situations that trigger repressed childhood material to spill over into current functioning.

Freud also conceptualized five **psychosexual stages** from birth through adolescence for the development of libido. These stages have a crucial effect on personality development, in that a healthy personality cannot develop without their successful resolution. They are as follows:

1. In the **oral stage,** the first year or so of life, the infant receives pleasure from sucking and biting and develops trust. This is a pleasurable stage, and people whose oral needs were gratified tend to have a more positive view of the world in later life.

2. In the **anal stage,** around the second and third years of life, the child receives pleasure from stimulation of the anal erogenous zone and experiences the power of retention and excretion, as well as the negative feelings that accompany that power. The child shows a great deal of interest in bodily processes, and in smelling, touching, and playing with feces.

3. In the **phallic stage,** the next few years, the child receives pleasure from the stimulation of the genital region and begins to develop love/hate relationships with others. During this period, the child experiences oedipal longings: intense, erotic desires for the parent of the opposite sex and hostile, competitive feelings toward the parent of the same sex (the **Electra complex** in girls, the **Oedipal complex** in boys). Girls may manifest **penis envy** during this stage, as boys gain more privileges through their identification with their apparently "freer, more powerful" father. Freud believed that later neurosis involved the repressed wishes of the Oedipal period, and that this stage laid the foundation for adult sexual relationships.

4. In the **latency stage,** from around 6 to 12 years, the child appears to lose interest in sexual fantasies and genital stimulation. This is a quiet phase, when the child focuses on socialization, directing most of his or her energy toward school and the outside world.

5. In the **genital stage,** which begins at puberty, the adolescent begins to focus his or her concerns and gratifications on others rather than on the self and begins to develop heterosexual relationships.

According to the Freudian school, neuroses can be traced to a fixation at any one of the psychosexual stages. Thus, adult problems involving distrust in relationships, low self-esteem, inability to recognize and express negative feelings, or inability to accept one's own sexuality and sexual feelings can result from impeded development in one of these psychosexual stages. Until an event or situation occurs in adulthood to cause symptoms of distress, one might not be aware of early developmental impairment.

The following are the major Freudian psychoanalytic constructs:

1. Human behavior is determined by unconscious forces (biological and instinctual needs and drives).

2. Sex drives are the principal determinants of behavior and underlie the dynamic conflicts, such as competition and jealousy, arising from early childhood.

3. Adult behavior is greatly influenced by early childhood experiences of the psychosexual developmental stages.

4. There is a fixed quantity of libido stored in the id.

5. Problems arise from intrapsychic conflict represented by anxiety and caused by past occurrences. This conflict results in the excessive use of defense mechanisms, which uses up an inordinate amount of libido. Thus, little libido is available for effective functioning in current life.

Jungian Theory

Other psychodynamic views are not as negative as Freud's. Carl Jung focused on the role of *purpose* in human development, presenting a more creative, optimistic view of humankind. He believed that a person had more energy than that derived from sexual drives and that one was always developing toward wholeness and self-fulfillment (individuation), using energy to be "creatively purposeful" and searching for a balance among body, mind, and spirit. Jung believed that the "transcendent function" (use of the energy to integrate and transcend conflict) mediates the relations between the conscious and the unconscious.

Jung differentiated between the personal unconscious (painful, threatening experiences repressed or ignored) and the collective unconscious (buried memories based on the wisdom of the ancestral past). This differentiation helps in understanding and interpreting unconscious material—that is, symbols. Through his construct of the collective unconscious, Jung paid more attention than did Freud to the role of culture in the development of the human personality. In time of war, for example, one can imagine the forces of the collective unconscious causing people to unite in aggression.

Other major Jungian concepts include the **persona** (public mask or social facade one displays in various situations), the **animus** (masculine side), the **anima** (feminine side), **extroversion** (orientation toward the outer, objective world), and **introversion** (orientation toward the inner, subjective world).

These concepts led to Jung's postulation of four types of people: thinking, feeling, sensing, and intuiting. In distinguishing among these psychological types, Jung pointed out that persons with different types communicate with great difficulty. For example, an intuitive person will be impatient with the workaday practicality of the sensation-oriented person. The thinking type will have trouble with the feeling type, and vice versa. All these types, in varying degrees of extroversion and introversion, exist within every human; however, one type tends to be more pronounced than the others.

Jung was not as deterministic as Freud. He postulated spiritual development throughout adult life, focusing particularly on one's capacity in midlife to integrate unconscious and conscious aspects of personality in order to become an authentic, spiritual individual.

Adlerian Theory

Alfred Adler, like Carl Jung, differed with Freud's biological, deterministic viewpoint. He viewed humans from a nondeterministic, social-psychological perspective. He emphasized the social determinants of personality and focused more on the conscious than on the unconscious, more on the future than on the past, and on people's power to control their destinies. Contrary to Freud or Jung, Adler believed that people have social, creative, decision-making capacities with which to reach their selected life goals. Today many include Adler among cognitive theorists because of this focus on decision making. For Adler, the focus is on the individual within social contexts. He highlights future rather than past orientation, although he explores clients' childhood memories and experiences to help them gain self-understanding so that they can correct mistaken beliefs and assume social responsibility.

Adlerian personality theory includes the following concepts:

1. *Teleology:* Behavior is purposeful, goal oriented, and consciously selected.

2. *Inherent inferiority:* Humans strive for perfection, significance, and superiority to compensate for their basic **inherent inferiority** feelings.

3. *Compensation:* While striving for power to overcome inferiority, people attempt to compensate—to translate weakness into strength or find a particular area of competence that will overshadow weakness.

4. *Lifestyle:* Each individual develops a unique **lifestyle** early in childhood as a way of compensating for inferiority and weakness.

5. *Birth order:* One's **birth order** (status) in one's family of origin strongly influences one's childhood experiences and the development of one's lifestyle.

6. *Social interest:* Interpersonal relations and community involvement are major life tasks.

In Adlerian theory, maladaptive behavior occurs when an individual develops inappropriate strategies to overcompensate for the feelings of inferiority that emerged during childhood. Through understanding and **psychoeducation,** therapy aims to develop social interest, change faulty thinking, help clients overcome feelings of inferiority and discouragement, and motivate them become to participate fully in social systems.

Ego Psychology

In the mid-1900s, ego psychologists such as Anna Freud, Heinz Hartmann, and Erik Erikson differed from Freud by paying more attention to the influence of the environment on personality development and to the ego's capacity to transcend the instincts of the id. Erikson proposed eight stages of development, which extend Freud's psychosexual stages throughout the life span and include psychosocial dimensions. Each stage provides the opportunity to resolve a core crisis and strengthen the ego.

1. *Infancy:* trust versus mistrust, based on parent–infant relationship
2. *Early childhood:* autonomy versus shame and doubt, based on separation from parent and independence experiences
3. *Preschool age:* initiative versus guilt, based on initiative and competence opportunities
4. *School age:* industry versus inferiority, based on learning skills and achievement experiences
5. *Adolescence:* identity versus role confusion, based on individuation and lifestyle choice opportunities
6. *Young adulthood:* intimacy versus isolation, based on peer relationship experiences
7. *Middle age:* generativity versus stagnation, based on helping younger people
8. *Later life:* integrity versus despair, based on reasonable satisfaction with one's life experiences

For ego psychologists, identity is associated with ego development, which is a lifelong process. At each stage throughout life, there is a core developmental crisis. Experiences in earlier stages affect one's resolution of a crisis in a later stage. Problems arise when there is a conflict between the ego and adaptation to society.

Object Relations and Self Psychology

Contemporary psychoanalytic thinkers (primarily Melanie Klein, Ronald Fairbairn, Donald W. Winnicott, Harry Guntrip, Margaret Mahler, Heinz Kohut, and Otto Kernberg) emphasize the ego and interpersonal relationships rather than the id and innate biological drives as the basis of personality development.

A person's primary drive from birth is considered to be for relationship contact, as opposed to the discharge of tension from sexual and aggression drives. The focus is on the relationship between an individual and real people, between an individual and his or her mental image or representation of real people, and between an individual's mental images or representations from early significant relationships and current significant people. Attachment theories inform object relations theories; in order for the ego to develop, secure, consistent attachment experiences are particularly essential in the first few years of life (Bowlby, 1988).

The crucial development of personality begins with the infant's earliest relationship with the primary caregiver, usually the mother, rather than with the father during the Freudian Oedipal phase. Mother becomes the infant's first love object. In the first stages of infancy, when the infant cannot differentiate self from other, the infant ego's ability to develop a sense of security within itself and the environment depends on the identification the mother feels with her infant and on her capacity to empathize and nurture. If the infant's needs are not met during this **symbiotic** phase, the infant's ego splits, withdrawing and hiding to avoid the anxiety resulting from not having primary essential needs consistently met. The ego splits into what Winnicott (1965) calls the true self and the false self. The true self is at the core of human existence and is able to relate to itself and to others. The false self arises as a protection for an undernourished, insecure ego. It hides from the outer world and relationships. Thus, shortcomings or failures in early maternal nurturance lead to false selves and inhibit the development of a whole ego. Aggression is viewed by these theorists as a response or reaction to frustrating relationships rather than as an instinct.

The ego passes through many stages or positions during infancy and early childhood, from the symbiotic relationship with the mother on through the separation and individuation stages. The quality of the infant's experiences of attachment and separation in the **object relations** of early years shapes the development of the ego, which includes the potential capacity to love and relate to others. **Splitting** and **projection,** the defenses one uses because of faulty object relations, disturb healthy ego development and can contribute to such pathologies as narcissistic character disorders, borderline states, and **psychoses.**

Psychodynamic Theory's Major Principles of Helping

The purpose of psychoanalytic treatment is to make the client conscious of unconscious material and to restructure his or her personality in order to attain a healthy balance of energy. To fulfill this purpose, Jungians stress the need for a restructuring of basic character, while Adlerians stress the need to change the client's self-concept and restructure his or her development, lifestyle, and social situation. Ego psychology and object relations practitioners stress the nurturing quality of the therapeutic relationship, to provide the object constancy lacking in early infancy and to allow the ego to reintegrate and develop.

Psychoanalysis is a moderately **directive therapy** within an interview format. It uses techniques such as questioning, interpretation, dream analysis,

free association (stream of consciousness), **recall,** and the analysis of **resistance, transference,** and **countertransference.** Some of these techniques (for example, questioning and interpretation) are directive; others (for example, free association and recall) are nondirective.

The four major phases of psychodynamic psychotherapy are (1) the opening phase, (2) the development of transference, (3) the working-through of transference, and (4) the resolution of transference. Transference is an integral part of the helping relationship. It occurs when the client revives emotions and attitudes, positive or negative, originally present in the parent–child relationship and directs them toward the therapist. For example, a client may see the therapist, either male or female, as his father with his father's attributes and feelings, and may experience powerful feelings toward the therapist based on that perception. The client may be able to work through his unresolved conflicts with his father by means of this transference relationship. Further, analysis of transference can help a client understand how he or she misperceives, misinterprets, and therefore misresponds to people in the present in terms of past relationships.

The working-through phase involves interpretation of material generated by the client through free association, reporting of dreams, and recall. The goal is to help the client achieve insight and a corrective emotional experience by means of **abreaction** (the expression and discharge of repressed emotions via catharsis).

In psychoanalysis, the client is encouraged to experience crises, resistance, and transference in order to work through impasses and unconscious material. Psychoanalysts and psychodynamically oriented psychotherapists emphasize the past (attempting to connect the past to the present), the exploration of causality, and the confrontation of client discrepancies.

Countertransference occurs when the therapist develops feelings toward or views about the client that stem from the therapist's conflicts rather than the client's. Countertransference can take the form of positive (love or excessive attachment) or negative (dislike or hostility) feelings and can result in distorted interpretations. However, the psychoanalyst is trained to be objective and to work through his or her own conflicts in order to avoid personalizing feelings projected by the client.

Classical Freudian psychoanalytic theory postulates a directive, authoritarian relationship between the helper and the helpee. The relationship is not reciprocal; the helper is an expert authority figure and remains detached, objective, and completely neutral, so that transference will develop without contamination by the therapist's personhood. However, Adler introduced the concept of empathy into the psychoanalytic helping relationship, and today, buttressed by the focus on empathic relationships by object relations theorists, therapists of this school are encouraged to demonstrate natural warmth and empathy as important components of the helping relationship.

More and more contemporary psychodynamic practitioners include and integrate relationship and intervention elements from a wider variety of psychotherapy theories. They recognize the need for brief, problem-solving treatment and are challenged by the need to adapt and integrate their psychodynamic principles with brief models.

Implications of the Psychodynamic
Approach for Helpers

To practice this type of therapy, the helper must undergo many years of rigorous training, so this approach is not directly relevant for counselors and helpers in other than traditional clinical settings. However, it does have important implications for nonpsychoanalytic helpers. Helpers need to recognize that there are motivating forces within people that are not wholly conscious; they need to know how people defend themselves from internal and external threats with defense mechanisms and resistance; and they must understand the significance of early childhood experiences and the possible implications of the concept of transference for any relationship.

The focus of classical psychodynamic approaches on the development of an autonomous self conflicts with recent theories of gender and multicultural development. For example, the research of Nisbett (2000) and his colleagues at the University of Michigan indicates that Asians and Americans have different thinking styles. This knowledge challenges some of our understanding about the universality of thought processes. This research, along with our recognition of the impact of sociocultural factors on the lives of individuals, suggests that those psychodynamic approaches that incorporate environmental perspectives and social frameworks may be more applicable to women, to people of color, and to people from non-Western cultures.

PHENOMENOLOGICAL THEORY

The **phenomenological** theories of helping focus on the uniqueness of each person's internal perspective, which determines one's reality. This approach emphasizes the here and now rather than what was or what will be, and how people perceive and feel about themselves and their environment rather than their adjustment to prevailing cultural norms. It also emphasizes affective rather than cognitive or behavioral domains.

The three most widely used phenomenological approaches are (1) existential psychotherapy, developed by Rollo May, Viktor Frankl, James Bugental, and Irvin Yalom; (2) person-centered (client-centered) theory, developed by Carl Rogers; and (3) the Gestalt theory advanced by Fritz Perls. Although we will focus more on the theories of Rogers and Perls, a brief description of the existential approach provides a glimpse of the philosophical framework that underlies these theories.

Existential Theory

Existential theory, a philosophical orientation that stems from the thinking of 19th-century European philosophers, was developed into a therapeutic approach by European analysts. They were reacting to the determinism of psychoanalysis and behaviorism. Thus, the existential view of human nature is that it is subjective and ever changing. Meaning is whatever one uniquely experiences. Human beings are always in the process of becoming. They have the capacity for awareness and the freedom and responsibility to make choices. They are always striving for identity, meaning, and relationship to others.

The goal of therapy is to enable clients to recognize the full range of their choices and to take responsibility for whichever option they select. Anxiety, an inevitable part of the human condition, emanates from the awareness of death, freedom, isolation, and meaninglessness, and can lead to excessive use of defense mechanisms and lack of authenticity. (Existentialists refer to authenticity as the congruent, genuine, integrated sense and expression of self.) The existential therapist serves as a model and a companion in the client's search for awareness, responsibility, and meaning. The relationship with the client is important. There are no specific techniques in this approach; rather, existential therapists choose interventions from different approaches. Thus, the humanistic nature and philosophy of the helping relationship are the most critical therapeutic variables. Carl Rogers elaborates on the ingredients of this crucial person-to-person relationship.

Person-Centered (Client-Centered) Theory

The person-centered approach, established during the 1930s and 1940s by Carl Rogers, was largely a reaction to the rigidity of the psychoanalytic school that dominated the helping professions in the United States during that period.

Person-Centered Theory's Major Principles of Helping   Contrary to the psychoanalytic view, person-centered theory assumes that human beings are rational, good, and capable of assuming responsibility for themselves and making the choices that can lead to independence, self-actualization, and autonomy. Further, it proposes that people are constructive, cooperative, trustworthy, realistic, and social. The theory does admit that negative emotions such as hate and anger exist, but it holds that they exist mainly as responses to frustrated needs for love, security, and a feeling of belonging, which are basic human needs. This is a "self" theory, based on a belief that people act in accordance with their **self-concept** and that their self-concept is heavily influenced by their experiences with others. It is phenomenological in that it is concerned with the client's perception of his or her self and situation, not the helper's or the outside world's perception of the client. This theory is not concerned with causes of behavior or with changing behavior; rather, it focuses on the individual's current experiences, feelings, and interactions.

This theory emphasizes the self, the environment, and the interaction of the two. The aware, self-actualizing organism is constantly experiencing in a phenomenal field. The part of that field that one accepts or experiences as separate from the rest becomes the self. Since the self, by nature, strives toward integration and actualization of potential, the self-concept becomes increasingly harmonious and increasingly consistent with experience, continually accepting and integrating experience as a part of the self-structure. An individual's experiences, feelings, and interactions may either be integrated into the self from the environment to become part of the self-concept or remain part of the environment, not yet integrated into the self.

The following are the major person-centered constructs:

1. Self-concept comprises the individual's perceptions of himself or herself based on interactions with others.

2. The phenomenal field is the individual's reality and consists of his or her self-concept and perceptions of his or her world.

3. Individuals behave in whatever ways will enhance their self-concept.

4. Problems arise out of incongruencies between the individual's self-concept and life experiences that become threatening and cause the individual to use defenses such as denial or distortion of experiences. These incongruencies lead to disorganization and pain.

5. Only by receiving unconditional positive regard (acceptance) from a significant other can persons be open to their experiences and develop more congruence between self-concept and behavior.

The foundation of person-centered therapy is the creation of an empathic relationship between therapist and client that will encourage the client's self-exploration and experience of spontaneity, genuineness, and here-and-now feelings. (The focus on the relationship as the vehicle for change is similar to the object relations and self psychology view about the process of change.) The goals of this therapy are self-actualization and self-realization. These goals can be achieved if the counselor can understand and empathize with the unique experiential world of the client and convey that understanding to the client, be genuine in the relationship, and provide unconditional positive regard. This type of therapy requires the therapist and the client to participate fully.

The person-centered helper uses minimal leads such as "Mm-hmm," "I see," and "Yes" (connoting acceptance); reflection (a verbal statement mirroring the client's statement); clarification (which explores and develops a client's statement); summarization (which synthesizes a number of the client's statements); and confrontation (a verbal statement that nonjudgmentally challenges a client's statement). Note that the client does all of the leading and directing, while the counselor follows the client's lead. Thus, there are no "techniques" in this form of helping. The helper is effective by being genuine and not playing the role of a "helper."

Carl Rogers's early work (1940–1950) mainly advocated use of nondirective parroting, or paraphrasing, of client statements in a permissive environment. He saw the therapist as a clarifier who should remain fairly distant and apart. Over time, Rogers began to advocate a degree of self-disclosure and sharing of attitudes on the part of the counselor, and some interpretation of feelings.

Thus, Rogers came to advocate that counselors experience themselves as persons in relation to clients. Rogerian counselors today are more active and involved with their clients than were early Rogerian helpers, and they have added questions and feedback to their verbal response repertoires.

More than any other helping approach, person-centered therapy focuses on the counseling relationship, which is nondirective and emphasizes the communication of respect, understanding, and acceptance by the helper. The goal is an affective, warm relationship that reduces clients' anxiety and frees them to experience, express, and explore their feelings. The helper is presented as an equal, a coworker of the helpee, not an expert or authority. The client experiences the helping relationship as one that allows him or her to take responsibility for determining goals and for taking action toward those goals.

Implications of the Person–Centered and Existential Approaches for Helpers The focus of these theories on the process rather than the content of verbal behavior is a major contribution to counseling psychology, and has provided the foundation for counselor training programs and research. Over the years, the focus on the primary significance of the therapeutic relationship has extended to other models. Because person-centered and existential therapy emphasizes relationships based more on empathic and accurate listening and openness than on techniques, the counselor's authentic self or "being" (attitude) is seen as more important than his or her acts or "doing." Helpers are encouraged to expand their own awareness at the same time that they are encouraging helpees to develop their self-awareness.

In the current climate of managed care and accountability, however, these approaches are seen to have several drawbacks, including lack of measurable outcome goals and unlimited time requirements. Furthermore, the focus on self-determination and individualism, as well as the inattentiveness to the impact of sexism, racism, discrimination, and oppression on healthy development and functioning, could limit their applicability to minority or nondominant helpees.

Gestalt Theory

The Gestalt approach to helping is based on the perceptual learning theory developed by Kurt Koffka, Wolfgang Kohler, and Max Wertheimer. The application of this theory as therapy was developed by Fritz Perls in the late 1940s.

Gestalt is a German word meaning "configuration." All human behaviors and experiences are organized into Gestalts, into configurations or patterns, in which the whole is greater than the sum of its parts. Individuals form meaningful wholes (patterns) out of their experiences, and their needs determine whether parts of their experience (events) become dominant or background material. Likewise, individuals and their behaviors must be perceived as wholes. The organism is contained within his or her environment by an ego boundary.

The environment is the source of activities, people, and experiences to fill the individual's needs. It is up to the self-aware individual to take responsibility for seeking from the environment what he or she needs to become more self-supportive and psychologically stable.

Like person-centered therapy, this approach is phenomenological in that it focuses on the present, the here and now, and on the client's perspective, rather than on the problem's original cause. Its concern is with increasing understanding and emotional and physical awareness of and by the client, which leads to integration of the parts of self and experience—eliminating any discrepancies—into a unified whole. Thus, Gestalt therapy is experiential (it emphasizes doing and acting out, not just talking), existential (it helps people to make independent choices and be responsible), and experimental (it encourages trying out new expressions of feelings).

Gestalt Theory's Major Principles of Helping   Gestalt theory holds that one can be responsible for one's actions and experiences and can live as a fully integrated, effectively functioning individual. The difficulty in assuming this responsibility results from a developmental impasse in one's past, a block that keeps one from living fully in the present and understanding the *how* and *what* (not the *why*) of behavior. Impasses, or inconsistencies, between the organism and its environment create conflict—that is, avoidance of contact and denying, negating, covering up a present experience rather than accepting it, and emphasizing what is not present rather than what is present.

Gestalt theory emphasizes the whole person (mind and body are seen as the same, not separate), and it regards the self as a total organism as it responds to the environment. One can reminisce about the past and daydream about the future, but one must live in the present to be a fully functioning individual. The individual must develop self-awareness, acceptance, wholeness, and responsibility in order to achieve **organismic** balance. Feelings are considered to be energy. A person gets into trouble by not expressing feelings and by accumulating **unfinished business,** which results in tension and somatic (physical) difficulties and does not allow problems to be solved.

The major constructs of Gestalt theory are the following:

1. Maturity (wholeness) is achieved when persons are able to be self-supportive rather than environment-supported, when they are able to mobilize and use their own resources rather than manipulate others, and when they are able to accept responsibility for their own behaviors and experiences.

2. Awareness reduces avoidance behavior by allowing one to face and accept previously denied parts of one's being in order to become whole.

3. Change occurs when people assume responsibility for themselves and when they terminate unfinished business (which usually consists of unexpressed feelings related to past events that currently interfere with one's functioning, thus preventing one from acting in the present).

4. The focus of therapy is on the individual's current feelings and thoughts; on exploring all of his or her sensations, fantasies, perceptions, and dreams; and on encouraging him or her to take responsibility for them and "own" them in order to achieve integration.

5. The individual is encouraged to trust his or her intuitive sense rather than adjust to society.

Gestalt therapy uses a workshop approach to helping, with one-to-one relations being developed within a group setting, although the techniques can be applied on an individual basis. Major techniques of Gestalt therapy include the use of exercises and games. Their goal is to interrelate mental activity, feelings, bodily sensations, and actions. Awareness of body language is as important as awareness of patterns of verbal language. Many of the awareness exercises in this book emanate from Gestalt theory.

In Gestalt therapy, the therapist acts as a catalyst in that he or she directs, challenges, and frustrates clients so they may develop awareness of their whole (Gestalt). As previously mentioned, vehicles for expression include acting-out exercises and games—that is, acting out conflicts in the present through exaggeration and role reversals. When Gestalt therapists ask clients to engage in role-playing exercises, they direct the clients to focus on certain details and feelings in order to push for client responsibility. The Gestalt therapist refuses to allow clients to avoid present experiences by intellectualizing ("talking about"), escaping to the past, or daydreaming about the future. The therapist's interventions involve asking "what" and "how" questions (never "why"!) to help expand the individual's sense of responsibility (owning the problem) and awareness and make the implicit explicit through the exaggeration of behavior.

Like person-centered therapy, Gestalt therapy focuses on the individual and an authentic helping relationship in the here and now, rather than on interpretation. Unlike person-centered therapy, the Gestalt approach is directive in that the therapist is like the director of a play.

Implications of the Gestalt Approach for Helpers   In Gestalt therapy, the therapist is involved in a learning situation with clients and has the skill to teach them how to learn about themselves and become aware of how they function. This awareness leads to greater self-responsibility. The focus in Gestalt therapy is on both verbal and nonverbal techniques. Warmth and empathy are not emphasized as in person-centered helping relationships, but unless the client has faith in the therapist's potency (skill and ability to help), it is unlikely that Gestalt therapy will be effective, because the client will resist the therapist's suggestions and directions to carry out specific exercises.

The Gestalt therapist is confrontational, and this attitude can lead to frustration on the part of the client. For example, the therapist often asks the client to "stay with this feeling," which is frustrating for the client who wants to avoid that particular feeling. In this way, the Gestalt therapist encourages the client to analyze and reintegrate the unpleasant feeling with his or her whole self. The Gestalt therapist attends to the client's body language and looks for incongruencies in awareness and attention. Emphasis is on the "what" and "how" of behavior rather than the "why."

There are several Gestalt principles that helpers without extensive training in Gestalt therapy can use. For instance, they can point out clients' body (nonverbal) language as well as verbal language and attempt to integrate these into a whole. They can also emphasize clients' responsibility for their feelings, thoughts, and actions in the here and now; use techniques to encourage clients' self-awareness and self-reliance; and recognize the effect of "unfinished business" on current functioning. Gestalt therapy de-emphasizes abstract intellectualization and provides a dramatic, quick methodology for enhancing self-awareness.

Corey (2005) points out that Gestalt techniques can present some risks because of their manipulative power and their de-emphasis of cognition. Clients may experience immediate or delayed intense emotional reactions, which will require follow-up discussion. The techniques may need to be modified in order to be effective with clients from differing cultures. For example, the dramatic emphasis on expressiveness may be contrary to some cultures' preference for verbal constraint and containment. Direct verbal messages and direct eye contact are also viewed differently among cultural groups.

BEHAVIORAL THEORY

Unlike the psychodynamic and phenomenological approaches, which were developed from clinical practice, the behavioral approaches to helping were developed in psychological laboratories. The ethos of behavioral approaches arose from the inability of scientists to measure and evaluate the outcomes of psychoanalytic and phenomenological approaches to helping and from a need to predict and measure outcomes of helping based on specific, observable, objective, and measurable variables (overt cognitive, motor, and emotional behaviors). The reasoning went that we cannot see, therefore we cannot measure, feelings or thoughts, so we must concern ourselves only with behavior in order to be truly accountable as helpers.

In the 1960s, behavior therapy was considered the clinical application of classical and operant **conditioning** theory. Gradually, it incorporated various other approaches, such as applied behavior analysis, stimulus–response approaches, behavior modification, and social learning theory. Today, behavior therapies are integrated with cognitive therapies into cognitive-behavioral approaches. In this text, however, we will focus on the basic, common concepts that distinguish behavioral theory from other helping theories. This will make it easier for you to see the relationship between thinking and behavior, which has become the predominant focus of cognitive-behavioral approaches.

Behavioral Theory's Major Principles of Helping

According to behavioral theory, human behavior is determined by its immediate consequences in the environment (**reinforcement**). Therefore, it is learned from situational factors, not from within the organism. All behavior is learned and, thus, can be unlearned. Difficulties occur when learned, maladaptive behavior results in anxiety; the anxiety is learned as a contingency of the learned maladaptive behavior. This view assumes that people have no internal control over their behavior, no self-determinism; all behavior is determined by environmental variables. The human being is viewed as an organism capable of being manipulated. Values, feelings, and thoughts are ignored; only concrete, observable behaviors are considered. As a result, all behavioral theories are committed to a rigorous scientific method, with emphasis on behavioral analysis and treatment evaluation.

The major constructs of this theory are the following:

1. All behavior is caused by the environment (stimuli).
2. Behavior is **shaped** (the **principle of gradation**) and maintained by its consequences (responses).
3. Behavior is determined by immediate rather than historical antecedents.
4. Behavior that is reinforced by either **concrete reinforcement** or **social reinforcement** is more likely to recur than behavior that is not reinforced.
5. **Positive reinforcement** has more conditioning **potency** than negative reinforcement.
6. Reinforcement must follow immediately after the behavior has occurred.
7. Reinforcement may be either concrete or social.
8. Behavior can be extinguished by the absence of reinforcement.
9. Behaviors can be shaped by reinforcing successive approximations of the desired behavior.

The behavioral helping approaches are specifically directive and controlled; they rely on learning processes and cognitive mechanisms. The helper identifies unsuitable stimulus–response bonds (causes and effects of the target behaviors) and arranges to interfere with or to extinguish these unsuitable bonds. The helper then sets up conditions for teaching new, more desirable stimulus–response bonds so that more appropriate behaviors will be learned.

These principles of reinforcement allow for both **discrimination** among stimuli and **generalization** of learning from one situation to another. The four general behavior modification approaches are (1) imitative learning (modeling), which teaches new behaviors through actual or simulated (video- or audiotape) performing of desired behaviors by models; (2) cognitive learning, which teaches new behavior through role playing, rehearsals, verbal instructions, or **contingency contracts** between helper and helpee that spell out clearly what the helpee is to do and what the consequences or reinforcement of this behavior will be (**token economy**); (3) emotional learning, such as **implosive therapy** (massive, exaggerated exposure to highly unpleasant stimuli in imaginal form to **extinguish** associated anxiety), systematic desensitization (counterconditioning to reduce anxiety by pairing negative events with complete physical relaxation—a positive event to extinguish the negative quality), or covert sensitization (the pairing of anxiety-producing stimuli with those that have pleasant associations); and (4) **operant conditioning,** whereby selected behaviors are immediately reinforced and systematic **schedules of reinforcement** have been consciously determined in advance. The goal of behavior therapy is to change behavior in general by increasing or decreasing specific behaviors, using empirically based treatments.

Implications of the Behavioral Approach for Helpers

Originally, the direct helping relationship was not considered important to the behavioral approach; the human relationship is not a variable in changing behavior unless, for some reason, the helper has tremendous reinforcement value to the helpee. The helper was seen more as a behavior engineer: objective, detached, and professional. In fact, the helper often served merely as a consultant and did not have direct contact with the helpee, except perhaps for initial observation. There are even cassette tapes available for specific behavioral techniques. Where there is verbal contact, the helper is trained to use systematically concrete, verbal reinforcement. The helper is also trained in observational and evaluation skills. Because of the focus on observable, overt behavior, the behavioral helper is able to determine what interventions have been effective and when to terminate therapy by noting the presence or absence of specific target behaviors. Thus, the helper is active and directive, often functioning as a teacher or consultant/trainer. More recently, however, behaviorists with direct contact with helpees have realized that an effective helping relationship improves the client's compliance and motivation to practice new behavioral skills. There is growing realization about the complexity of human beings, that what occurs in the laboratory may not apply to real people. In other words, recent neuroscience research shows that there is a relationship between environmental factors, learning processes, and biological factors.

Because the behavioral approaches are specific and relatively open to measurement and evaluation, they have helped to move counseling and helping from the "art" end of the continuum toward the "science" end. Focusing on behavioral outcomes appears to lessen dependency relationships and results in shorter-term treatment. As helpers, we can: focus on observable behavior (rather than talk about feelings and thoughts, which are difficult to measure); use techniques that enable us to evaluate the results of our interventions; specify goals, strategies, and outcomes of helping, and thus be more accountable and avoid running the risk of imposing our subjective values and attitudes on helpees; focus on what the helpee is doing and can do as opposed to what the helpee cannot or should not do, thereby emphasizing the positive rather than negative aspects of individual behaviors; and deal only with observable behaviors and avoid risking questionable interpretations of subjective data. In order for these approaches to be useful with diverse cultures, one must be familiar with different cultural values and attitudes. Behavioral assessment needs to be culturally relevant.

COGNITIVE AND
COGNITIVE-BEHAVIORAL THEORIES

Cognitive and cognitive-behavioral approaches to helping deal with rationality, the thinking processes, and problem solving. They focus on the helpee's appraisals, attributions, belief systems, and expectancies, as well as the effects of those cognitive processes on emotions and behaviors. They are instructive, directive, and verbally oriented (as opposed to an approach like Gestalt, which is more nonverbally oriented). Many vocational counseling approaches fall into this domain, with an emphasis on testing, synthesis of a variety of collected data, and rational decision making. The major philosophical assumption of cognitive-behavioral theory is that by changing people's thinking one can change their belief system, which in turn changes their behavior and emotions.

Three major representatives of cognitive-behavioral theory are rational-emotive behavior therapy (REBT), reality therapy (RT), and cognitive-behavioral therapies (CBT).

Rational-Emotive Behavior Therapy

The rational-emotive behavioral approach to helping was developed by Albert Ellis in the mid-1950s and is based on his belief that people need to change their way of thinking (**cognitive restructuring**) to correct faulty (irrational) thinking.

Rational-Emotive Behavior Therapy's Major Principles of Helping

Ellis believes that people must take full responsibility for themselves and for their own fates. He maintains that although people are influenced by biological and environmental factors, they are not controlled by them. Rather, their thought processes mediate between those factors and their emotions. People perceive, think, feel, and behave simultaneously. They can learn to control what they feel and do, to a great extent. Ellis further posits that people are born with a tendency to be both rational and irrational, with both self-sabotaging and self-actualizing capacities. They are greatly affected by social conditioning, so although there are biological, genetic determinants of rational and irrational thinking, people primarily teach themselves to become more and more irrational by incorporating the world's irrationality into their belief systems.

Ellis originally postulated an A-B-C theory: A = the activating experience that the client wrongly believes causes C = emotional or behavioral consequences; B = the client's belief system, either rational or irrational, which is the intervening variable really causing C. More recently he has added D and E, so it is now an A-B-C-D-E theory. D = disputation of the helpee's irrational thoughts and beliefs, and E = the new, more rational emotion or effect. It is B, the client's belief system, that needs to be restructured. Ellis identified four evaluative thinking dysfunctions and 12 irrational ideas (listed in Chapter 7) that people keep repeating to themselves that cause faulty thinking.

The following example demonstrates faulty thinking:

Because it would be highly preferable if I were outstandingly competent, I absolutely should and must be. It is awful when I am not, and I am therefore a worthless individual. Because it is highly desirable that others treat me considerately and fairly, they absolutely should and must, and they are rotten people who deserve to be utterly damned when they do not. And because it is preferable that I experience pleasure rather than pain, the world absolutely should arrange this, and life is horrible and I can't bear it when the world doesn't.

Ellis claims that these are the kinds of things we tell ourselves that make us upset—but we can learn to give ourselves different messages.

The major constructs of this theory are the following:

1. Problems are caused by irrational beliefs that result in dysfunction.

2. People are capable of changing their belief systems by learning how to refute their irrational beliefs.

3. People are biologically and culturally predisposed to choose, to create, to relate to others, and to enjoy, but they also have inborn propensities to be self-destructive, evasive, selfish, and intolerant.

4. Emotional disturbance results from people's continual irrational thinking, their refusal to accept reality, their insistence on having things the way they think they should be, and their self-absorption.

Rational-emotive behavior therapy is a teaching approach that helps people achieve a change in thinking in order to take control of how they experience their emotions, either healthily or unhealthily. By instructing, giving information, teaching **imagery techniques,** and assigning homework, the therapist helps change the helpee's irrational belief system. Thus, the technique is both cognitive (teaching) and behavioral (role playing, homework assignments). REBT techniques are designed to change behavior by changing thinking, which, in turn, will help the client to feel better. Clients are taught to understand themselves, to understand others, to react differently, and to change their basic life philosophy by correcting faulty thinking.

Implications of the Rational-Emotive Behavior Therapy Approach for Helpers   In this approach, the helping relationship is cognitive and directive in that helpers exhort, frustrate, and command helpees to get them to analyze their thoughts and learn to rationally restructure their belief systems. The helping relationship depends on the potency of helpers and on their ability to communicate that power to helpees, rather than on warm, empathic, reciprocal relationships. REBT therapists accept clients as fallible humans without necessarily giving personal warmth. They criticize and point out behavioral deficiencies and encourage clients to use more self-discipline. They discourage dependency and often use impersonal, highly cognitive, active-directive homework assigning and discipline-oriented techniques such as didactic discussion, bibliotherapy, and audiovisual aids. Helpees who have experienced discrimination and oppression due to their gender, race, ethnicity, class, or sexual orientation may find these impersonal, confrontational techniques offensive. They may feel that they are being "blamed" for their feelings. This approach pays little attention to the impact of social forces on individuals' psychological well-being.

The rational-emotive behavioral approach teaches helpers to integrate the cognitive domain with the behavioral and affective domains. Helpers recognize the interrelation of reason, emotion, and behavior to foster clients' responsibility for acknowledging and reassessing their own internalized belief systems. The REBT methodology quickly exposes the linear relationship of feelings, thoughts, and behavior.

Reality Therapy

Like rational-emotive behavior therapy, this branch of cognitive-behavioral theory, developed by psychiatrist William Glasser, is rational, logical, and learning oriented. Reality therapy explores the client's values and behavioral choices, exposing inconsistencies and enforcing responsibility for those choices. Glasser's more recent work has stressed helping people take more effective control of their lives by helping them choose effective, responsible behaviors to fulfill the following needs: survival, belonging, power, fun, and freedom. These five needs are genetically determined, and our behavior is designed to control our environment in ways that will satisfy them. Thus, current reality therapy theory is based on control theory. There are two fundamental ways to control the world to meet our needs: (1) to perceive what in the world can possibly satisfy needs—input, and (2) to act upon or control what is perceived to satisfy needs—output.

Reality Therapy's Major Principles of Helping   The theory is interpersonal in that one must be involved with others in order to meet the needs delineated above. The goal of reality therapy is to assist people to make responsible choices (involving consistency between value systems and behavior) and to meet the basic psychological needs without depriving other people of the opportunity to fulfill their own needs. People are seen as capable of assuming responsibility for themselves and capable of rational thought and behavior. They have the ability to judge that their behavior is not helping as well as the ability to make a commitment to change. They have no excuse for not exercising these attributes. The focus is on what they are able and willing to do, not on what they may "try."

The practice of reality therapy involves a candid, human relationship through which helpers teach helpees to accept responsibility for themselves by analyzing inconsistencies among their goals, values, and behaviors. Reality therapy is a direct approach; it deals with the present. It is based on eight steps:

1. Make friends and ask clients what they want.
2. Ask clients what they are choosing to do to get what they want.

3. Ask if their behavioral choice is working.

4. If it is not, as is almost always the case, help them to make better choices.

5. Get a commitment to follow the better choices that have been worked out in the previous planning phase.

6. Do not accept excuses for failure to carry out the plan; if the plan is impracticable, replan.

7. Do not punish, but ask clients to accept reasonable consequences for their behavior.

8. Do not give up.

The acronym WDEP has been adopted by Glasser (1998, 2000) and Wubbolding (2000) to clarify the major procedures of reality therapy. W refers to the exploration of wants, needs, and perceptions; D refers to the focus on current behavior, direction and doing. E refers to evaluation, asking questions such as "Do you know what you are doing?" and "Is this behavior likely to get you where you want to go?" P refers to the last phase of therapy, planning and commitment to a written plan.

Implications of the Reality Therapy Approach for Helpers   The reality therapist encourages, suggests alternatives, praises positive behavior, confronts inconsistencies openly and directly, and cares enough about the helpees to reject behaviors that prevent them from meeting their basic psychological needs. Helpers are concerned about present behavior, what helpees are currently doing, and what the consequences of alternative choices might be. They refuse to engage in self-defeating conversations about negative experiences and symptoms. The focus is on helping clients to recognize irresponsible behaviors and contracting with them for responsible behaviors.

The relationship between the reality therapist and the client is crucial; it must be a warm, honest, personal involvement. Through this relationship, the client learns to feel loved by the therapist, learns to love the therapist, and learns to feel worthwhile because the therapist focuses on what the client is doing, on the client's approach behaviors rather than on avoidance behaviors. (This process is similar to the psychoanalytic concept of transference, although it is not acknowledged as such.) This relationship differs from the person-centered relationship in one major aspect: the helping relationship in reality therapy is indeed judgmental, in that the reality therapist judges the value of the client's behavior in terms of the therapist's perceptions of reality. For example, if the client persists in self-defeating behavior, the therapist may say, "That behavior is ridiculous because it will keep you from getting what you say you really want."

The major implication of reality therapy for helpers is that honest, intense involvement of the helper and the helpee is required for success. Helpers must examine the inconsistencies between clients' actions and their values and needs, focus on action (what clients are doing rather than what they are thinking or feeling), and insist on clients' assuming responsibility for their choices and the consequences of those choices. Helpers facilitate clients' meeting their needs and gaining control of their world.

Reality therapy is proving quite popular in Asian and Middle Eastern countries as a short-term movement different from the conventional psychodynamic model. The concepts of "reality" can be culturally defined.

Cognitive-Behavioral Therapies

The approaches of the cognitive-behavioral therapies combine the learning theories of behaviorism with a new emphasis on constructs such as thinking, feelings, motives, plans, purposes, images, and knowledge. They were formulated to preserve the best of clinical behavioral interventions while recognizing an individual's inner cognitive processes. Cognitive-behavioral therapies represent a major theoretical orientation today and are the treatment of choice for many because of the current sociocultural constraints on providing mental health services.

Cognitive-Behavioral Therapies' Major Principles of Helping   Beck's (1976) cognitive therapy focuses on the systematic errors in reasoning that underlie psychological problems. Beck postulates three major components of a theory of emotional disorders:

1. Negative, automatic thoughts that disrupt one's mood and cause further thoughts to emerge in a downward thought/affect spiral
2. Distorted reality based on systematic logical errors, such as
   a. Arbitrary inference: inferring a conclusion from missing, false, or irrelevant evidence
   b. Overgeneralization: concluding from one specific negative event that another is therefore more likely
   c. Selective abstraction: focusing on certain aspects of a situation and ignoring others
   d. Magnification or minimalization: thinking the worst of every situation or else refusing to acknowledge its importance
   e. Personalization: relating an external circumstance to oneself when there is no basis for that relationship
   f. Dichotomous thinking: all-or-nothing extremism
3. Depressive schemas in which one's assumptions about the world represent the way one organizes past experience and are the system by which incoming information about the world is classified

For Beck, problems arise from distortions of reality based on faulty premises and assumptions. These distorted appraisals lead to specific emotions and, therefore, one's emotional response is consistent with the distortion, not with reality.

The three major stages of cognitive therapy are (1) eliciting thoughts, self-talk, and the client's interpretations of them; (2) gathering with the client evidence for or against the client's interpretations; and (3) setting up experiments (homework) to test the validity of the client's interpretations and to gather more data for discussion. This is an active therapy in which the therapist collaborates with the client in the here and now. It is a verbal therapy, and each session establishes an agenda, structures the therapy time, summarizes periodically what is happening, questions the client, assigns homework, and asks the client to sum up the session. Beck emphasizes the necessity of accurate empathy, warmth, and genuineness in the helping relationship; he says rapport, collaboration, and mutual understanding are important. Some specific techniques are cognitive rehearsal, questioning, searching for alternatives, monitoring thoughts, reality testing, thought substitution, and teaching coping skills and self-control techniques.

Meichenbaum's (1977) cognitive-behavior modification is based on the belief that psychological stress and difficulties are self-induced by our internal verbal dialogues. These internal self-instructions can be altered to change behavior. By teaching people to think aloud, we can help them learn to recognize their faulty thinking. They then can change this thinking by cognitive restructuring, by learning new self-statements. This cognitive restructuring can be taught through modeling or direct instruction.

Implications of Cognitive–Behavioral Therapies for Helpers   As previously suggested, cognitive-behavioral therapies are the preferred modality for managed care organizations, particularly for patients with mild to moderate disorders. The therapies have been proven effective with a wide variety of affective and adjustment disorders. These approaches have an impressive array of empirical validation and training manuals for helpers.

Pragmatic and concrete, the cognitive-behavioral techniques demystify the therapy process and are readily teachable. Although variations exist among cognitive-behavioral schools, they are all unified by a belief in the central role played by mediating knowledge structures or thinking processes in explaining and changing human behavior. To differing degrees regarding which is more significant, they acknowledge the interaction of cognition and emotion and they utilize both cognitive and behavioral techniques to effect change.

Because they are collaborative, educative approaches, these therapies may be particularly effective with multicultural clients: they can focus on individuals' belief systems within cultural contexts and emphasize cognition and action as well as relationship. The therapist's awareness of cultural contexts is crucial because a primary emphasis on changing thoughts may keep clients adjusting to an unhealthy status quo. Furthermore, some diverse clients may find it difficult to challenge and change values and thoughts that may be culturally based or culturally different from those of the helper. The helper must take care in how these changes are proposed. The minimization of unconscious processes and the downplay of emotion, however, may limit the effectiveness of these approaches with people who have chronic and/or major disorders.

EXERCISE 5.2 ■ This exercise was suggested by Amy Bernstein, a student at the University of North Carolina–Greensboro, although I've added some questions. After studying this chapter, answer the following questions about psychodynamic, phenomenological, behavioral, and cognitive-behavioral theories:

1. What is the theory's view of people?
2. What does the theory deal with?
3. What meaning is attached to the theory?
4. What does the theory leave out?
5. How attuned is the theory to diversity?
6. For what kinds of people, in what kinds of situations, would this theory apply?

EXERCISE 5.3 ■ Now review what you wrote in Exercise 5.2. Which elements of these theories appear to be a good fit for you at this time? Consider your relationship and communication styles, your views about human behavior and human development, the kinds of work you want to do, and what does and does not make sense to you. Do you think there are discrepancies between what you think you should believe, what you say you believe, and what you actually do? How would you describe your actual theory-in-action?

SUMMARY

This chapter stresses the need to become aware of one's personal theory of helping and to develop a style of helping that is consistent with that theory. One's personal theory of helping will inevitably influence one's perception and assessment of the major formal theories of helping that we have presented in brief overview: psychodynamic (Freudian, Jungian, Adlerian, ego psychology, and object relations), phenomenological (existential, person-centered, and Gestalt), behavioral, and cognitive (rational-emotive behavior therapy, reality, cognitive-behavioral). Table 5.1 compares these major theories in schematic fashion; the following summary should also help to clarify the broad outlines of each approach.

1. The psychodynamic approach emphasizes unconscious causes of behavior and early childhood experiences; it focuses on content more than on process.

2. The phenomenological approach emphasizes process more than content and stresses the helping relationship as a vehicle for change. This helping relationship provides a climate in which clients can explore their own feelings, thoughts, and behaviors to achieve both insight and behavioral change. This approach focuses on the present, as opposed to the past.

TABLE 5.1 Comparison of major theories of helping

	Psychodynamic	Phenomenological Person-Centered	Phenomenological Gestalt	Behavioral	Cognitive-Behavioral
Major principles	1. People have no free will	1. People have free will	1. People have free will	1. People have no free will	1. People have free will
	2. Behavior is determined by biological and environmental factors	2. Locus of behavioral determinism is internal	2. Organism works as whole within environment	2. Behavior is caused by environment and shaped by consequences	2. Behavior is determined by logical thinking and responsibility
	3. Neurosis stems from repressed infantile conflicts	3. Neurosis stems from incongruence between self-concept and environment	3. Neurosis stems from impasse between organism and environment	3. Neurosis results from maladaptive learning	3. Neurosis stems from irrational thinking and irresponsible choices
Therapy process	1. Directive	1. Nondirective	1. Directive	1. Directive	1. Directive
	2. Diagnosis and past experience important	2. Here-and-now experience important	2. Here-and-now verbal and body awareness important	2. Present behavior and reinforcement history important	2. Present behavior, thinking, and values important
	3. Verbal	3. Verbal	3. Verbal and nonverbal; games	3. Verbal; activities	3. Verbal; activities
	4. Transference in relationship important	4. Empathic relationship important	4. Honest, trusting, and supportive but confrontative relationship	4. Analytical, conditioning relationship	4. Instructional, involved relationship

(continued)

TABLE 5.1 Comparison of major theories of helping (*continued*)

	Psychodynamic	Phenomenological Person-Centered	Phenomenological Gestalt	Behavioral	Cognitive–Behavioral
Requisite therapist behaviors	1. Therapist neutral, benign, objective, but also empathic	1. Therapist honest, congruent, empathic, nonjudgmental, capable of unconditional positive regard	1. Therapist honest, open, confrontative but basically supportive	1. Therapist analytical, objective, observational, evaluative	1. Therapist involved and judgmental; confronts illogical thinking and irresponsibility
	2. Interprets transference, resistance, and unconscious material	2. Needs ability to communicate the above qualities	2. Provides experience via verbal and nonverbal games	2. Analyzes goals, directs strategies, evaluates, provides positive reinforcement, arranges environmental contingencies	2. Rejects illogical thinking and irresponsible behavior
	3. No contracts	3. No contracts	3. No contracts	3. Explicit contracts	3. Explicit contracts
Domain	Affective/cognitive	Affective	Affective	Behavioral	Cognitive/behavioral

3. The behavioral approaches emphasize environmental consequences of behavior as determinants of behavior; they focus on the learning of new behaviors and the extinction of maladaptive behaviors. The process is one of identifying dysfunctional behaviors, planning new behaviors, and systematically arranging valued reinforcements for these new behaviors.

4. The cognitive-behavioral approaches are concerned with teaching new ways of thinking and with exploring and examining discrepancies between values and behaviors. They also function in the present, rather than in the past.

REFERENCES AND FURTHER READING

General

Brammer, L. M., & MacDonald, G. (2003). *The helping relationship: Process and skills* (8th ed.). Boston: Allyn & Bacon.

Corey, G. (2005). *Theory and practice of counseling and psychotherapy* (7th ed.). Belmont, CA: Brooks/Cole.

Ivey, A. E., D'Andrea, M., Ivey, M. B., & Simek-Morgan, L. (2002). *Intentional interviewing and counseling: Facilitating client development* (4th ed.). Pacific Grove: Brooks/Cole.

Nisbett, R. E. (2000, August 6). *Relationship schemas and cultural style.* Presentation at the meeting of the American Psychological Association, Washington, DC.

Psychodynamic Theory

Classical Psychoanalytic

Adler, A. (1927). *The practice and theory of individual psychology.* New York: Harcourt Brace Jovanovich.

Alexander, F. (1963). *Fundamentals of psychoanalysis.* New York: Norton.

Erikson, E. H. (1963). *Childhood and society* (2nd ed.). New York: Norton.

Erikson, E. H. (Ed.). (1968). *Identity: Youth and crisis.* New York: Norton.

Erikson, E. H. (1982). *The life cycle completed.* New York: Norton.

Freud, A. (1946). *The ego and the mechanisms of defense.* New York: International Universities Press.

Freud, S. (1943). *A general introduction to psychoanalysis.* Garden City, NY: Doubleday.

Freud, S. (1949). *An outline of psychoanalysis.* New York: Norton.

Hall, C. (1954). *A primer of Freudian psychology.* New York: Mentor.

Jung, C. (1928). *Contributions to analytic psychology.* New York: Harcourt Brace Jovanovich.

Jung, C. (1933). *Modern man in search of a soul.* New York: Harcourt Brace Jovanovich.

Jung, C. (1933). *Psychological types.* New York: Harcourt Brace Jovanovich.

Object Relations

Bowlby, J. (1988). *A secure base: Parent-child attachment and healthy human development.* New York: Basic Books.

Fairbairn, W. R. D. (1954). *An object relations theory of personality.* New York: Basic Books.

Guntrip, H. (1979). *Psychoanalytical theory, therapy, and the self.* New York: Guilford.

Kernberg, O. (1968). The therapy of patients with borderline personality organization. *International Journal of Psychoanalysis, 49,* 600–619.

Klein, M. (1932). *The psychoanalysis of children.* London: Hogarth Press.

Kohut, H. (1971). *The analysis of self.* New York: International Universities Press.

Mahler, M., Pine, F., & Bergman, A. (1975). *The psychological birth of the human infant.* New York: Basic Books.

Winnicott, D. W. (1965). *The family and individual development.* London: Tavistock.

Phenomenological Theory

Person-Centered

Carkhuff, R., & Berenson, B. (1967). *Beyond counseling and therapy.* New York: Holt, Rinehart & Winston.

Combs, A. (1989). *A theory of therapy: Guidelines for counseling practice.* Newbury Park, CA: Sage.

Combs, A., Avila, D., & Purkey, W. (1977). *Helping relationships: Basic concepts for the helping process* (2nd ed.). Boston: Allyn & Bacon.

Farber, B. A., Brink, D. C., & Raskin, P. M. (Eds.). (1996). *The psychotherapy of Carl Rogers: Cases and commentary.* New York: Guilford Press.

Gendlin, E. T. (1996). *Focusing-oriented psychotherapy: A manual of the existential method.* New York: Guilford Press.

Hart, J. (1970). *New directions in client-centered therapy.* Boston: Houghton Mifflin.

Rogers, C. (1951). *Client-centered therapy.* Boston: Houghton Mifflin.

Rogers, C. (1961). *On becoming a person.* Boston: Houghton Mifflin.

Rogers, C. (1980). *A way of being.* Boston: Houghton Mifflin.

Rogers, C., & Dymond, R. (1954). *Psychotherapy and personality change.* Chicago: University of Chicago Press.

Existential

Bugental, J. F. T. (1987). *The art of the psychotherapist.* New York: Norton.

May, R. (1961). *Existential psychology.* New York: Random House.

May, R. (1983). *The discovery of being: Writings in existential psychology.* New York: Norton.

Van Deurzen-Smith, E. (1997). *Everyday mysteries: Existential dimensions of psychotherapy.* London: Routledge.

Yalom, I. (1980). *Existential psychotherapy.* New York: Basic Books.

Gestalt

Fagan, J., & Shepherd, I. (Eds.). (1970). *Gestalt therapy now.* Palo Alto, CA: Science and Behavior Books.

Hycner, R., & Jacobs, L. (1995). *The healing relationship in Gestalt therapy.* Highland, NY: Gestalt Journal Press.

Koffka, K. (1935). *Principles of Gestalt psychology.* New York: Harcourt, Brace.

Perls, F. (1969). *Gestalt therapy verbatim.* Lafayette, CA: Real People Press.

Perls, F., Hefferline, R., & Goodman, P. (1951). *Gestalt therapy.* New York: Dell.

Yontef, G. (1993). *Awareness, dialogue and process: Essays on Gestalt therapy.* Highland, NY: Gestalt Journal Press.

Behavioral Theories

Bandura, A. (1969). *Principles of behavior modification.* New York: Holt, Rinehart & Winston.

Bandura, A. (1977). *Social learning theory.* Englewood Cliffs, NJ: Prentice-Hall.

Bandura, A. (1986). *Social foundations of thought and action: A social cognitive theory.* Englewood Cliffs, NJ: Prentice-Hall.

Franks, C., Wilson, G., Kendall, P., & Brownell, K. (1982). *Annual review of behavior therapy: Theory and practice* (Vol. 8). New York: Guilford Press.

Kazdin, A. E. (1994). *Behavior modification in applied settings* (5th ed.). Pacific Grove, CA: Brooks/Cole.

Krasner, L., & Ullman, L. (Eds.). (1965). *Research in behavior modification.* New York: Holt, Rinehart & Winston.

Krumboltz, J. (Ed.). (1966). *Revolution in counseling: Implication of behavioral sciences.* Boston: Houghton Mifflin.

O'Leary, K. D., & Wilson, G. T. (1987). *Behavior therapy: Application and outcome* (2nd ed.). Englewood Cliffs, NJ: Prentice-Hall.

Spiegler, M. D., & Guevremont, D. C. (1998). *Contemporary behavioral therapy* (3rd ed.). Pacific Grove, CA: Brooks/Cole.

Wolpe, J. (1958). *Psychotherapy by reciprocal inhibition.* Palo Alto, CA: Stanford University Press.

Wolpe, J. (1990). *The practice of behavior therapy* (4th ed.). Elmsford, NY: Pergamon Press.

Cognitive-Behavioral Theories

Alford, B. A., & Beck, A. T. (1997). *The integrative power of cognitive therapy.* New York: Guilford Press.

Beck, A. T. (1976). *Cognitive therapy and the emotional disorders.* New York: International Universities Press.

Beck, A. T., Rush, J., Shaw, B., & Emery, G. (1979). *Cognitive therapy of depression.* New York: Guilford Press.

Beck, A. T., & Weishaar, M. E. (1995). Cognitive therapy. In R. J. Corsini & D. Wedding (Eds.), *Current psychotherapies* (4th ed., pp. 285–320). Itasca, IL: F. E. Peacock.

Beck, J. S. (1995). *Cognitive therapy: Basics and beyond.* New York: Guilford Press.

Dobson, K. S. (Ed.). (1988). *Handbook of cognitive-behavioral therapies.* New York: Guilford Press.

Ellis, A. (1962). *Reason and emotion in psychotherapy.* New York: Lyle Stuart.

Ellis, A. (1973). The no cop-out therapy. *Psychology Today, 7,* 56–62.

Ellis, A. (1994). *Reason and emotion in psychotherapy revised.* New York: Carol.

Ellis, A. (1999). *How to make yourself happy and remarkably less disturbable.* San Luis Obispo, CA: Impact.

Ellis, A., & Harper, R. (1997). *A guide to rational living* (3rd ed.). North Hollywood, CA: Wilshire.

Ellis, A., & Whiteley, J. (Eds.). (1979). *Theoretical and empirical foundations of rational-emotive therapy.* Pacific Grove, CA: Brooks/Cole.

Freeman, A., & Dattilio, R. M. (Eds.). (1994). *Comprehensive casebook of cognitive therapy.* New York: Plenum.

Glasser, N. (Ed.). (1989). *Control theory in the practice of reality therapy: Case studies.* New York: Harper & Row.

Glasser, W. (1965). *Reality therapy.* New York: Harper & Row.

Glasser, W. (1981). *State of the mind.* New York: Harper & Row.

Glasser, W. (1994). *The control theory manager.* New York: Harper & Row.

Glasser, W. (1998). *Choice theory: A new psychology of personal freedom.* New York: HarperCollins.

Glasser, W. (2000). *Counseling with choice theory.* New York: HarperCollins.

Kuehlwein, K. T., & Rosen, H. (Eds.). (1993). *Cognitive therapies in action.* San Francisco: Jossey-Bass.

Meichenbaum, D. (1977). *Cognitive-behavior modification.* New York: Plenum Press.

Meichenbaum, D. (1985). *Stress inoculation training.* New York: Pergamon Press.

Wubbolding, R. E. (2000). *Reality therapy for the 21st century.* London: Routledge.

Visit the book companion site at www.thomsonedu.com to access tutorial quizzes.

6

Current Theoretical
Perspectives

At the end of the 20th and the beginning of the 21st centuries, questions have been raised about the assumptions of the major theories of helping presented in Chapter 5. Some of these questions concern the universality of the theoretical principles and values, as well as their disregard of the significant impact of sociocultural, economic, and political variables on human development. In this chapter, we present the integrative constructivist, feminist, multicultural, and ecological systems perspectives. These are inclusive viewpoints that transcend the basic theoretical models, but they are likely to be integrated with one's theory-of-use in current practice.

INTEGRATIVE THEORETICAL
APPROACHES

Most helpers use principles, concepts, and techniques from a variety of different theoretical viewpoints and, therefore, have an integrated or pluralistic approach to helping. This approach requires some flexibility and versatility as it is not guided by a single theoretical construct. It requires the helper to appreciate that each theory has limitations as well as something of value regarding the understanding of human behavior.

A helper who uses an integrated approach must always strive to be consistent and comprehensive in integrating the different approaches and must be clear about how the approach is or is not related to the theory from which it is derived. Obviously, the helper must carefully select strategies that are appropriate for the client he or she is helping. Thus, an integrated approach requires heightened self-awareness, so that helpers understand why certain viewpoints and approaches appeal to them and others do not. Furthermore, it is necessary for helpers to understand mind–body connections so as to consider the reciprocal influence of somatic and psychological conditions.

The integrated approach, then, presupposes that helpers are continually open to and searching for new understanding of human behavior and for more effective techniques. This implies that they are actively involved in continual professional training. The current professional literature indicates a major shift toward integration and pluralism in the practice of counseling and psychotherapy (Alford & Beck, 1997; Arkowitz, 1997; Corey, 2005; Ivey, D'Andrea, Ivey, & Simek-Morgan, 2002; Lazarus, 1995; Moursund & Erskine, 2004; Norcross & Goldfried, 1992; Preston, 1998; Prochaska & Norcross, 2003; Sharf, 2000; Sue & Sue, 2003). Most authors caution against a "sloppy eclecticism" and urge an integration of theory based solidly on supportive empirical study.

CONSTRUCTIVISM

Constructivism, a more recent cognitive-behavioral theory, focuses on the interdependence of thinking, feeling, and behavior, rather than on the supremacy of thinking. This theory is phenomenological in that it focuses on one's subjective view of self, of others, and of the world. It differs from other cognitive-behavioral theories in its attention to the internal meaning-making processes and to the involvement of early attachment experiences as a context for cognitive development. In other words, constructivists recognize unconscious processes, consider past development, and explore the relationships of thinking, feeling, and doing in the past, present, and future.

Constructivist theorists (Goldfried, 1988; Greenberg & Safran, 1989; Kelly, 1991a, 1991b) believe that people are active creators and construers of their own realities. They focus particularly on how people process new information to adapt to environmental demands and how they derive meaning from their experiences. The issue is not what objective "reality" is, but whether one's constructed view of the world is pragmatic enough to foster adaptation to the environment. Family systems constructivist theorists (Anderson, 1991; Breunlin, Schwartz, & MacKune-Karrer, 1997; Gergen, 1991; White, 2006) have developed narrative therapy to help families deconstruct and reconstruct new stories about who and how they are.

Constructivism's Major Principles of Helping

In constructivism, the emphasis of therapy is on exploring the origin and maintenance of clients' most fundamental core assumptions. The goal is modification and reorganization of these bold core schemas about self and self-in-relation to others and the world. If deep structural changes of self and how one experiences the world are to occur, unconscious, unspoken levels of personal knowledge structures must be brought into consciousness. Thus, the focus of therapy is on exploring the developmental process of how people have made and continue to make meaning of their life experiences. It is from these early, continuing, and newer attachment experiences with primary and other significant caretakers that one's constructs of self, others, and the world evolve.

Constructivism's major principles of helping are:

1. The client, rather than the therapist, is seen as the expert. The therapist collaborates with the client, empowering the client to challenge his or her core assumptions through metaphor, narratives, and responses to direct questions.

2. Alternative outcomes and choices are considered. The client is encouraged to develop his or her own voice and goals, to take risks to achieve these goals, to accept consequences of choices, and to acknowledge his or her capacities for change.

3. The major vehicle for change is the collaborative deconstruction of defeating core assumptions and co-construction of empowering, positive constructs in a warm, collaborative helping relationship.

Implications for Helpers

In these approaches, helpers consider the objective and subjective, conscious and unconscious thinking and information processing of clients. Since helpers place equal value on clients' feelings and behaviors as well as on their thoughts, clients become aware of how their thoughts, behaviors, and feelings influence one another. This can help clients recognize connections of which they have been unaware, develop alternatives for thinking and action, and explore and reconstruct their patterns of thinking and feeling.

A sensitive helper can encourage clients to examine the complex influence their multiple experiences and beliefs have had on their present constructs. These influences include the client's early and current environments, gender, race, ethnicity, class, religious beliefs, and sexual orientation. This multiperspective approach, based on the client's meanings of language, can be integrated with other major theories and can be used with many different kinds of clients.

FEMINIST THERAPIES

A variety of approaches, rather than a unified theory, feminist therapies cut across the different schools of theory. Feminist therapists focus on understanding gender as both a cause and a consequence of women's experiences in a male-dominated culture. They challenge and question the attitudes toward women of the prevalent psychological theories, which have largely been developed and practiced by male theorists and therapists. Feminist therapists believe that those theories advocate maintaining the status quo of a male-dominated, hierarchical society. Instead, feminist therapists value women's self-development in relation to others (interdependence) differently from men's autonomous development of self as a self-sufficient individual (independence). A study by Moradi and others (2000) found that feminist therapists subscribe to the notion that the personal is political, and they pay attention to issues of oppression (sexism, racism, heterosexism) and socialization inherent in a hierarchical society. The "third wave" of feminism (Gillis, Howie, & Munford, 2004) addresses community and national and international oppressive variables as areas of concern and targets for intervention.

There are several major differences between feminist theories and more traditional theories, particularly in the way feminists incorporate issues of gender and power. Theorists such as Bem (1993), Chodorow (1989), Gilligan (1982), and Miller (1976, 1991) have written about how gender shapes development and thinking. Their theories have led to research on the impact of sociocultural variables on both female and male development, and this research has led to better understanding of gender differences and similarities. Current theoretical debate concerns the nature/nurture dichotomy as neuroscience studies suggest gendered brain structure and process differences (Ballou & Brown, 2002).

Major Principles of Helping Among
Feminist Therapies

Close examination by feminist theorists of the influence of sociocultural context on the development of self-identity, views of others, goals and aspirations, and psychological well-being laid the groundwork for later multicultural approaches. Feminist therapies are based on a collaborative relationship of equality between helper and helpee. Women's problems are viewed as being inseparable from society's oppression. Feminist therapists emphasize social, political, and economic action as a major aspect of the helping process.

As summarized by Corey (2005, pp. 350–352), the major principles of feminist theory are these:

1. The personal is political.
2. Personal and social identities are interdependent.
3. Women's perceptions and experiences are valued.
4. Definitions of distress and mental illness are reformulated.
5. Feminist therapists use an integrated analysis of oppression.
6. The counseling relationship is egalitarian.

Feminist therapists believe in stating their values at the beginning of the helping relationship and using those values deliberately in modeling and interpreting. They respect helpees' diverse worldviews and emphasize that assessment and treatment formulations must take into account these varying perspectives.

The kinds of helping goals commonly ascribed to feminist therapies include awareness and desirability of androgyny (the complementary coexistence of feminine and masculine characteristics within both males and females), equal-in-power relationships between men and women, acceptance of diversity within groups, acceptance of one's worldview, acceptance of one's body image "as is," and career choice unbiased by sex (Brown, 1994; Brown & Ballou, 1992; Enns, 2004; Miller & Stiver, 1997; Mirkin, Suyemoto, & Okun, 2005; Okun & Ziady, 2005; Worell & Johnson, 1997).

Feminist theories range on a continuum from cultural to radical feminism. The former focuses on gender differences and the belief that each individual helpee needs to determine for herself or himself what sex-role options represent the best personal choice—that helpees should be exposed to feminist values but that the choice of values should be the free and individual choice of the client. Radical feminism minimizes gender differences and advocates active social and political analysis and change strategies as part of the helping process. Feminist therapies cut across the affective, cognitive, and behavioral domains.

In her comprehensive review of feminist counseling and therapy, Enns (2004) summarizes that contemporary feminist theorists examine the interaction of internal and external influences on women's life-span development. Emotional distress is viewed as emanating primarily from disrupting environmental influences on a woman's normal development. Miller (1976) clearly addresses the power of context and the power of a patriarchal culture on women's development. Relational-cultural theory, currently developing at the Stone Center (Jordan, Hartling, & Walker, 2004), focuses on the necessity of human connection to foster growth and resiliency.

Implications for Helpers

It is essential that helpers of all persuasions acknowledge the impact of gender role socialization on the identity and development of females and males, the impact of privilege or lack of privilege on an individual's access to power and opportunity, and the impact of subtle and not-so-subtle sexism on individuals in the family, school, workplace, and community. This acknowledgment allows helpers to consider a client's distress from sociopolitical and cultural perspectives.

The formation of an egalitarian, mutual relationship, in which women's unique attributes—their skill at connection, their individual aspirations, intuitive thinking, and transformed perspectives—are valued, is fundamental to this approach. The focus on **empowerment** and advocacy interventions helps to strengthen clients' sense of efficacy and broaden their options and opportunities.

MULTICULTURAL MODELS

As noted above, current feminist therapies and other integrative therapies also incorporate elements of multicultural models. Multicultural models do not subscribe to any one theoretical model but strongly question the relevance of theories based on Eurocentric values to clients of different cultural backgrounds. Multicultural models are based on the theoretical premises that (1) sociocultural conditions are responsible for the problems for which people seek help, (2) each culture has meaningful ways of coping with problems, and (3) counseling in the United States and Europe is predominantly a Western cultural invention (Pedersen, 2003). Although substantive research conclusions are lacking, some elements of the major clinical theories may be universal while others may be specific to cultural groups. A culturally aware helper is appreciative of cultural diversity, the impact of socialization on minority cultures, acculturation issues, and the culture-specific variables of counseling theory and strategies. He or she is open to multiple perspectives (Corey, 2005; Ivey et al., 2002; Okun, 1996, 2004; Okun, Fried, & Okun, 1999; Pedersen, 2000; Sue, 1992; Sue, Ivey, & Pedersen, 1996; Sue & Sue, 2003).

Corey (2005) points out that while there is a growing movement toward creating a separate multicultural theory of counseling, each current theory can and should be expanded to incorporate a multicultural component in order for therapists to work effectively with culturally diverse populations. A major objective of helping professional associations is to recruit and train more helpers from culturally diverse backgrounds.

Implications for Helpers

It is important for helpers to learn about and value diverse worldviews. They need to be aware of emerging models of racial and ethnic identity development (Suyemoto & Kim, 2005; Delgado-Romero, Galvan, Maschino, & Rowland, 2005). For example, feminist and multicultural theorists question the assumption of traditional theories that the most advanced stage of self-development is autonomy. Theories of women's development and studies of Latino and Asian cultures recognize that interconnectedness and relatedness may represent levels of development equally as valuable as autonomy. In fact, the concept of autonomy may be understood differently, if considered at all, in a number of other cultures. Problems are viewed from a person/environment perspective, and major counseling goals include empowerment and racial and ethnic identity development.

Helpers need to be sensitive to cultural differences in clients' sense of self, and how they view relationships, family, and the world. They must be accepting of clients' use of language and their verbal and nonverbal styles; their comfort with space, time, and distance; and their differing sense of the permissibility of expressing emotions (see Okun et al., 1999). In addition to understanding differences between cultural groups, helpers must acknowledge intragroup differences—individual, gender, class, generational, and regional differences within any one cultural groups.

The development of an empathic relationship is critical to accurately perceiving and responding to another's views in the affective, cognitive, and behavioral domains. Helpers must be aware of how their own identity development has been shaped by racial, ethnic, gender, class, regional, religious, and generational influences. This awareness is necessary to their development of multicultural sensitivity.

MULTIMODAL THEORY AND THERAPY

As developed by Arnold Lazarus (1986, 1989, 1992, 1995, 1996b, 1997a), multimodal therapy is a comprehensive, systematic, eclectic approach. Lazarus is perhaps the most articulate spokesman for a technically eclectic view. He describes a flexible, personalized approach to helping in which the helper uses a combination of techniques from different theoretical approaches without necessarily subscribing to their principal beliefs. The selection of techniques fits the treatment to the needs and individual characteristics of each client.

Theoretically, the multimodal therapy approach is based on social learning principles, the reciprocal interaction between personal and environmental variables. Lazarus (1986) believes that personality is formed, maintained, and altered through many processes: classical and operant conditioning; modeling and vicarious learning; thoughts, feelings, images, and sensations; and unconscious processes such as interpersonal distortions and avoidances and metacommunications.

Multimodal therapy postulates seven specific, interrelated aspects of human personality to which the helper must attend. Together they form the acronym BASIC ID:

1. Behavior—overt actions, observable and measurable

2. Affect—emotions, moods, strong feelings

3. Sensation—seeing, hearing, touching, tasting, smelling

4. Imagery—created mental pictures

5. Cognition—ideas, values, opinions, attitudes

6. Interpersonal relationships—interactions with others

7. Diet/drugs—exercise, nutrition, drugs

The helper covers as many of these modalities as possible, using techniques from whichever approaches focus on them. For example, phenomenological techniques may deal with the affect modality, whereas cognitive restructuring can deal with the cognition modality. The effectiveness and durability of therapeutic results are directly proportional to the number of modalities addressed, according to Lazarus.

Lazarus is really proposing a *technical* eclecticism rather than a *theoretical* eclecticism. He believes that helpers can successfully use techniques from different models without having to subscribe to the theories from which these techniques are derived. It is the effectiveness of the technique in treating a client's particular problem that is the therapist's concern, not the theoretical viewpoint about the cause and meaning of the client's problem (Lazarus, 1989).

Major Principles of Helping

The multimodal approach allows helpers the freedom to select techniques from whichever approaches address the specific concern of the helpee. Adhering to the BASIC ID affords breadth of exploration as opposed to depth. Although helpers prioritize the modality to be addressed, they focus on outcome. For example, if the helpee's relationship difficulties suffer from her rigid expectations, the helper may find the cognitive-behavioral strategy of cognitive restructuring useful; this is a strategy in which the person's beliefs and assumptions are challenged.

In later work, Lazarus (1997a, 1997b) specifies what should be emphasized in this brief, comprehensive therapy: conflicting or ambivalent feelings, maladaptive behaviors, misinformation, missing information, interpersonal pressures and demands, external stressors, severe traumatic experiences, and biological conditions. The active, teaching, consultative, and role-modeling functions of helpers are core to Lazarus's helping principles. Therapists have a broad repertoire of relationship styles and techniques that are constantly adjusted to the issues and needs of the helpee. Clients learn to use the strategies offered by the helper, continuing them after treatment concludes.

Implications for Helpers

Multimodal therapy is clear and concrete and can be learned and mastered relatively quickly. It can be used in a variety of settings—particularly schools and residential settings—and relies on observable outcomes of behaviors. The techniques and breadth of issues enable helpers to obtain an overall holistic assessment of clients and to formulate clear, prioritized goals and objectives. Helpers appreciate the flexibility and openness of this approach and can incorporate it into working with resistant as well as willing clients.

ECOLOGICAL SYSTEMS PERSPECTIVE

No survey of helping theory is complete without reference to the ecological systems perspective, which provides a larger context within which to help an individual. This perspective evolves from family systems theories, which were the first to assert that individuals cannot be considered outside the context of their primary family relationship system. The ecological systems perspective carries these principles into larger social systems (see Chapter 1, Table 1.1). Its major premises are these:

1. An individual is a system, comprised of interacting components or subsystems such as the cognitive, affective, and physiological arenas.

2. An individual is also a component of past and current family systems, which in turn are components within larger social systems such as school, workplace, and community.

3. An individual's problems are likely to derive as much from a poor person/ environment fit as from internal pathology alone.

The ecological perspective is thus multicontextual. An individual's problems have meaning to the larger social system. All behavior is relational and communicative, and there are mutually reciprocal influences among one's problems, one's life circumstances, and the interactional patterns of family, school, workplace, and community. It is important for helpees to consider the part that environmental variables play in the creation and maintenance of their problems. For example, if a freshman in college is excessively homesick and becomes depressed enough to need to go home, the problem may be that the student feels responsible for ensuring that her parents' marriage survives, and thinks that if she goes home she can be the stabilizing "third leg" in a shaky two-person relationship. The focus of the helping process in this case would be more on the dysfunctional family (interpersonal relationships) than on the individual's "sickness." Other contributing variables may be the environment in the dormitory, which, for this particular student, could be adding to her distress. Perhaps she is unaccustomed to the self-discipline and organization required to study without parent-imposed structure. Perhaps she comes from a culture in which the oldest girl is supposed to stay home and help care for the younger siblings, rather than pursue higher education.

Thus, the identification and clarification of an individual's problems require consideration of both individual and system contributing factors. An individual's problems affect his or her family, just as the family affects the individual (see Figures 1.1 and 1.2). If, for example, an individual has distorted thinking that affects his or her feelings, those feelings will affect interpersonal relationships with family or colleagues that, in turn, may cause problems that reinforce and intensify the distorted perceptions. This is the notion of **circular causality** (events are related through a series of interacting loops or repeating cycles and codetermine each other). It differs from the notion of linear causality (events are related through sequential development, and preceding events influence later events) underlying the major theories of helping. The ecological perspective emphasizes the social/political/economic/cultural variables that impact individual development. It suggests an approach that empowers clients to take action and advocates **change agentry**—that is, political and social action.

Ecological systems theories, based on the work of Bronfenbrenner (1979) and Knoff (1986), provide two important tenets for helpers to keep in mind: (1) that a change in one component of a system (within the individual or the larger social system) will effect changes elsewhere in the systems, and (2) that the needs and goals of a larger system take precedence over those of a subsystem or component. How an individual functions and makes choices is greatly influenced by internal and external systems such as internal thinking, affective and physiological systems, and family, school, and other social influence systems. Likewise, any growth or change in the individual has an impact on the social systems within which he or she functions.

The ecological systems perspective serves as a framework within which to consider individual development, functioning, and behavior change embedded in the primary family context, which in turn is embedded in larger sociocultural contexts. The impact of gender, class, ethnicity, race, and sexual orientation on these contexts is crucial.

Implications for Helpers

Helpers familiar with the ecological systems perspective can no longer view the individual out of context. They must decide where to access and work with the problem(s), and there may be simultaneous types of helping. For example, one might meet with an individual child, the child with siblings, the parents alone, or the entire family; the helper might participate in school meetings, social services meetings, medical meetings, or others. The helpers become a team, and the primary therapist takes responsibility for contact and coordination of other team members. The goal is to improve the functioning of the interacting systems while at the same time empowering individuals to improve their relationships and interactions with other systems. The focus is on active systems change, not on pathologizing an individual or blaming others: What is needed to get unstuck and move on? Popular strategies include coaching, role modeling, and helping an individual to take action, such as making a phone call or requesting services. The basic thesis is that we are all working together to improve the environment/person fit.

From an ecological or a family systems perspective, it is important not to lose sight of an individual's power and participation. The focus is on shared responsibility and participation, with particular sensitivity to the power of external and internal variables.

EXERCISE 6.1 ■ This exercise, suggested by Amy Bernstein, a student at the University of North Carolina–Greensboro, is a continuation of Exercise 5.2. After studying this chapter, answer the following questions about constructivist, feminist, multicultural, multimodal, and ecological systems perspectives:

1. How are people viewed within the theory?

2. What does the theory deal with?

3. What meaning is attached to the theory?

4. What does the theory leave out?

5. How attuned is the theory to diversity?

6. To what kinds of people, in what kinds of situations, would this theory apply?

EXERCISE 6.2 ■ Now review what you wrote in Exercise 6.1. Which elements of these theories appear to be a good fit for you at this time? Consider your relationship and communication styles, your views about human behavior and human development, the kinds of work you want to do, and what does and does not make sense to you. Do you think there are discrepancies between what you think you should believe, what you say you believe, and what you actually do?

SUMMARY

This chapter emphasizes the newer, postmodern perspectives of the helping relationship and psychological processes of human development and change. Table 6.1 compares these perspectives in schematic fashion and can be considered in conjunction with Table 5.1. The broad outlines of each perspective follow:

1. The constructivist approach focuses equally on the reciprocal relationships of thinking, feeling, and behaving. Integrating past and current human development, conscious and unconscious thinking and information processing, constructivism emphasizes the co-construction of new and optional meanings and perspectives.

2. The feminist approaches stress gendered development within sociocultural and political contexts. They utilize egalitarian, empowering helping relationships focused on transforming traditional roles, functions, and views, along with political and social action and change agentry.

3. The multicultural approaches demand sensitivity to and awareness of inter- and intracultural differences about lifestyles and values. They focus on the culturally different meanings of self, relationships, life values, beliefs, and attitudes, as well as the helping process.

4. The multimodal perspective is an integrative approach that values the unique contributions of differing therapies. It combines various helping approaches according to clients' situations and needs.

5. The ecological systems perspective focuses on interpersonal relationships—that is, interactions—in contexts. An individual's symptoms both reflect and control interpersonal relationships, which in turn reflect and are controlled by larger sociocultural systems.

Perhaps the reason we have so many different approaches to helping is the great diversity that exists among people and their problems. No single theory answers all questions or satisfies all conditions. At best, theories are approximations of knowledge—guidelines that are constructed to help us make sense out of the complexity of human nature and development. As helpers seek approaches and viewpoints that are consistent with their personal

TABLE 6.1 Comparison of current theoretical perspectives

	Constructivism	Feminist Therapy	Multicultural Therapies	Ecological Systems
Major principles	1. People have free will	1. People have free will but men have more power	1. People's view of whether they have free will is culturally determined	1. People have no free will
	2. Knowledge is subjective	2. Intuitive knowledge is valued	2. Knowledge is culturally determined	2. Knowledge is subjective
	3. Behavior is shaped by people's emotional and cognitive meaning-making	3. Behavior is shaped by societal gender-role expectations	3. Behavior is shaped by cultural traditions and influence on identity and values	3. Behavior is shaped by socio-cultural institutions and ide-ologies; individual is embedded in family that is in turn embedded in sociocultural systems
	4. Psychological distress ema-nates from current mainte-nance of distorted emotional and cognitive beliefs	4. Psychological distress comes from internalization of bias of patriarchal values and pre-scriptions	4. Psychological distress may occur due to clashes between dominant and nondominant cultures	4. Psychological distress stems from misfit between person and environment
Therapy process	1. Collaborative	1. Collaborative	1. Empathic attunement to cultural norms and values of client	1. Consultative
	2. Past emotional cognitive and behavioral development explored	2. Past and present gender socialization	2. Interrelationship between self and culture	2. Interactions with systems and interpersonal connections
	3. Verbal	3. Verbal empowerment	3. Verbal encouragement to maintain cultural identity while living in other dominant culture	3. Verbal and action
	4. Exploration and co-construction of new narratives in empathic helping relationship	4. Egalitarian helping relation-ship modeling change agentry and advocacy	4. Flexible helping relationship adapted to client's culture and needs	4. Collaborative coaching, advocacy, empowering helping relationship

(continued)

	Constructivism	Feminist Therapy	Multicultural Therapies	Ecological Systems
Prerequisite therapist behaviors	1. Therapist is empathic, supportive, collaborative, exploring, open to other perspectives 2. Therapist and client co-construct options and narratives	1. Therapist is strong role model 2. Analyzes power; advocates actions; is transtheoretical	1. Therapist sees multiple realities; is sensitive, flexible 2. Has knowledge of and is open to cultural differences	1. Therapist is supportive, pluralistic; empowers, reframes, and uses change agentry 2. Collaborates to plan and implement systems changes
Domains	Affective/cognitive domains	Affective/cognitive/behavioral domains	Affective/cognitive/behavioral domains	Affective/cognitive/behavioral domains

theories and their personalities, they must constantly refine existing approaches and create new ones. Feminist and multicultural therapies provide increasingly significant approaches to the helping relationship. It is critically important that we consider gender, racial, ethnic, and sexual orientation differences in our appraisal of helping theory and application, and in our support of research about the process and outcomes of the helping relationship.

The ecological systems perspective is an example of a nontraditional adaptation of conventional major approaches. This perspective deals with the identification of systemwide problems rather than individual problems. Thus, the client is a system, such as a family, hospital, school, or correctional institution, rather than an individual within a system. The helper looks at the communication patterns as well as the structures (roles, rules, boundaries) of the system in order to understand the reciprocal influences of individuals and the contexts in which they function. Strategies derived from this approach include **advocacy** and change agentry. Human relations skills are essential in applying these strategies, because effective relationships between helpers and individuals within the system are crucial.

As the helping professions expand and mature, there is an increasing tendency toward a more open, multifaceted view of the major traditional theories and the currently emerging integrated theories. This integration will allow helpers to consider all the aspects of human development, behavior, and change at different levels in different situations and will, ideally, enable us to provide helping services to a greater variety of people in confusing, complex situations. And in today's health care climate, the basic tenets of the major theories must be reformatted into briefer periods of time.

REFERENCES AND FURTHER READING

The following reading list will help you further explore these views and approaches.

Integrative Theories

Alford, B. A., & Beck, A. T. (1997). *The integrative power of cognitive therapy.* New York: Guilford Press.

Arkowitz, H. (1997). Integrative theories of therapy. In P. L. Wachtel & S. B. Messer (Eds.), *Theories of psychotherapy: Origins and evolution* (pp. 227–288). Washington, DC: American Psychological Association.

Ivey, A. E. (1991). *Developmental strategies for helpers: Individual, family, and network interventions.* Pacific Grove, CA: Brooks/Cole.

Lazarus, A. A. (1976). *Multimodal behavior therapy.* New York: Springer.

Lazarus, A. A. (1997). *Brief but comprehensive psychotherapy: The multimodal way.* New York: Springer.

Moursund, J. P., & Erskine, R. G. (2004). *Integrative psychotherapy: The art and science of relationship.* Pacific Grove: Brooks/Cole.

Norcross, J. C., & Goldfried, M. R. (Eds.). (1992*). Handbook of psychotherapy integration.* New York: Basic Books.

Okun, B. F. (1990). *Seeking connections in psychotherapy.* San Francisco: Jossey-Bass.

Preston, J. (1998). *Integrative brief therapy: Cognitive, psychodynamic, humanistic and neurobehavioral approaches.* San Luis Obispo, CA: Impact.

Prochaska, J. O., & Norcross, J. C. (2003). *Systems of psychotherapy: A transtheoretical analysis* (5th ed.). Pacific Grove, CA: Brooks/Cole.

Sharf, R. S. (2000). *Theories of psychotherapy and counseling: Concepts and cases.* Pacific Grove, CA: Brooks/Cole.

Sue, D. W., & Sue, D. (2003). *Counseling the culturally different: Theory and practice* (4th ed.). New York: Wiley.

Constructivism

Anderson, T. (1991). *The reflecting team: Dialogues and dialogues about the dialogues.* New York: Norton.

Breunlin, D. C., Schwartz, R. C., & MacKune-Karrer, B. (1997). *Metaframeworks: Transcending the models of family therapy.* San Francisco: Jossey-Bass.

Corey, G. (2005). *Theory and practice of counseling and psychotherapy* (7th ed). Belmont, CA: Brooks/Cole.

Gergen, K. (1991). *The saturated self.* New York: Basic Books.

Gergen, K. (1999). *An invitation to social construction.* Thousand Oaks, CA: Sage.

Goldfried, M. R. (1988). Personal construct therapy and other theoretical orientations. *International Journal of Personal Construct Psychology, 1,* 317–327.

Greenberg, L. S., & Safran, J. D. (1989). Emotion in psychotherapy. *American Psychologist, 44,* 19–29.

Guidano, V. F. (1991). *The self in process.* New York: Guilford Press.

Kelly, G. (1991a). *The psychology of personal constructs: Vol. I. A theory of personality.* London: Routledge. (Original work published 1955)

Kelly, G. (1991b). *The psychology of personal constructs: Vol. 2. Clinical diagnosis and psychotherapy.* London: Routledge. (Original work published 1955).

Mahoney, M. J. (1991). *Human change processes.* New York: Basic Books.

Meichenbaum, D. (1997). The evolution of a cognitive-behavior therapist. In J. K. Zeig (Ed.), *The evolution of psychotherapy: The third conference* (pp. 96–104). New York: Brunner/Mazel.

Neimeyer, R. A. (1993). Constructivism and the cognitive psychotherapies: Some conceptual and strategic contrasts. *Journal of Cognitive Psychotherapy, 7*(3), 159–171.

White, M. (2006). *Narrative practice with families and their children.* Dulwich, Australia: Dulwich Center.

Feminist Therapies

Ballou, M., & Brown, L. S. (2002). *Rethinking mental health and disorders.* New York: Guilford Press.

Bem, S. (1993). *The lenses of gender.* New Haven, CT: Yale University Press.

Brown, L. S. (1992). The future of feminist therapy. *Psychotherapy, 29*(1), 51–57.

Brown, L. S. (1994). *Subversive dialogues: Theory in feminist therapy.* New York: Basic Books.

Brown, L. S., & Ballou, M. (Eds.). (1992). *Personality theory and psychopathology: Feminist reappraisals.* New York: Guilford.

Chodorow, N. J. (1989). *Feminism and psychoanalytic theory.* Berkeley: University of California Press.

Corey, G. (2005). *Theory and practice of counseling and psychotherapy* (7th ed). Belmont, CA: Brooks/Cole.

Enns, C. Z. (2004). *Feminist theories and feminist psychotherapies: Origins, themes, and variations.* (2nd ed.). Binghamton, NY: Haworth.

Gilligan, C. (1982). *In a different voice.* Cambridge, MA: Harvard University Press.

Gillis, S., Howie, G. & Munford, R. (2004). *Third wave feminism: A critical exploration.* New York: Palgrave Macmillan.

Jordan, J.V. (Ed). (1997). *Women's growth in diversity: More writings from the Stone Center.* New York: Guilford Press.

Jordan, J.V., Hartling, L. M., & Walker, M. (Eds.). (2004). *The complexity of connection: Writings from the Stone Center's Jean Baker Miller Training Institute.* New York: Guilford Press.

Jordan, J.V., Kaplan, A. G., Miller, J. B., Stiver, I. P., & Surrey, J. L. (Eds.). (1991). *Women's growth in connection: Writings from the Stone Center.* New York: Guilford Press.

Landrine, H. (Ed.). (1995). *Bringing cultural diversity to feminist psychology: Theory, research, and practice.* Washington, DC: American Psychological Association.

Miller, J. B. (1976). *Toward a new psychology of women.* Boston: Beacon Press.

Miller, J. B. (1991). The development of women's sense of self. In J.V. Jordan, A. G. Kaplan, J. B. Miller, I. P. Stiver, & J. L. Surrey (Eds.), *Women's growth in connection* (pp. 11–26). New York: Guilford Press.

Miller, J. B., & Stiver, I. P. (1997). *The healing connection: How women form relationships in therapy and in life.* Boston: Beacon Press.

Mirkin, M. P., Suyemoto, K. L., & Okun, B. F. (2005). (Eds.). *Psychotherapy with women: Exploring diverse contexts and identities.* New York: Guilford Press.

Moradi, B., Fischer, A. C., Hill, M. S., Jome, L. M., & Blum, S. A. (2000). Does "feminist" plus "therapist" equal "feminist therapist"? *Psychology of Women Quarterly, 24*(4), 285–296.

Okun, B. F., & Ziady, L. G. (2005). Redefining the career ladder: New visions of women at work. In M. P. Mirkin, K. L. Suyemoto, & B. F. Okun (Eds.), *Psychotherapy with women: Exploring diverse contexts and identities* (pp. 215–236). New York: Guilford Press.

Suyemoto, K. L., & Kim, G. S. (2005). Journeys through diverse terrains: Multiple identities and social contexts in individual therapy. In M. P. Mirkin, K. L. Suyemoto, & B. F. Okun (Eds.), *Psychotherapy with women: Exploring diverse contexts and identities* (pp. 9–41). New York: Guilford Press.

Worell, J., & Johnson, N. G. (Eds.). (1997). *Shaping the future of feminist psychology: Education, research, and practice.* Washington, DC: American Psychological Association.

Worell, J., & Remer, P. (2003). *Feminist perspectives in therapy: Empowering diverse women.* New York: Wiley.

Multicultural Models

Carter, R. T. (2005). *Handbook of racial-cultural counseling and psychotherapy: Theory and research.* New York: Wiley.

Delgado-Romero, E. A., Galvan, N., Maschino, P., & Rowland, M. (2005). Race and ethnicity in empirical counseling and counseling psychology research: A ten-year review. *Counseling Psychologist, 33*(4), 419–448.

Ivey, A. E., D'Andrea, M., Ivey, M. B., & Simek-Morgan, L. (2002). *Counseling and psychotherapy: A multicultural perspective* (5th ed.). Boston: Allyn & Bacon.

Okun, B. F. (1996). *Understanding diverse families: What practitioners need to know.* New York: Guilford Press.

Okun, B. F. (2004). Human diversity. In R. Combs (Ed.), *Family therapy review: Preparing for comprehensive and licensing examinations* (pp. 122–153). Mahwah, NJ: Erlbaum.

Okun, B. F., Fried, J., & Okun, M. L. (1999). *Understanding diversity: A learning-as-practice primer.* Pacific Grove, CA: Brooks/Cole.

Pedersen, P. A. (2000). *A handbook for developing multicultural awareness* (3rd ed.). Alexandria, VA: American Association for Counseling and Development.

Pedersen, P. A. (2003). Increasing the cultural awareness, knowledge, and skills of culture-centered counselors. In F. D. Harper & J. McFadden (Eds.), *Culture and counseling: New approaches* (pp. 252–284). Needham Heights, MA: Allyn & Bacon.

Ponterotto, J. G., & Pedersen, P. B. (1993). *Preventing prejudice: A guide for counselors and educators.* Newbury Park, CA: Sage.

Sue, D. W. (1992). Culture-specific strategies in counseling: A conceptual framework. *Professional Psychology, 21,* 424–433.

Sue, D. W., Ivey, A. E., & Pedersen, P. (1996). *A theory of multicultural counseling and therapy.* Pacific Grove, CA: Brooks/Cole.

Sue, D. W., & Sue, D. (2003). *Counseling the culturally different: Theory and practice* (4th ed.). New York: Wiley.

Wehrly, B. (1995). *Pathways to multicultural counseling competence: A developmental journey.* Pacific Grove, CA: Brooks/Cole.

Multimodal Therapy

Lazarus, A. (1971). *Behavior therapy and beyond.* New York: McGraw-Hill.

Lazarus, A. (1976). *Multimodal behavior therapy.* New York: Springer-Verlag.

Lazarus, A. (1986). Multimodal therapy. In J. C. Norcross (Ed.), *Handbook of eclectic psychotherapy* (pp. 65–93). New York: Brunner/Mazel.

Lazarus, A. (1987). The need for technical eclecticism: Science, breadth, depth, and specificity. In J. K. Zeig (Ed.), *The evolution of psychotherapy* (pp. 164–178). New York: Brunner/Mazel.

Lazarus, A. (1989). *The practice of multimodal therapy.* Baltimore: Johns Hopkins University Press.

Lazarus, A. (1992). Multimodal therapy: Technical eclecticism with minimal integration. In J. C. Norcross & M. R. Goldfried (Eds.), *Handbook of psychotherapy integration* (pp. 231–263). New York: Basic Books.

Lazarus, A. (1995). Different types of eclecticism and integration: Let's be aware of the dangers. *Journal of Psychotherapy Integration, 5*(1), 27–39.

Lazarus, A. (1996a). Some reflections after 40 years of trying to be an effective psychotherapist. *Psychotherapy, 33*(1), 142–145.

Lazarus, A. (1996b). The utility and futility of combining treatments in psychotherapy. *Clinical Psychology: Science and Practice, 3*(1), 59–68.

Lazarus, A. (1997a). *Brief but comprehensive psychotherapy: The multimodal way.* New York: Springer.

Lazarus, A. (1997b). Can psychotherapy be brief, focused, solution-oriented, and yet comprehensive? A personal evolutionary perspective. In J. K. Zeig (Ed.), *The evolution of psychotherapy: The third conference* (pp. 83–94). New York: Brunner/Mazel.

Lazarus, A., & Beutler, L. (1993). On technical eclecticism. *Journal of Counseling and Development, 71*(4), 381–385.

Ecological Systems Perspectives

Bronfenbrenner, U. (1979). *The ecology of human development.* Cambridge, MA: Harvard University Press.

Knoff, H. (1986). *The assessment of child and adolescent personality.* New York: Guilford Press.

McAndrew, F. T. (1993). *Environmental psychology.* Pacific Grove, CA: Brooks/Cole.

Trickett, E., Watts, R., & Birman, D. (Eds.). (1994). *Human diversity: Perspectives on people in context.* San Francisco: Jossey-Bass.

Visit the book companion site at www.thomsonedu.com to access tutorial quizzes.

7

Introduction
to Strategies

During the transition between the overlapping stage 1 (development of the relationship) and stage 2 (strategy planning, implementation, and evaluation) of the helping process, the helper and helpee explore the goals and objectives of the helping relationship; they then focus on specific helping requirements and finally agree on their goals. Before this transition can be successfully completed, helper and helpee must define the problem(s) to be solved and the nature of the help to be generated. This occurs within the helping context—number of sessions allowed, length of session, likelihood of further authorized sessions, and so on.

After the problem has been defined, it is possible to choose the appropriate strategy or combination of strategies to use in solving it. Variables of timing, setting, and the nature and contexts of the presenting problem(s) will affect both how the transitional period is handled and which strategies are chosen to resolve the problem. It is important to remember that a client's presenting problem needs to be addressed regardless of whether the resolution of more complex, underlying, or environmental problems becomes a goal of the helping relationship. For example, if an employee is referred to a counselor for chronic tardiness, that issue needs to be resolved behaviorally immediately (so the employee won't be fired—unless he or she wishes to be); then the counseling process can focus on the employee's underlying or higher-order issues that may be being expressed through chronic tardiness. Likewise, if a person is distraught because he or she is unable to pay bills due to an unexpected employment layoff, the first order of business is to locate resources for survival (e.g., unemployment insurance) and strategies to deal with the feelings of help-lessness and insecurity that such a layoff engenders.

STRATEGIES AND THE THREE MAIN
PROBLEM AREAS

When speaking of strategies in the helping relationship context, we are talking about overall approaches to achieving general or long-term goals. Strategies reflect the concepts and premises of specific theories or models for certain classes of problems. The techniques are specific applications of the strategies. Figure 7.1 illustrates how therapeutic strategies are derived from theoretical approaches and in turn, how specific intervention techniques are derived from these therapeutic strategies. Certain strategies and corresponding techniques work best in a particular type of situation. And although certain techniques may represent only one strategy, other techniques may be used in several different strategies. The strategies selected will depend on the helper's theoretical beliefs about the situation.

Helping strategies can be categorized according to whether they deal with the affective, cognitive, or behavioral domains. Table 7.1 shows how the various strategies of the major helping theories address those areas. Awareness of these three domains aids in determining appropriate strategies for dealing with individual, interpersonal, and person/environment difficulties.

Affective problems are those dealing with emotion—with self-awareness and awareness of others' feelings (for example, feelings of inadequacy or

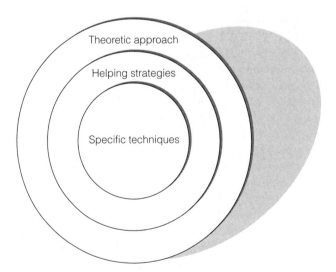

Theoretic approach

Helping strategies

Specific techniques

FIGURE 7.1 Specific techniques are derived from therapeutic strategies, which in turn are derived from the theoretical approach

TABLE 7.1 The application of strategies and techniques to the three problem areas according to their theoretical framework

	Problem Areas (Domains)			
	Affective (Emotion/Feelings)	**Cognitive (Understanding/Thinking)**	**Behavioral (Action/Doing)**	**Multiple Contexts**
Helping strategy	Person-centered	Reality therapy	Behavioral	
	Gestalt	Rational-emotive therapy		
	– – – – – – – – – – – – – – –Multimodal– →			
	– – – – – – – – –Feminist, Multicultural, Ecological/Systems– – – – – – – – – – – – →			
	Psychoanalytic (Freudian, Jungian, Adlerian, Object relations)			
	– – – – – – – – – – – – – – – – –Identity Awareness – – – – – – – – – – – – – – – – →			
	Gestalt experiments		Assertiveness training	
	Responsive listening– – – – – – – – –decision making– – – – – – – – –Reinforcement			
	Imagery		Contracts	
			Modeling	
Representative techniques	Sensory awareness		Systematic desensitization	
	Free association – – – – – – – – – – – –Psych. Education – – – – – – – – – – – – – →			
	Dream analysis – – – – – – – – – – – –Reframing – – – – – – – – – – – – – – – →			Empowerment
	Interpretation	Cognitive restructuring		Change agentry
		Reality therapy contracting		Advocacy
		Cognitive analysis and validation		

(continued)

TABLE 7.1 The application of strategies and techniques to the three problem areas according to their theoretical framework (*continued*)

Problem Areas (Domains)

	Affective (Emotion/Feelings)	Cognitive (Understanding/Thinking)	Behavioral (Action/Doing)	Multiple Contexts
Theoretical framework	Phenomenological	Cognitive-behavioral	Behavioral	
		– – Integrative/Pluralistic – – – – – – – – – – – – – – – →		
	Psychodynamic			
		– – – Feminist, Multicultural, Ecological/Systems – – – – – – – – →		
		– – – Interpersonal adjustment – – – – – – – – – – – – →		
		– – – Developmental conflicts – – – – – – – – – →		
Kinds of problems	Anxiety			Behavioral problems
	Personal adjustment			
	Self-esteem	Problem solving		Person/
		Decision making		Environment
			Coping/Mastery	Conflicts

inferiority, or not being in touch with what and how you and others are feeling, or the impact of your behaviors on others). For these kinds of problems, experiential strategies focusing on imagery, sensory awareness, and verbal and nonverbal expressions of feeling are effective.

Cognitive problems involve thinking (for example, how you interpret situations and events, make decisions, and solve problems). People who always seem to make the wrong decisions or who are afraid to make decisions or who refuse to accept responsibility for their actions can use help in this area. The didactic (instructional) strategies, which focus on step-by-step verbal processing of decision making, analyzing, and problem solving, are effective for such people. Other important cognitive strategies include reframing and cognitive restructuring; assessment and instruction of client appraisal of self, of others, and of events; and training in coping skills.

Behavioral problems involve actions (for example, stopping smoking or some other habit, learning to be more assertive, or changing self-defeating behavior into behavior that elicits increased rewards). Behavioral strategies involve verbal and action-oriented instructions that arrange for environmental rewards and elicit behavior change.

Affective-cognitive-behavioral problems involve a broad variety of symptoms: they may be evidenced by depression, eating disorders, uncontrollable temper, specific behavioral disorders, and interpersonal and work-related difficulties. Cognitive-behavioral strategies include psychoeducational and verbal techniques that challenge one's core assumptions.

Person/environment problems may involve the feelings, thoughts, and behaviors one has when experiencing alienation and discrimination. For example, women, people of color, gays and lesbians, or others who deviate from mainstream norms may experience anxiety and depression from feelings of inadequacy, and doubt about self-worth. Ecological/systems strategies include consciousness raising, reframing, and change agentry. The helper serves as an active advocate.

These classes of problems and strategies are not always discrete—they may overlap or coincide. The nature of the problems, the nature of the helping relationship and situation, and the competence and skill of the helper all influence the choice of strategies and specific techniques.

There are times when the problem falls clearly into the cognitive, affective, or behavioral domain and the range of strategies that can be used is apparent. For example, if the presenting problem is chronic tardiness, a behavioral problem, the strategy may be behavioral and the technique may be contracting. Often, however, the presenting problem is in a different domain from the underlying problem or problems, such as tardiness requiring also the cognitive technique of cognitive restructuring.

For example, a client was once referred to one of us (BFO) by another counselor for the specific behavioral counseling technique called systematic desensitization. This client was unable to swallow solid foods; medical examinations revealed no organic cause for this condition. After several sessions of establishing a relationship and attempting to meet the client's expectations for systematic desensitization (which will be described later in this chapter), it became apparent that her suffering was rooted more in the affective domain than in the behavioral domain. She was unable to express any anger toward anyone, and she had accumulated a great deal of anger because of a recent broken engagement. She was losing weight rapidly and was endangering her health because she was eating only liquefied foods. Many sessions of phenom- enological person-centered and Gestalt strategies were necessary for this client to be able to acknowledge her feelings and to begin to express them appropri- ately. Eventually, she was able to swallow solid foods and to improve her inter- personal relationships. This is an example of the underlying problem (expression of anger) requiring a strategy quite different from the presenting problem (inability to swallow).

In another situation, a 34-year-old female medical technician was becom- ing more and more irritable and depressed. She came from a family in which the expression of anger was discouraged, so she turned her resentments inward, perceiving herself as "inadequate" and "unworthy." When the helper tried to discern the roots of her anger, the helpee began to talk about her work situa- tion, how male technicians with less training and experience were being paid more and promoted more readily, and how she was expected to "get the coffee" and be "grateful" for being there. This woman needed to have her feelings of outrage validated; she then was able to benefit from empowerment strategies. She was encouraged to network with other female employees, study human resource policies, and, eventually, devise a workable plan for assertively seeking a raise and access to further opportunities.

The following sections provide a brief overview of strategies and their techniques in each of the three major problem areas (affective, cognitive, and behavioral) and in the areas where they overlap (affective-cognitive and cognitive- behavioral). Please note that some of these strategies are more appropriate for experienced professionals than for beginning helpers and generalist human services workers. This introduction to the strategies will give you some idea of where your interests and inclinations lie and perhaps will suggest some direc- tions for further study. Each section includes examples and exercises, and a reading list appears at the end of the chapter. As you work through the exer- cises, see which techniques are most comfortable and seem to make the most sense to you.

AFFECTIVE STRATEGIES

The theoretical rationales for affective strategies come from Carl Rogers's client-centered therapy and the Gestalt theory underlying Gestalt therapy. The focus is on self-awareness and experiencing feelings.

Rogerian person-centered therapy has contributed the basis for responsive listening communication skills. The helper, by communicating empathy, hon- esty, congruence, genuineness, and acceptance of the helpee, is able to create a nonthreatening climate in which helpees can explore their own feelings, thoughts, and behavior and gain some understanding of themselves and their world. Remember, Rogerian theory insists upon these environmental variables for the helpee to develop a positive self-concept. For this technique to be effective, the helpee must be able to perceive these feelings and attitudes on the part of the helper. The technique of responsive listening may suffice as the only strategy needed in a helping relationship.

Gestalt strategies, on the other hand, specifically focus on awareness. Many helpers with theoretical orientations other than Gestalt nevertheless use Gestalt strategies to help clients achieve awareness. The purpose of Gestalt strategies is to reintegrate attention and awareness so that helpees can take responsibility for the *what* and *how* of their present behaviors.

Some of the rules for conducting Gestalt therapy are as follows:

1. Use the phrase "here and now" to focus on the present and on people who are here.
2. Use direct language, such as "I" instead of "it" and "I won't" instead of "I can't."
3. Allow no gossiping. The client should not talk about a person who is not present but instead should talk directly to the absent person by role playing.
4. Insist that clients own their own feelings, thoughts, and actions by using "my" and "I" and "I take responsibility for. . . ."
5. Direct the client to take action instead of imagining and thinking.

Games such as "Dialogue," "I Take Responsibility," and "Reversals" encourage present-oriented and responsibility-oriented verbal styles. In these games clients deal with an absent person by role playing, take both roles in a dialogue, and play all the roles, including inanimate objects from a dream.

The verbal techniques of Gestalt strategies are aimed at keeping the helpee in constant contact with what is going on. The following are the rules of verbal techniques:

1. Keep communication between helper and helpee in the "now" through the use of the present tense. Emphasize what is happening now. Use questions such as "What are you feeling now?" and "Are you aware that . . . ?"
2. Use the words "I" and "thou" to personalize and direct communication toward, not at, the listener.
3. Use the word "I" so that the helpee assumes more responsibility for his or her own behavior by substituting "I" for "it" (for example, instead of "The noise in the dormitory kept me from doing my homework" substitute "I did not do my homework").
4. Pursue the *what* and *how* instead of the *why* (for example, "What are you aware of now?" and "What are you experiencing now?" instead of "Why do you feel . . . ?"), which helps lead the client away from endless explanations, speculations, and interpretations.

5. Don't gossip. This rule promotes the expression of feelings and encourages the helpee to deal directly with people. If the people he or she is discussing are not present, the client is encouraged to talk directly with them using the **empty seat** or some other device.

6. Change questions into statements, which helps prevent manipulative games and encourages the helpee to take responsibility for and deal directly with issues.

The preceding rules are based on the following guidelines (Levitsky & Perls, 1970):

1. Live now; be concerned with the present rather than with the past or future. We spend too much time daydreaming about the past or future, and this habit distracts and detracts our energies and awareness from the present.

2. Live here and deal with what is present rather than what is absent. One of many avoidance strategies we use is to focus on what is missing rather than on what we have, on who is missing rather than who is here.

3. Stop imagining, and experience the real. Imagining takes us away from what *is* and blocks our experiencing and awareness. We sometimes lose sight of what is real for us.

4. Stop unnecessary thinking, and taste, see, and feel. When was the last time, for example, that you ate an orange without thinking about the concept of orange but just sensing every feeling, taste, and smell? We have allowed thinking to block out our senses, and we need to take the time to get back in touch with our senses.

5. Express rather than manipulate, explain, justify, or judge. Learn to express yourself directly, to ask for what you want, to accept yourself and others for what they are, not for their verbal competencies.

6. Expand your awareness by giving in to unpleasantness and pain as well as pleasure. True awareness includes negative experiences as well as pleasurable ones, and if we use our energies to block out the negative, we will also lose some of our ability to sense the positive.

7. Accept no "should" or "ought" other than your own, and follow no idol. The words "should" and "ought" have caused more difficulties than just about any other words in the English language. We must assume responsibility for our rules and practices and our own behaviors.

8. Take full responsibility for your actions, feelings, and thoughts. This is the essence of maturity in Gestalt thought. We must stop blaming others and situations and take full advantage of our autonomy and the choices that do exist within any situation.

9. Surrender to being you as you are. Accept yourself for who you are and what you are and not what you or others think you should be.

The following excerpt is an example of the application of a Gestalt strategy:

Client: I'm upset with my fiancé because he decided where we would live next year without talking it over with me. We're going to Des Moines, and that's over a thousand miles away!

Helper: You feel angry because he is making important decisions without consulting you.

Client: Well, yes. I don't want to go so far away. My mother lives all alone here, and we're very close. If I go so far away, I won't be able to see her, and she needs me.

Helper: Are you aware that your right hand is tightly clenched?

Client: Oh . . . yes, I guess I'm more upset than I realized.

Helper: Let's try something to see if we can find out what this is all about. How about letting your right hand be the Pam who doesn't want to go away from your mother and your left hand be the Pam who wants to go with your fiancé. See if you can have your two hands talk to each other.

Client: Well, I'll try. (*shaking right fist*) Listen, you, you know you're afraid to leave your mother . . . she won't be able to manage without you and you don't really know if you can get along without her.

Helper: Now be the other Pam.

Client: Come on, now. I'm a big girl, and I certainly can make it on my own. Besides, I love Ron and I want to marry him, and that means I go where he goes.

Helper: See if you can talk directly to your other hand. Tell her what you feel.

Client: (*still the Pam who wants to go*) I'm annoyed at you for always getting in my way. You're a scaredy-cat, and you always foul things up by getting angry when you don't want to do something. (*now the right-hand Pam, who doesn't want to go*) I don't want to go. I've never been that far away before.

Helper: What are you feeling now, Pam?

Client: I'm feeling scared, but also a little bit excited about the possibilities of a new life.

This short dialogue experiment helped Pam become aware of the range and depth of her feelings and the real issues she is struggling with. Although there is reason for Pam to deal with and work through her feelings about her fiancé, it became clear that the underlying problems dealt with Pam's dependent/ independent relationship with her mother.

The technique demonstrated in the preceding example is called the *dialogue game*. It can take place between two "aspects" of the helpee or between the helpee and another person with whom he or she is experiencing some kind of continued conflict. Other Gestalt techniques involve the use of imagery and sensory awareness, focusing on the relationship between verbal and nonverbal behavior ("You say you are angry, yet you are smiling"), acting out fantasies (playing all the roles of animate and inanimate parts of a fantasy), repeating and exaggerating verbal or nonverbal behaviors ("Can you stay with that feeling? Exaggerate your leg swing and repeat what you just said in a louder voice . . . louder . . . louder"), playing out projected roles by doing to others what one does to oneself, and completing unfinished business through active role playing.

Gestalt therapists also ask helpees to play out dreams in the same way that they might play out fantasies. Any part or piece of the dream or fantasy is considered an aspect of the helpee, a metaphor to understanding what is happening in the here and now. Important Gestalt questions include "What are you experiencing now?" "Where are you now?" "What do you want to do?" "What are you doing now?" and "What are you avoiding?" Helpees are encouraged to use "I" messages by completing such statements as "I am aware that . . ." "Now I feel that . . ." and "I notice that . . ." Examples of directives that Gestalt helpers use include "Say *I* instead of *it*"; "Get a sense of your strong part"; "Be more specific"; "Say this again . . . again . . . now exaggerate it"; "Tell your strong part what it should do"; "Act stupid"; and "Act as if you don't care." Frequently, the Gestalt therapist will share his or her experiencing of what the client is doing at the moment—for example, "I'm aware that you're jiggling your foot while you talk about this" or "My hunch is that you're feeling scared, as if you want to run away and hide." The goals of the affective strategies are to develop feelings and self-awareness, using techniques of responsive listening and Gestalt experiments. The focus is on the present and the here and now.

When to Use Affective Strategies

Strategies that use responsive listening and focus on the development of a genuine, empathic relationship are appropriate for individuals who are unable to express their feelings and are unable to have close, meaningful personal relationships with family or friends. The technique of responsive listening may suffice as the sole strategy in a helping relationship whose goal is the development of self-concept in the helpee. If a helpee who has difficulties with interpersonal relationships is able to develop an honest, close, meaningful relationship with the helper, the experience will have a lasting effect. And once having attained this type of relationship with one person, the helpee will be better able to achieve a close relationship with another. The responsive listening approach is also appropriate for informal and short-term relationships, when having someone listen to and understand one's concerns is helpful in and of itself.

Gestalt techniques are particularly effective for people who lack awareness of the *how* and *what* of their present behavior, people who refuse to take responsibility for themselves and their lives, people who interact rigidly and in a ritualized manner with their environment, people who dwell on past unfinished business or on future rehearsing, and people who seem split in two because they deny or exclude part of themselves. Gestalt techniques are also effective with children, who are more in touch with their fantasies and imagination than are older people. These techniques are generally not effective with people who do not want to develop awareness of their feelings, people who need information in order to make immediate decisions cognitively, people who have experienced a sudden crisis, and those who are unable to imagine and fantasize sufficiently to participate in the games and experiments.

To use Gestalt techniques effectively, it is important for you to have actually participated in Gestalt games and experiments and thereby developed some confidence in your own capacities for self-awareness and taking responsibility. Try some of the following exercises to see how you feel about Gestalt techniques. You may wonder if people you are helping would think you were odd for using these techniques, but you will find that if you have an effective, trusting helping relationship, helpees are usually willing to engage in novel techniques. (Actually, some of the communication skills exercises in Chapter 4 are Gestalt exercises, so you have already tried a few.)

EXERCISE 7.1 ▪ An effective beginning Gestalt exercise involves a group sitting in a circle; each person begins a three-minute monologue with "Now I am aware that . . ." Try to get in touch with as much of yourself in the here and now as you can. Personalize pronouns and begin each sentence with "I" in order to focus on your self-awareness. For example, you might say, "Now I am aware that I am sitting in a hard chair with a pillow at my back. My legs are crossed, and I am typing this manuscript. My fingers are deftly moving over the keyboard, my eyes are on the draft, my shoulders are sort of slumped . . ." and so forth. (This exercise can also be performed in pairs.)

EXERCISE 7.2 ▪ Fantasizing is very much a Gestalt technique. In this exercise, each person in a small group is asked to think of a place where he or she feels especially comfortable, to visualize all the details of those surroundings, to get in touch with the sights, smells, and noises as well as the thoughts and feelings associated with this special place. Then, each person takes turns relating his or her scene in the present tense, personalizing pronouns. Other people in the group may ask "what" and "how" questions and may also ask the person sharing the fantasy to act out different aspects of it, playing out the animate and inanimate roles. For example, a person who describes a scene at the beach may be asked to be the water, to be the sand, to be the sun.

EXERCISE 7.3 ▪ "Shuttling" is an extension of Exercise 7.2. Spend some time in your special place and then "shuttle" to the here and now and get in touch with the details of where you are right now, the sights, smells, noises, and other people. Then return to your special place. Shuttle back and forth between reality and fantasy and spend several minutes in each place. How hard is this shuttling? What do you feel? Where do you want to be? What have you become aware of while doing the exercise?

EXERCISE 7.4 ▪ "Dialoguing" is a useful Gestalt technique. Imagine that one of your parents is sitting facing you. Describe this scene as precisely as you can, relating the emerging feelings as you face this parent. Then begin to talk aloud to this parent, using the first and second persons ("I" and "you"). Say whatever comes to your mind. Stay with the feelings that are emerging, then switch seats when you choose and be your parent talking back to you. Go back and forth between your seat and your parent's seat until you feel as if you are ready to stop. If possible, share your feelings with your group and see if you have learned something about your feelings and relationship with this parent. If you are having a difficult time getting started, begin in your parent role, introducing you. Tell who you are and how you feel about your offspring and you.

EXERCISE 7.5 ▪ Try a variation of the preceding exercise by playing two different aspects of yourself. For example, you might be "strong" in one seat and "weak" in the other. First, choose the aspects that are most comfortable for you and verbally share your thoughts, feelings, and experiences in one seat. When you finish, switch to the other seat and share your conflicting thoughts, feelings, and experiences from that perspective. Continue verbalizing and acting out this conflict until you feel you have some understanding (and perhaps experience some integration) of your different parts. This technique is termed "empty chair" by Gestalt therapists. It is a stimulating method of facilitating self-knowledge.

AFFECTIVE-COGNITIVE STRATEGIES

The theoretical basis for affective-cognitive strategies is developmental psychodynamic theory. The primary goal is to bring unconscious material into the conscious realm so as to strengthen the ego in order for behavior to be based more on conscious thinking than on unconscious instincts. The personality becomes restructured by the achievement of insight (emotional awareness and cognitive understanding). The objective is to eliminate the crippling effects of internal anxiety, which both causes and results from repression, so that the client can live more fully in the present with inner peace and self-understanding. This enables clients to achieve more productive relationships and to function more effectively at work.

Techniques

The major techniques of psychodynamic helpers include free association, dream analysis, and interpretation. These are verbal techniques that allow helpees to proceed at their own pace to develop a transference relationship with the helper and work through unconscious conflicts. The purpose of free association and dream analysis is to allow helpees to become gradually aware of deeply unconscious material. The focus is on childhood experiences, to enable clients to understand the connections between the past and their current functioning.

The transference phenomenon focuses on the transfer of feelings, attitudes, and conflicts experienced in the past to current situations and relationships (Cashdan, 1988; Okun, 1990; Watkins, 1983). By recognizing the possibility of this phenomenon, helpers can become more aware of its impact on the helping process. Watkins posits five major transference patterns commonly found in the counseling relationship. The counselor may be perceived and treated as (1) ideal, (2) seer, (3) nurturer, (4) frustrater, or (5) nonentity.

The perception of each type will affect client attitude and behaviors as well as the counselor's experience of the relationship. For example, if the client experiences and treats the counselor as a seer, he or she will expect expert advice and solutions, and the counselor may experience feelings either of omnipotence or of incompetence for being unable to come up with the answers. In such a case, the counselor needs to use strategies that address the client's past dependency needs and past relationships with "authority figures," and to focus on helping the client gain self-esteem and independence.

When to Use Affective-Cognitive Strategies

Psychodynamic techniques are useful for people who have persistent, deep-seated problems requiring restructuring of the personality. They are particularly effective for fragile survivors of chronic trauma or childhood neglect and deprivation. Unless you pursue formal psychoanalytic training, it is likely that you will use these techniques only when you provide support to this type of helpee, perhaps as a psychiatric aide in an inpatient facility.

The following exercises will help you experience free association and what it can mean to and for you.

EXERCISE 7.6 ■ In pairs or small groups, allow 10 minutes for each person to look at a list of words (such as *red, blue, black, pink, white*) and say whatever comes to mind as a result of the stimulus word. After each person has spent 10 minutes on this task, he or she can share reactions and observations. Other members of the group can then ask the person questions and share their reactions.

EXERCISE 7.7 ■ With a partner, recall every verbal slip you've made in the past two weeks. Then you and your partner should brainstorm all the possible unconscious meanings of those slips. See if you can help each other get in touch with what the slips symbolized.

EXERCISE 7.8 ■ Recall a recent dream. Allow yourself to focus on one particular aspect of or character in the dream and attempt some free association. See what you can learn about the possible meaning of your dream.

EXERCISE 7.9 ■ Look around the class and allow your gaze to rest on the person for whom you have the strongest dislike. Does this person remind you of someone else? Allow yourself to free-associate and see if you can achieve some insight about this transference. Now repeat the exercise and look at the person that you like the most.

EXERCISE 7.10 ■ Recall the significant authority figures in your life, such as parents, teachers, doctors, and employers. Think of one you idealized and then think of another you experienced as frustrating or rejecting. Can you separate feelings and behaviors that were appropriate from those that were overreactions and projections? Do these people remind you of anyone else? Are there patterns in the way you perceive, feel about, and behave toward authority figures? How do current relationships mirror your past experiences? What kinds of feelings does this exercise elicit?

COGNITIVE STRATEGIES

Cognitive strategies emphasize rationality, thinking processes, meaning, and understanding. The theoretical foundations are cognitive, including rational-emotive and reality therapy concepts.

Techniques

Decision-making techniques are used in the cognitive problem area because decisions are cognitive processes. It is important to help people learn decision-making skills so they will have more freedom and control over their lives. We make decisions from the moment we get up in the morning to the moment we retire.

Although there are different models for decision making, the basic process recommended for helping relationships consists of the following steps:

1. *State the problem clearly.* Be sure that you have identified the problem that is causing difficulty. For problem solving to be effective, the problem must be accurately identified.

2. *Identify and accept ownership of the problem.* Unless the decision maker believes that he or she has a problem and has some power to effect a decision, the decision-making process is futile. People do not invest energy in decision making unless they have a stake in the outcome.

3. *Propose every possible alternative to the problem* (**brainstorming**). Often our options are limited. Brainstorming enables us to consider all possible options without judging them. It gives us more to choose from.

4. *Evaluate each proposed alternative in terms of implementation realities and hypothesized consequences (value clarification).* Here we have the opportunity to

evaluate each of the alternatives proposed in step 3. Some we will automatically discard, either because they are impractical or because they violate our value system. Before discarding any item, however, we try to hypothesize its consequences.

5. *Reassess the final list of alternatives, their consequences, and the risks involved.* We review our final list, and for each alternative we review the steps involved and the likely consequences. We may eliminate additional alternatives in this step.

6. *Decide to implement one alternative.* Based on our previous assessments, we choose one alternative. We may even list some backup alternatives.

7. *Determine how and when to implement the plan.* Here we spell out exactly what is needed to implement this decision: who needs to do what, when, where; what materials are required; and so forth. Decisions are often not carried out because of failure to work through this step.

8. *Generalize to other situations.* This may or may not be a necessary step, but it involves exploring the effect that the decision and its implementation may have on situations other than the immediate one.

9. *Evaluate the implementation.* This is a crucial step for determining whether the implementation plan and the decision choice were satisfactory. Too often, we call a choice poor when in fact the implementation is what was lacking.

Helpers can facilitate the preceding process by clarifying, providing information, and suggesting alternatives in the brainstorming step. In instances such as vocational and educational planning, information from tests may be used in the decision-making process. The gathering and synthesizing of pertinent information provide a valuable tool in cognitive decision making.

In addition to test interpretation and dissemination of appropriate information, helpers can use value clarification exercises, observation, and didactic teaching to aid helpees in learning to understand and to apply data obtained from tests, written and verbal information, and observation. These data, in turn, can aid helpees in clarifying and explaining their values, attitudes, and beliefs as well as their assets and liabilities. It is the helpee who makes the final decision; the helper provides invaluable assistance.

The following excerpt gives an example of decision-making techniques used in cognitive strategy.

Client: I'm having a hard time figuring out how to deal with the tardiness in my department.

Helper: It's frustrating, isn't it? Sounds as though you're being held accountable for it.

Client: Oh, yes. As department head, I get blamed when the boss calls up in the morning and the secretaries aren't there to answer the phones and give him the information he wants.

Helper: So it becomes your problem. What kinds of things have you thought about doing?

Client: Oh, I don't know . . . docking people's pay, sending notes up to Human Resources to be put in their files, making people make up lost time, rescheduling.

Helper: Sounds as though you've thought of some options. Let's jot them down. Can you think of any others?

Client: I don't know. I suppose I could just ignore it and see what happens.

Helper: Have you thought about holding a department meeting and discussing it there? Maybe you could get some more ideas from your staff.

Client: Hmm . . . I don't know. We never seem to get anywhere when we discuss these kinds of issues.

Helper: Hmm. Maybe if you told them that your problem is that you're being held responsible for their tardiness. . . . Anything else we can put down as possible options?

Client: Wait a minute. I think before I can really consider different possibilities, I ought to see what my own staff has to say. Sort of put the shoe where it fits.

In this particular excerpt the decision-making process is not completed; rather, the helpee decides to get some more information before making a final decision. This is indeed appropriate, as sometimes decisions are made too quickly, before all the necessary data are collected.

When to Use Cognitive Strategies

Cognitive decision-making strategies are effective for educational and vocational planning and for problem solving and decision making in just about any life situation. Some categories of decisions require cognitive information, and others need information about attitudes and beliefs.

The following exercises will help you to recognize how you make everyday decisions in your life and how other people can help.

EXERCISE 7.11 ▪ The purpose of this exercise is to put you in touch with your decision-making processes. Think back over the past 24 hours and write down every decision you made, such as what time you got up yesterday morning, what you had for breakfast, what you wore, and when you brushed your teeth. See how many decisions you made in that time span, and then go over your list and classify your decisions according to the following code: A = major decisions; B = commonplace, but not everyday, decisions; C = routine, everyday, taken-for-granted decisions. What does your list look like? Compare it with others'.

EXERCISE 7.12 ▪ In small groups, take a few minutes to jot down all the variables that influenced your decision to be where you are right now: in class, on a job, or wherever. See if you can go back to the very beginning of your decision-making process and identify a problem clarification point. Discuss your findings with your group and note similarities and differences.

EXERCISE 7.13 ▪ Divide into groups of six. Pick something that you all agree is a problem in your setting (for example, too much noise in the cafeteria or too few parking places). Try to decide how to solve the problem by going through the first seven steps of the decision-making process. Be sure you discuss each of the steps together.

COGNITIVE-BEHAVIORAL STRATEGIES

Cognitive-behavioral strategies are approaches that deal with both the thinking and the behaving processes. They are based on the premise that faulty thinking must be changed before effective behavior change can occur. The theoretical bases come from Ellis's rational-emotive behavior therapy, Glasser's reality therapy, Beck's cognitive therapy, Meichenbaum's cognitive-behavior modification, and constructivism, as well as from behavioral theory. Rationality and responsibility are key concepts in these approaches.

Techniques

Cognitive-behavioral techniques are largely verbal and require homework outside of the helping relationship to facilitate the transformation of new thinking into action or behavior.

The rational-emotive behavior therapy model has contributed an effective strategy called cognitive restructuring, which means replacing faulty thinking with new, rational thinking. This strategy includes the didactic techniques of teaching, persuading and confronting, and assigning homework. The purpose of cognitive restructuring is to aid helpees to control their emotions by teaching them more rational, less self-defeating ideas and convincing them of the illogic of the irrational ideas identified by Albert Ellis (1962).

Ellis (1998) describes four types of evaluative thinking dysfunctions:

1. Demandingness—demands and shoulds about self, others, the world
2. Awfulizing—exaggerating consequences of past, present, and future behaviors
3. Discomfort intolerance—can't stand-it-itis
4. Rating, judging and overgeneralizing a person's weakness to think the person is a bad person

The helper who uses cognitive-behavioral techniques continually unmasks helpees' faulty thinking by bringing it to their attention, showing them how irrational thoughts are the basis of their problems, demonstrating the A-B-C-D-E links (explained in the following paragraph), and teaching helpees how to rethink and restate their preceding and similar sentences in a more logical, self-helping way. Thus, helpers directly contradict and deny the faulty statements that helpees repeat to themselves, and they demand that helpees become involved in some kind of activity (homework) that will act as a "counterpropagandist" force against the faulty belief system.

In the A-B-C-D-E system, A stands for activating event, B stands for belief system, C stands for consequences, D stands for disputing irrational ideas, and E stands for new emotional consequence or effect. An added F refers to further action.

The following excerpt demonstrates this system.

Client: I'm really upset. I just did a job for a person and it didn't come out right. I can't stand it when things don't go right, and I just don't understand how it happened. It's really terrible!

Helper: Wow, you seem to believe that everything should always go right and that if it doesn't, you're no good. You're really doing a job on yourself.

Client: Well, I don't understand when things don't turn out right and I've done the right thing. I'm really upset.

Helper: I know you're upset. But you're upset because of what you're thinking about a job not coming out right, because you believe that everything should go right and if it doesn't, you're no good. Let me draw you something. See this A? That's the activating event, the job that didn't come out right. This B is your belief that everything should go right and that if it doesn't, you're no good. The C, upset feelings, is the result of B. Come on now, what kinds of things do you think you're telling yourself in B that are resulting in you feeling upset?

Client: I'm not sure. I guess I'm telling myself that I should always do well and that it's terrible when I'm not perfect.

Helper: That's really unreasonable. How about telling yourself that you did the best you could, that it's OK when everything does not always work out, and that you don't have to be perfect?

The homework in a case like this may consist of the helpee practicing new sentences, such as those suggested by the helper in the preceding example, every time he or she begins to feel upset when things don't go well. Helpees report back on their homework assignments. In conformance with Ellis's approach, the following kinds of rational ideas are taught:

1. It is not a dire necessity for one to receive love or approval from all significant others. One can concentrate on loving rather than on being loved.

2. It would be better not to determine self-worth according to external ideals of competence, adequacy, and achievement, but to focus on self-respect and winning approval for performance.

3. Wrongdoers ought not to be blamed or punished, but should be considered merely unaware or ignorant or emotionally disturbed.

4. One's unhappiness is caused or sustained by the view one takes of things rather than by the things themselves.

5. If something is dangerous, one should face it and try to make it nondangerous, not make a catastrophe out of it.

6. The only way to solve difficult problems is to face them squarely.

7. It is usually far better to stand on one's own feet and gain faith in oneself and one's ability to meet difficult circumstances of living than to depend on someone else.

8. One should accept oneself as imperfect with general human limitations and specific fallibilities.

9. One should learn from one's past experiences but not be overly attached to or prejudiced by them.

10. Other people's deficiencies and weaknesses are largely their problems, and putting pressure on them to change is unlikely to help them do so.

11. People are usually happiest when they are actively and vitally absorbed in fulfilling pursuits outside themselves.

12. One has enormous control over one's emotions if one chooses to work at learning new, rational kinds of thoughts.

Needless to say, pointing out and disputing faulty thinking once is not likely to result in permanent behavior change. Rather, the helper must keep pounding away at the faulty belief system, time and time again, by reframing, playing the devil's advocate, using a catastrophe scale, **disputing** double standards, and so on. Helpers must insist on the completion of homework assignments that will demonstrate some behavior change.

The following is an excerpt from a rational-emotive behavior therapy training session.

Mr. Whittier is 66 years old, retired, and widowed. He is currently living alone in his apartment of 40 years. He has three grown sons who live in other towns. He's been referred to a counselor at the community center because of continued moping and self-pity.

Mr. Whittier: I'm all alone now. The boys, they've gone off, and they don't really bother with me now. I suppose I should move to a smaller apartment, but all the memories are here. Where have all the years gone to?

Helper: Mr. Whittier, you seem to think that your boys should be more attentive to you.

Mr. Whittier: Yes . . . why not? What are children for? We all had some good years together.

Helper: It certainly would be nice if your boys did pay more attention to you, but the fact that they don't doesn't mean you have to stop living, you know.

Mr. Whittier: What do you mean?

Helper: You keep acting as if you can't live without them. You go around here telling everyone how terrible it is that your sons don't write more, don't visit and call more. But you are healthy and you are living, and things don't always have to be the way you want them to be.

Mr. Whittier: What kind of talk is this? Things *don't* always have to be the way I want them to be . . . um . . . let me think.

Helper: Isn't that what you keep on telling yourself?

Mr. Whittier: (*long pause*) Maybe, maybe you have something.

Helper: Let me help you think it out. There are some new sentences you can learn to say over and over to yourself every time you feel yourself getting upset with your sons. If, instead of telling yourself over and over again how terrible it is that your boys don't call, write, and visit more, you could learn to say instead, it's too bad those boys don't call, visit, write more—we could have good times together—but I'm making friends of my own here at the center, and I'm going to manage and live anyway. . . .

In this case the helper had gotten to know Mr. Whittier over several years at the community center, so she felt comfortable confronting him with his irrational thinking.

Reality Therapy   Reality therapy uses different techniques in the cognitive-behavioral domain. Involvement between helper and helpee is crucial to reality therapy techniques, which involve eight steps:

1. Get involved; be personal and communicate "I care about you" by words and actions.

2. Stay in the here and now; avoid references to the past and avoid dwelling on feelings. What the person does with them is more important than the feelings themselves.

3. Evaluate behavior; ask the helpee to evaluate his or her own behavior and ask, "Is what I did appropriate?" "Is it helping me? . . . others?" If the client cannot evaluate his or her behavior to your satisfaction, it is necessary to return to step 1. The helpee must decide whether to change his or her behavior.

4. Plan to change behavior; ask "What do you think would be a better way to do things?" Help the client formulate a plan. Let the client choose; the helper offers suggestions but does not provide the plan. The plan should be minimal, specific ("How and when will you do this?"), positive rather than negative or punitive, and have a high probability of success.

5. Contract to seal the plan. If necessary, write out a contract and have the helpee sign it. Follow through with a check on how it is going and support success. This contract is between the helper and the helpee.

6. Accept no excuses for failure to fulfill the plan. If the contract is not fulfilled, ask "When will you do this?" not "Why didn't you do this?" If unsuccessful, follow through with the natural consequences of not having followed the plan, and then go back and make a new plan.

7. Make sure the helpee knows and is involved with making the rules. Use natural consequences (results when the rules are broken) rather than punishment.

8. Never give up.

A helper using reality therapy techniques will become very involved with the helpee, who can then begin to evaluate his or her own behavior and see what is unrealistic. Helpers confront clients with reality and ask them again and again to decide whether or not they wish to take the responsible path. Helpers then ask clients to make specific plans and to take responsibility for implementing them. Helpers can reject unrealistic behavior but still accept helpees and maintain respect for them. Helpers teach helpees better ways to fulfill their needs without hurting themselves and others. Helpees assume responsibility for their behavior, work in the present, learn to assess the morality of their behavior, and learn more effective ways of behaving.

An example of this approach follows.

Client: I don't want to finish school. I hate the teachers, I can't learn anything from them, and it's no use going back there.

Helper: What's going on in school? What are you doing?

Client: I'm always getting sent to the office. My English teacher is a real nag. She picks on me for everything, and I know she has it in for me.

Helper: What are *you* doing?

Client: Nothing much. I just sit there . . . sometimes I mess around a little.

Helper: What's "messing around"?

Client: Oh, you know, talking to other guys, fooling around . . .

Helper: Do you think this is appropriate behavior?

Client: Aw, I don't know. Most of the guys do it.

Helper: Let me ask you something. If you don't go back to school, what will you do?

Client: I'll get a job. I want to go up north and work at a ski resort. I can be an instructor.

Helper: You think you can get that kind of job without a high school diploma?

Client: I think so . . . I don't know. Why would a ski instructor need a high school diploma?

Helper: Well, it might help. It will certainly give you more choices for the rest of your life.

Client: I'm sick of school. I really don't want to go back.

Helper: It's up to you to decide what you want to do. I think you should think about what you're doing and whether it is going to get you what you want in this world.

This excerpt shows the implementation of steps 2 and 3 (step 1 had been started in previous sessions). As mentioned earlier, reality therapy uses a teaching strategy that deals directly with choices of the helpee. The basic philosophy is that the helpee can decide whether or not to be troubled.

Beck's Cognitive Therapy   Beck's form of cognitive therapy uses a wide range of core strategies incorporating cognitive and behavioral techniques. Many of these resemble Ellis's cognitive restructuring. Some of Beck's strategies include cognitive rehearsal to identify roadblocks in thoughts, associating feelings with behaviors by imagining situations in every detail during the session, many types of reality testing such as finding alternative responses to negative thoughts, task assignment, and actively testing out negative thoughts and assumptions.

Helping the client to become aware of and distanced from faulty thinking may prevent similar future errors. Beck (1976) outlines seven steps of a reality testing technique that illustrates his application of strategy.

1. Identify thoughts and statements made by the client that are negative or associated with bad feelings.

2. Ask the client how much he or she believes that the statement or thought is true or how likely it is that the negative event will occur.

3. Check the client's feelings associated with the statement—for example, "When you say that to yourself, how do you feel?"

4. Leaving the validity of the statement as an open question, gently probe the evidence: past outcomes of similar situations, alternative outcomes and their frequency, times when the same situation has had better or worse consequences than presently imagined, and so on.

5. Rate the possibility of catastrophes in the future—for example, "How probable is it that you will never find another friend like him? One in 10? One in 100?"

6. Continually challenge thoughts with reality.

7. Check how much the client believes the original statement is true after going through these steps.

Note that cognitive-behavioral techniques include evaluation and judgment on the part of the helper, who labels the helpee's thinking and behavior as rational or irrational, responsible or irresponsible. Helpers do not arbitrarily impose their value systems on helpees; rather, they examine and evaluate the helpee's values. In other words, helpers challenge helpees but do not punish them or reject them for not having the "right" values or beliefs. This approach does differ, however, from the phenomenological strategies, which are both nonjudgmental and nonevaluative.

Meichenbaum's Cognitive Behavior Modification Meichenbaum's *stress inoculation approach* includes verbal self-instructions and relaxation strategies. The helpee learns a programmed sequence of new verbal self-instructions that allow more rational decision making about responses to stimuli. The sequence suggested by Meichenbaum and Goodman (1971) covers an education phase, a skill acquisition phase, and application training.

1. Trainer models the task and talks out loud while helpee observes. (*overt cognitive modeling*)
2. Helpee performs tasks, instructing himself aloud with overt, external guidance from trainer.
3. Helpee performs task aloud with no assistance from trainer.
4. Trainer models same statements but now in a whisper. (*faded overt modeling*)
5. Helpee performs task whispering to himself. (*faded overt self-guidance*)
6. Trainer performs task using silent verbalizations. (*covert modeling*)
7. Helpee performs task using silent verbalizations.

An example of this approach follows.

Client: She pushes my buttons and I just let loose. I don't know why she doesn't understand that I just need to blow off steam. She gets mad and doesn't talk to me for days.

Helper: When you begin to feel your anger rising—you said you feel it in your gut—try to learn to put the fingers of your right hand on your left wrist (pulse), take some deep breaths, and say to yourself, "I will not get hooked into a fight." Try that right now.

Client: Is this right? (*puts fingers on pulse and takes some deep breaths*) I will not get overexcited and hooked. It takes two to fight.

Helper: Great! Now keep doing that and visualize your heart and pulse slowing down rather than speeding up.

Client: I will not react. I will stay calm.

Helper: (*puts fingers on pulse and takes deep breaths*) I will stay calm and not get drawn into a fight. (*whispers*)

Client: (*continuing pulse taking and deep breathing*) I will stay calm and not fight. (*Helper and Client continue silent pulse taking and deep breathing.*)

This strategy enables the client to become more aware of his physiological stress reactions so that he can monitor and control his reactions.

When to Use Cognitive-Behavioral Strategies

These approaches have been used with a wide variety of the population, in schools, hospitals, industry, and correctional institutions. The rational-emotive behavior therapy approach might not be effective with helpees who are not intelligent enough to follow a rational analysis or for those who are so caught up in emotion that they cannot attend to this logical procedure. The reality-therapy approach involves much straightforward common sense and has also been used with a broad spectrum of the population. Beck's cognitive therapy has been particularly effective with depressed clients and is now applied to a wide array of disorders. This therapy, as do other cognitive approaches, requires verbal ability and the motivation for change on the part of the client. Meichenbaum's approaches have been used with noncompliant medical patients, impulsive children and adults, hyperactive youngsters, and helpees who want to manage stress.

The following exercises will provide you with opportunities to question your own belief system and to design a reality therapy contract.

EXERCISE 7.14 ▪ In triads, share the last strong negative feeling each of you has experienced. Describe the circumstances, and help each other to analyze irrational thinking via the A-B-C-D-E system. Which of the four types of evaluative thinking dysfunctions or 12 irrational ideas does the faulty belief system come from? What kinds of new sentences can you teach yourself to refute the old sentences you've been telling yourself? Prepare a homework assignment for yourself and report back to your triad in one week.

EXERCISE 7.15 ▪ In groups of six, reverse roles such as masculine/feminine, supervisor/supervisee, and black/white, depending on the makeup of your group. Role-play a scene and then discuss the assumptions and conceptions you've become aware of while playing an unfamiliar role and observing others playing a role familiar to you. What irrational beliefs have you uncovered? What do they mean to you?

EXERCISE 7.16 ▪ In small groups, construct a reality therapy contract for at least one member of the group in accordance with the eight steps previously discussed. Stick to specific behaviors and identify the logical consequences of meeting and not meeting the contract. What did you find functional or dysfunctional for you in this process? How well were you able to identify responsible and/or irresponsible behavior?

EXERCISE 7.17 ▪ Imagine being in a situation that would probably upset you. Perhaps you can think of something that has actually occurred in the past week or is likely to occur in the next few days. Imagine that you are experiencing this right now, with its whole range of accompanying negative thoughts and feelings. Now tell a partner what the situation is and share those negative thoughts and feelings. See if you can recapture your internal verbalizations, what you said to yourself. Together, attempt to brainstorm resolutions for the situation. During or after generating some options, develop each possible course of action in great detail to discover possible roadblocks.

BEHAVIORAL STRATEGIES

Behavioral strategies are based on learning theory and focus on specific, observable behaviors as opposed to feelings and thoughts. The objectives of these strategies are to alter inappropriate behaviors and to teach appropriate ones. The assumption is that change in behavior results in changes in feelings and thoughts and that helpers can evaluate their effectiveness only by observing concrete, specific behavior changes.

Techniques

The many behavioral techniques require some skills of the helper. Some of those skills are the following:

1. Understanding of the concepts and principles of reinforcement, punishment, extinction, discrimination, shaping, successive approximations, and schedules of reinforcement
2. Ability to identify specific target behaviors that the helpee wishes to change
3. Ability to identify and assess the conditions preceding the helpee's target behavior
4. Ability to collect baseline data on the frequency and severity of the target behavior
5. Ability to identify and assess those conditions that both result from the target behavior and maintain (reinforce) it
6. Ability to determine reinforcements that are meaningful for the helpee
7. Ability to determine feasible and meaningful schedules of reinforcement
8. Sufficient knowledge of the theoretical framework, design, and application of different behavioral strategies
9. Ability to evaluate outcomes of behavioral strategies

It is beyond the scope of this book to teach you these skills, but you will find readings at the end of the chapter that cover this material. Behavioral strategies are being taught to teachers and parents and are increasingly being used in businesses, schools, and health organizations. Many generalist human services workers and beginning professionals are assisting in the implementation of these strategies. Some important behavioral techniques that we will discuss are modeling, contracting, assertiveness training, and systematic desensitization.

Modeling is based on the principle that people learn to behave in new ways by imitating the behavior, values, attitudes, and beliefs of significant others. Modeling may be accomplished through role playing, the use of media, and individual and group counseling relationships. Remember that the helper is a model, a very powerful model, in a helping relationship.

An example of role-play modeling follows.

Client: I always have a hard time at those dorm parties. I'm never able to go up and start a conversation with someone I don't know.

Helper: Um. Let's role-play. I'll be a stranger at a party, and you be standing by the wall with a beer.

Client: OK. (*rearranges self*) Ummmmm . . . hot, isn't it?

Helper: Yeh.

Client: Lots of people here . . . Oh darn! See, I can't do it; it just goes nowhere.

Helper: OK. Now let's reverse roles and see what happens. Hi, there. Some crowd here . . . it's difficult getting around. You struck me as someone interesting to talk to.

Client: I did? Oh, well, thanks. That's nice.

Helper: I was wondering what you're thinking about all this. (*gestures around the room*)

Client: I see what you did. You asked broader questions and I asked dumb ones that didn't need answering.

Helper: That's one thing. What were you feeling when we did this?

In modeling, it's important for the helper to be aware of his or her modeling influence on the helpee and of positive and negative models in other aspects of the helpee's life. The helper assists the helpee in identifying appropriate models. Sometimes helpers arrange for people to work or study together or in small groups, having definite models in mind. By the same token, helpers sometimes break up existing groups or cliques because of the effect of negative models.

Contracting is based on theories of reinforcement, which state that reinforced (rewarded) behavior tends to be repeated. A behavioral contract is a specific agreement between helper and helpee that breaks down the target behavior into its smallest parts and that provides for systematic reinforcements of the performance of the behavior.

Contracts may be informal (for example, "If you do X, I will do Y") or formal (written statements of specific behavior to be performed, the specific reward to be granted, and the specific responsibilities and conditions for implementing and monitoring the contract).

Contracts should still follow the basic rules proposed years ago by Homme (1970) in that they should (1) use reward liberally and immediately following performance, (2) be clearly understood by all parties, and (3) be expressed in positive terms, meaning that they should state what one is to do, not what one is not to do.

Here is an example of a formal contract drawn up between a residence adviser, a college student, and the student's girlfriend in a dormitory. The problem was that the student was in danger of failing a chemistry course because he was falling behind with homework assignments and getting low test scores. Tom, Mary Beth, and Len agreed to participate on the following terms:

If Tom reads one chapter of his chemistry text and completes the problems at the end of the chapter with 75 percent accuracy by 9:30 each evening, he will meet Mary Beth in the lounge for coffee between 10 and 11 P.M. Len will be available to correct the problems at 9:30 P.M. If Tom does not meet these terms, he will stay in his room the rest of the evening and not meet with Mary Beth. This contract will be reviewed after two weeks.

As in reality therapy contracts, there is no punishment or rejection for not meeting the terms of the contract; however, reinforcement is given only after performance of the target behavior, and it is important that this reinforcement not be available outside the terms of the contract. Contracts must be positive and within the realm of possibility. The target behavior is broken down into its smallest component parts, and an appropriate amount of reinforcement is administered for each small component behavior performed. For example, Tom may be far enough behind in his chemistry to warrant reading two chapters per night, but the contract begins with one chapter because Len and Tom know that Tom can definitely meet those terms. When the contract is reviewed, the terms may change.

The use of contracts in a helping relationship has the advantage of specifying in positive terms exactly what is expected from the helpees and what they will receive for fulfilling those expectations. Contracts enable some movement and growth in problem areas, resulting in higher self-esteem and thus permitting attention to be turned to other areas of concern. Contracts are ethical as long as they do not specify performance of immoral behavior and as long as all involved parties agree to the terms.

Assertiveness training is used in the cognitive as well as the behavioral domain. It can involve changing helpees' belief systems by teaching them that they should stand up for their own rights as long as they do not harm someone else or impinge on someone else's rights in the process. This kind of training reduces helpees' anxiety by teaching them to say what they want to say.

Methods of assertiveness training can involve role-playing **successive approximations** of the assertive response, modeling from media, and verbal instructions and illustrations.

Here is an example of assertiveness training for a 25-year-old divorcée.

Client: I've been in a terrible state all day. Since I left Russ, my parents have really been on my back. My dad called last night and announced they're coming up this weekend, and now I have to change all my plans. I've been unable to concentrate on anything all day.

Helper: Sounds to me like you're really uptight about this. You were unable to tell your parents that this weekend was inconvenient for you.

Client: Yes. I never can tell them what I feel. They get so upset and carry on so. But I hate myself for getting into this state.

Helper: I wonder what would happen if you called your dad tonight and told him you'd like to see him, but this weekend is inconvenient for you and you'll let him know when he can come up.

Client: I wish I could do that. I'd love it. I don't think I can.

Helper: Let's rehearse and see what happens.

They then role-played the same scene over and over, with the helper playing both roles at different times for modeling purposes. After the fifth rehearsal, the client reported that she felt less anxious. The next day she reported that she had phoned her father and felt relieved that she had been able to take this step. Her assertive responses did not contain a "You're no good, you have no right to interfere in my life" kind of message. She sent an "I" message, communicating her interest in seeing her father, but letting him know, clearly and firmly, that she had other plans and would let him know when it was all right for him to come up. As she continues to practice this kind of behavior, she will come to change her belief system and really believe that she has the right to her own life.

Systematic desensitization involves breaking down anxiety-response behaviors by exposing the helpee to the imagery of those behaviors while in a state of deep physical relaxation. The theory is that anxiety responses have been conditioned (learned) and can be counterconditioned (unlearned). One way to countercondition anxiety responses is to pair them with an incompatible state—in this case, a physiological state of relaxation, which inhibits anxiety. The anxiety stimulus eventually loses its potency, and the helpee no longer needs to expend energy on the anxiety response.

It is unlikely that many human services workers will actually apply complete systematic desensitization; but the first stage, that of inducing deep muscle relaxation, is often helpful in and of itself and is easy to learn to apply. It usually takes two to three sessions to effectively teach relaxation. Between sessions, helpees are asked to practice relaxation skills at least once a day. Helpees are taught to contract (tense) and then relax specific muscle groups for several minutes at a time until they learn to monitor their own relaxation.

Before beginning this training, the helper explains the process to the helpee. The helper explains that it is impossible to be both tense and relaxed at the same time and that once helpees learn relaxation, they can use this training whenever they are tense. This is skill learning and requires continual practice in order to be effective.

At the beginning of the training session, the helpee is seated in a comfortable chair that supports all body muscles. Eyes are closed (the helpee is asked to remove eyeglasses or contact lenses), the head is supported by the chair or wall, arms are on the armrests of the chair, and legs are uncrossed and firmly on the floor. Relaxation training commences after the helper demonstrates to the helpee the tensing and relaxing of each muscle group. It is a good idea to darken the room and reduce interfering noises.

The following is an example of relaxation instructions. (I [BFO] am indebted to Flora Hummel, R.N., for introducing me to this technique.)

Close your eyes now, lean back, and just get comfortable. Think about your body and what you're feeling now . . . now I want you to raise your hands and clench your fists as tightly as you can . . . feel those muscles pulling . . . tighter now . . . OK. 1 . . . 2 . . . 3 . . . 4 . . . now relax and let your hands fall into your lap. Now let's do that again . . . tighten those hands . . . 1 . . . 2 . . . 3 . . . 4 . . . now let them relax again . . . now raise your fore- arms and pull those muscles as tightly as you can . . . 1 . . . 2 . . . 3 . . . 4 . . . relax and let them fall into your lap . . . attend to the different feelings you get from relaxed and tense muscles . . . now let's do those muscles again . . . 1 . . . 2 . . . 3 . . . 4 . . . relax . . . feel your arms getting heavier as they become more relaxed . . . now pull in on your upper arm muscles by rais- ing your arms and flexing those muscles . . . harder, now . . . that's right . . . 1 . . . 2 . . . 3 . . . 4 . . . relax . . . your arms feel heavier and warm feelings are spreading down through your fingertips . . . now let's do that again . . . 1 . . . 2 . . . 3 . . . 4 . . . relax . . . we'll concentrate on your head muscles now . . . let your arms continue to grow heavier and relax more while you think about your head muscles . . . now raise your eyebrows and wrinkle up your forehead as much as you can . . . tighter . . . hold it . . . 1 . . . 2 . . . 3 . . . 4 . . . now relax, and feel that tension slipping out over your head, right over the top . . . let's do that again . . . hold it . . . 1 . . . 2 . . . 3 . . . 4 . . . relax . . . now scrunch up your eyes and feel them get as tight as possible . . . 1 . . . 2 . . . 3 . . . 4 . . . now do that again . . . 1 . . . 2 . . . 3 . . . 4 . . . relax and feel your eyelids getting heavier as everything gets darker . . . now scrunch up your nose as tight as you can . . . hold it . . . 1 . . . 2 . . . 3 . . . 4 . . . now relax . . . do it again . . . 1 . . . 2 . . . 3 . . . 4 . . . that's right, now relax and feel your breathing get clearer and easier . . . now stretch your mouth in an ear-to-ear grin and pull on your lip, jaw, and cheek muscles . . . come on, you can pull tighter than that . . . hold it . . . 1 . . . 2 . . . 3 . . . 4 . . . now relax . . . let your jaw hang loosely and your head lean right into the back of the chair . . . do that again . . . 1 . . . 2 . . . 3 . . . 4 . . . that's right, now relax . . . now think back over your arm muscles and let your head rest heavier and heavier . . . you're getting more and more relaxed and all you're thinking about is your muscles getting more and more relaxed . . . now pull in your neck and throat muscles . . . feel that tension . . . hold it . . . 1 . . . 2 . . . 3 . . . 4 . . . now pull in your neck and throat muscles . . . feel that tension . . . hold it . . . 1 . . . 2 . . . 3 . . . 4 . . . relax . . . let your neck and head slump into the chair . . . how about repeating that . . . 1 . . . 2 . . . 3 . . . 4 . . . relax and feel your neck get looser and looser . . . now raise your shoulders and pull those muscles tightly . . . hold it . . . 1 . . . 2 . . . 3 . . . 4 . . . that's right, now relax and let those shoulders slump . . . let those warm, tingly, relaxed feelings connect up from your shoulders down your arms . . . that's right . . . repeat that . . . 1 . . . 2 . . . 3 . . . 4 . . . relax . . . feel those relaxed feelings get- ting deeper and deeper . . . now tighten up your upper back muscles by arching your back as much as you can . . . 1 . . . 2 . . . 3 . . . 4 . . . relax . . . slump down into your chair . . . do it again and tighten your chest muscles at the same time . . . 1 . . . 2 . . . 3 . . . 4 . . . relax . . . take a couple of minutes to feel more relaxed and go over your arm muscles and your head muscles . . . if any group of muscles starts to tighten up, pull them in, contract them and then relax them, like a rubber band . . . now pull your tummy muscles in as tightly as you can and feel that tension . . . hold them . . . 1 . . . 2 . . . 3 . . . 4 . . . relax . . . feel your stomach get looser . . . repeat that . . . 1 . . . 2 . . . 3 . . . 4 . . . relax . . . breathe deeply and slowly and with each breath in, feel more relaxed and with each breath out, feel that relaxation spreading throughout your body . . . now tighten your buttocks and hold them tight . . . 1 . . . 2 . . . 3 . . . 4 . . . relax . . . now do that again . . . 1 . . . 2 . . . 3 . . . 4 . . . relax and sink deeper and deeper into the chair . . . now we'll work on your leg muscles . . . tighten your thigh muscles . . . 1 . . . 2 . . . 3 . . . 4 . . . relax . . . do that again . . . 1 . . . 2 . . . 3 . . . 4 . . . feel your legs getting heavier and the warm, relaxed feelings spreading down . . . now tighten up your calves by pointing your toes away from your head . . . 1 . . . 2 . . . 3 . . . 4 . . . relax . . . repeat . . . 1 . . . 2 . . . 3 . . . 4 . . . that's right . . . the warm tingly feelings are spreading down your legs . . . now crunch up your toes and tighten those feet muscles . . . 1 . . . 2 . . . 3 . . . 4 . . . relax . . . now do that again . . . 1 . . . 2 . . . 3 . . . 4 . . . fine . . . now think back over all the muscle groups we've relaxed and see if they can become more and more relaxed . . . that's right . . . the arms . . . your head . . . your shoulders . . . back . . . stomach . . . buttocks . . . legs . . . take a few minutes to really get in touch with these warm, tingly feelings . . . now I'm going to count to 20 very slowly, and when I use an odd number, breathe in, and when I use an even one, breathe out (*counts to 20 very slowly*).

At this point either desensitization begins or, if relaxation is being used alone, after several moments the helper counts slowly to 10 and asks the helpee to open his or her eyes and slowly stretch.

If desensitization follows, it is in this relaxed state that the helper asks the helpee to call different scenes to mind: a neutral scene (like a blank screen), which does not arouse any feeling; a comfortable scene (like sitting in front of a fireplace or by the ocean), which arouses only comfortable feelings; or a scene that can arouse anxiety. Anxiety scenes are first introduced for 10 seconds and then followed by a neutral or pleasurable scene and more relaxation concentration; then they are introduced for 20 seconds, and again, after more pleasurable scenes, for 40 seconds. If anxiety occurs, the helpee signals the helper, and the length of the anxiety scenes is reduced. An anxiety item is considered successfully mastered when the subject can imagine it for three 40-second periods without experiencing any anxiety.

A desensitization hierarchy is constructed during the first two relaxation-training sessions. This hierarchy comprises a series of statements that describe anxiety-provoking stimuli, ranked from least to most anxiety-provoking.

A sample of a hierarchy used for test desensitization follows (stimulus number 1 causes the least anxiety; number 13, the most).

1. Walking to class.
2. Professor announces examination is two weeks away.
3. Copying classmate's notes for missed class.
4. Obtaining references to study.
5. Discussing class with friends.
6. Studying the week of the exam.
7. Studying the night before the exam.
8. Waking up the morning of the exam.
9. Walking to the classroom.
10. The exam is being handed out—you receive a copy.
11. While trying to think of the answer to an exam question you notice everyone around you writing quickly.
12. You come to a question you can't answer.
13. Professor announces that 40 minutes remain; you have one and a half hours of work to complete.

When the cause of anxiety is something that can actually be tested in the helping relationship, you can validate the client's desensitization to it. For example, I (BFO) once treated a client who had a driving phobia. After reducing her anxiety through systematic desensitization, we entered my car and found that she was able to drive for the first time in 18 years.

When to Use Behavioral Strategies

Behavioral strategies are effective with a wide population, especially those who have difficulty with verbal strategies. The implementation of these action strategies is usually shorter term than with other types of strategies.

In particular, modeling is effective for those who are unsure of themselves and need specific teaching examples. Contracting is helpful for the developmentally slow as well as "normal" populations and is particularly effective in families and organizations in which reinforcements can be immediately provided and monitored. Assertiveness training is helpful for shy, inhibited people. This technique has also been used in women's consciousness-raising groups. Systematic desensitization is helpful for those with phobic reactions such as fear of flying and fear of water.

The following exercises will give you some experience with the previously described behavioral techniques.

EXERCISE 7.18 ■ The purpose of this exercise is to check your ability to identify behavioral statements (statements that describe behavior that is observable and measurable). Which of the following statements are behavioral? (Answers are given at the end of the chapter.)

1. "That child is no good—he's stubborn and fresh."
2. "Johnny never sits down at his desk. He's always up walking around."
3. "I feel so guilty when I think of him all alone."
4. "Ms. Leonard came late to the board meeting."
5. "Ms. Leonard really isn't interested in this organization."
6. "Pam is so spoiled—she whines and complains a lot."
7. "My husband doesn't appreciate me."
8. "He's lazy, just like his father."
9. "He never seems to get anything done on time."
10. "I had a boring day today."
11. "I cleaned the house all day."
12. "She really is a good mother."
13. "My secretary is the fastest typist I've ever seen."
14. "He belongs to a gang."
15. "Gangs are roaming the streets at night."

EXERCISE 7.19 ■ Individually, write down five behaviors that you think an effective helper ought to use. Then, in small groups, agree on one list. Then all groups can share their lists. Do the lists all contain behaviors, or do some of the items represent attitudes and evaluations?

EXERCISE 7.20 ■ *Modeling:* Who are the most influential role models in your life? What are their most important characteristics, in your opinion? Discuss these questions in small groups, and see if you can draw up a list of effective model characteristics. Compare lists among the small groups.

EXERCISE 7.21 ■ *Reinforcement:* In triads or small groups, discuss what is reinforcing to each of you in your life. See if you can identify the major social reinforcers (from people, such as a smile, gesture, or visit) and concrete reinforcers (things, such as money, gifts, or purchases) that operate in your life at home, at work, and at leisure. See if they differ in the different settings. As you discuss each other's reinforcers, you will see that different people have different kinds of reinforcers, that what is reinforcing for one person may or may not be so for another.

EXERCISE 7.22 ▪ *Reinforcement:* Imagine yourself in a familiar setting, either at home, at work, or at school, and see if you can determine what kinds of reinforcements, both social and concrete, you give others and yourself. For example, "When I am at home and complete a housekeeping task I dislike, I usually reward myself by talking to a friend on the phone or having a cup of coffee with a neighbor." Share your responses in small groups.

EXERCISE 7.23 ▪ *Contracting:* In pairs, draw up contracts for each of you, listing your partner as monitor. This contract may be between you and your partner or between you and someone else. Select a target behavior (like losing so many pounds or getting to class on time), determine a time limit, and write out what you will do, when you will do it, and what you will receive for your performance. For example, "If I lose two pounds between today and next Thursday, I will buy myself a new shirt." It is essential that the reinforcement be something that is meaningful to the helpee, not to the helper.

EXERCISE 7.24 ▪ *Assertiveness training:* In each of the following situations, which response is the most assertive? (Answers are at the end of the chapter.)

1. Your mother telephones you long distance and wants to know why she hasn't received a letter from you all week.
   a. "It's hard for you to realize that I'm grown up now. I'll write when I can."
   b. "I'm sorry, Ma, I've just been too busy; I'll write tonight."
   c. "Oh, Mom, please stop bugging me. I'm not a baby, you know."

2. A coworker asks you to get him coffee. This is the umpteenth time, and you do not want to do it.
   a. "I guess so, since I'm going down there anyway."
   b. "Why can't you get your own coffee?"
   c. "I'd really feel better about our relationship if you would stop asking me to get your coffee."

3. Someone pushes in front of you at the box office line.
   a. "Who do you think you are?"
   b. "I'm ahead of you in this line. Please move."
   c. "Some people really have a nerve!"

4. Your boss asks you at the last minute to stay late to work on a report. You know it is not an emergency, and this is the third time this has happened this month.
   a. "OK. You're the boss."
   b. "But we're having company tonight, and I promised Marge I'd pick up some ice."
   c. "I do have other plans tonight, and I'm afraid it's too late for me to change them."

5. Your friend wants to borrow your car. Last time this happened, you promised your husband you wouldn't do it again.
   a. "I wish I could, but Paulo made me promise not to lend out the car."
   b. "I'd like to help out, but Paulo and I have agreed that we can be more accountable about the car if we don't let others drive it."
   c. "Oh dear, I think I'll need it when you want it."

6. The salesclerk tells you that the store does not accept returns or exchanges. If the merchandise is defective, you'll have to deal directly with the manufacturer.
   a. "That's ridiculous. I'm going to call the Better Business Bureau."
   b. "I insist that you refund my money, and I'm not budging until you do."
   c. "I'd like to see your manager, please. I intend to straighten this out here and now."

7. Your doctor tells you that there is nothing wrong with you, but he would like you to have some tests done anyway.
   a. "Before I have any tests, I'd like to know the reasons, costs, and just what's involved."
   b. "But why do I need these tests if there's nothing wrong with me?"
   c. "Is this another example of useless tests I keep reading about?"

8. Your friend pleads with you to go out to dinner, and you want to stay home alone and relax after a hard week.
   a. "I have a headache, so I want to go to bed early."
   b. "I'd really like to be alone tonight and relax. Some other time."
   c. "Well, why don't you come over here, and we'll fix something to eat?"

9. A neighbor calls you to complain about your son being a bully. This has happened before with this particular neighbor, and you have checked it out and determined that it is your neighbor's problem, not yours.
   a. "I'm sorry. Thanks for letting me know about this. I'll talk to him."
   b. "You really ought to find out about your own kids before you complain about mine."
   c. "I'd appreciate it if you'd check out both sides of the situation, as I will."

10. You've been sitting in a restaurant for almost an hour and you still have not been served, even though you told the waiter you had a curtain time to make.
    a. "Waiter! What's taking so long? I told you I have to be at the theater in half an hour."
    b. "Waiter! Curtain time is in 30 minutes. I expect to have finished eating by then."
    c. "Waiter! Will you please hurry? The service around here is terrible."

EXERCISE 7.25 ■ *Assertiveness training:* Arrange a line of seven or eight people, such as one sees at a grocery checkout counter, at the box office of a movie, or waiting to get on a bus. Those in your group who are not in line should try, one at a time, to break in and push ahead. See how each of you reacts, and then discuss those reactions in your group.

The purpose of the previous two exercises is to help you become aware of your own assertive behaviors or lack of them. In smaller groups, identify situations that require assertive (not aggressive) behaviors, and then role-play those situations in as many ways as you can.

EXERCISE 7.26 ▪ *Relaxation:* Using the relaxation-training example in this chapter, see if you can help one or more persons in your group to relax. Each time a set of ellipses appears in the example, allow several seconds to elapse. Keep your voice soft and soothing, and be careful not to rush. Experience the role of trainee as well as trainer, and share your feelings and reactions.

EXERCISE 7.27 ▪ *Problem solving:* To practice problem-solving behavioral strategies, pair students and have them come up with a real behavioral problem, such as biting fingernails, hitting the snooze button too often, or overeating in the evening. Each student takes a turn being the helpee and works with the helper to devise a plan: identifying the problem, setting measurable goals, and designing a plan after analyzing facets of the problem. Enact the plan over the next few days, and follow up with the helper in the next few classes to evaluate success and to fix elements of the plan that did not work. Modify goals as appropriate.

STRATEGIES THAT CUT
ACROSS DOMAINS

Cutting across the affective, cognitive, and behavioral domains are feminist and multicultural approaches, multimodal therapy, and ecological/systems strategies. These are pluralistic approaches in that they draw on many of the theoretical bases of the other approaches.

Pluralistic or integrated strategies can be used when the helpee's problem does not fall clearly into one domain; when it overlaps into two or three domains; and when the problems are individual, interpersonal, and/or related to the person's environment. For example, one may use a behavioral technique for modifying a particular behavior and, at the same time, attempt some cognitive restructuring (to change the client's thinking about the target behavior) and/or elicit the client's feelings by using affective techniques. Eclectic therapists believe that the more domains addressed, the stronger is the likelihood of change in the helpee.

The multimodal BASIC ID model discussed in Chapter 6 provides a specific, functional basis for selecting an eclectic group of techniques. For example, clients who are restricted in awareness and expression of their feelings may benefit from Gestalt as well as person-centered methods. Clients who are well aware of their thoughts and feelings might benefit by behavioral change techniques.

The BASIC ID paradigm allows helpers to prioritize helpee needs and goals. Microskills such as responsive listening and questioning are the helper's core tools. These techniques are particularly useful for life-span development issues across cultures.

Ecological/Systems Strategies

Systems strategies are selected when the objective is to improve helpees' observation and communication skills and their relationships within and outside their family. The focus is on interpersonal processes. An individual's problem is considered only in the context of his or her relational systems, regardless of how many people in the system come for help. Thus, the focus is on interactions between individuals and the assumption is that problems and problem solving involve all members of the system.

The aim of the intervention strategies is to resolve problems by rearranging the family (or other relationship) system (such as a classroom or workplace). This requires changing the communication and relationship patterns. The systems techniques used may include **reframing** the problem from a systems perspective (such as relabeling a child's behavioral problems as helpful and positive because they bring the parents together and interrupt their fighting); teaching verbal and nonverbal communication and problem-solving skills by providing feedback, new information, and coaching; assigning direct and indirect behavioral tasks; and *psychoeducation* (supportively providing guidance and new information by didactic teaching and bibliotherapy). Systems therapists often choose techniques from the other major models to implement their goals. Recent systems theories pay particular attention to the gender, race, and ethnic variables that affect interpersonal relationships. Specific techniques include the following:

1. Prescribing the symptom, such as telling a couple to fight more, not only because that will increase their caring but also because they are so good at expressing love by fighting

2. Family sculpting, a nonverbal experiential technique in which family members position themselves or are positioned by the therapist in a tableau that reveals their perceptions and feelings about family relationships

3. Drawing a genogram, a family map that spans several generations, to help understand the themes and patterns of the family's relationship style and lifestyle

4. Drawing an ecomap, a map that includes all of the community and larger sociocultural systems that impact one's life—health, professional associations, friends, extracurricular activities, religious community, legal services, government agencies, and many others—then coding the relative impact of each of the identified ecosystems

5. Circular questioning, asking nonparticipating members to speak for others or to hypothesize about the past or future in relation to the present

The following example illustrates a systems perspective.

Ms. Marsh, age 32, was referred for help by her neighborhood health center because of continuing headaches without any organic cause. She complained of irritability and persistent arguments with her 6-year-old son. A single parent on welfare, she had not worked steadily since the birth of her child. Her son seemed to be doing well in kindergarten. At the first session, the helper learned that Ms. Marsh's 26-year-old boyfriend, a cab driver, was putting pressure on her to let him move in with her. She said she was afraid of jeopardizing her welfare benefits. The mental health worker suggested that the boyfriend come in for a joint couple session.

During several couple sessions, it became clear that the headaches and irritability were symptoms of trouble in the couple system. Mr. Rich, the boyfriend, now wanted to become more involved with Ms. Marsh and her son; Ms. Marsh was fearful of this closeness due to the pain she had experienced in her brief relationship with the father of her son and in the abusive, alcoholic family from which she had run away. The couple were at an impasse. The level of their arguing was escalating. In tracking the pattern of this relationship, it emerged that every time one member of the couple wanted to move closer, the other became frightened and started arguments to create distance. Rather than continue this pursuer–distancer cycle, the couple contracted with the helper to learn to communicate their concerns more directly to each other and to engage in activities that would allow them to get closer to each other.

An ecological perspective emphasizes the fit between an individual and his or her environment. An important objective is to reframe from a multipart perspective the individual's perception of the problem so that he or she understands the influence of environmental variables. Many clients in nondominant groups assume blame and responsibility for their problems without recognizing the power of external variables. Systems interventions can be utilized to deal with larger social systems. Techniques include action-oriented advocacy and change agentry. The specific elements recommended by Steenbarger (1993) include these:

1. Empathy and validation of the helpee's plight

2. Recontextualization, which encourages the client to consider the wider role of the environment in the creation and maintenance of stress

3. Partnership, in which helper and helpee are active collaborators

4. Empowerment, whereby the helpee is encouraged to take action to effect systems change

5. Multiple change targets, meaning that the different facets of the helpee's context—family, school, peers, institutional policy, work—are targeted for change

An example of the ecological perspective in an initial interview follows.

Client: My husband is getting more and more depressed. He never thought, after 26 years of working for the same company, that he'd be laid off with no notice, and now he doesn't think he'll be able to find another job. And they replaced him with a younger person at half the salary. Just one week after a fabulous job review! They were so horrid and nasty the way they did it. Our health insurance runs out next month. I'm scared—I don't know what to do. We may not be able to get insurance because I had breast cancer five years ago.

Helper: It really is frightening to have the rug pulled out from under you. You both are experiencing real stress, and I can appreciate how helpless you feel.

Client: It's so unfair. I can't reassure him, because I'm not so sure he will find a comparable job. He really has been so responsible and so good. I just don't understand how this can happen.

Helper: Sounds like you guys need to find out more about your options.

Client: What do you mean? There's nothing we can do.

Helper: I'm not so sure. First of all, I'd talk to the unemployment people about possible benefits, talk to other people who've been laid off from that company and see if together you can find some patterns, and certainly talk to a lawyer about your rights—the state may have some laws about your right to health insurance. You may want to talk to the antidiscrimination people if there seems to be a pattern of ageism. There's a lot to find out about so you can decide what to do.

Client: I've been thinking of talking to some of the other wives. My husband doesn't want to make waves—he's frightened and terribly hurt.

Helper: Let's go slowly, but at least begin some exploration and see what's going on. He may find that taking some steps to learn more about his rights will help him feel better. At the same time, I'd suggest he see his doctor to be certain there are no medical issues contributing to his depression.

Client: Well, it can't hurt if I talk to a few people. And you're right, I never thought about talking to the unemployment people, and I know he hasn't even thought about applying for that. It seems so demeaning.

Helper: You've worked hard and responsibly all your lives. And this isn't your fault or his.

Client: It doesn't feel that way.

In the above example, the helper is validating the helpee's feelings while at the same time empowering her to take some active steps to find out more about possible options. The last interchange is critical in eliciting her automatic self-blame and then introducing her to the influence of environmental factors.

When to Use Ecological/Systems Strategies

The ecological and systems perspectives are important in all cases, in all settings that are human systems, because no one lives in a vacuum. Whether one works with an individual, a couple, or an entire family, with a student, a student and teacher, a classroom, or an entire school, one must consider how any individual's problem contributes to the systems in which the individual exists, and how the individual simultaneously is affected by these systems. It is the perspective, rather than any particular strategies or techniques, that is important. Thus, these approaches are effective when applied to interpersonal problems, to a bad fit between a person and his or her environment, and to people who experience devaluation, discrimination, or oppression due to race, gender, sexual orientation, physical appearance or disability, ethnicity, or some other type of societal oppression.

The following exercise illustrates some of the systems principles.

EXERCISE 7.28 ■ The purpose of this exercise is to facilitate your reframing a problem from a systems perspective. Try to remember a problem you had in your family growing up. What did it mean to you? To each other member of your family? Who benefited and who suffered from this problem? What were all of the ramifications of this problem? Then? Later? Now? Pick a partner in your class and share your thinking about your problem. Together, consider what you can learn about this problem from the systems perspective. What do you think about this problem now?

EXERCISE 7.29 ■ Now assess where you are as a helper in relation to the seven aspects of human personality addressed by multimodal therapy.

1. *Behavior:* Which helping behaviors do you want to learn, to increase, and/or to decrease?

2. *Affect:* What feelings do you experience most often as a helper (in class or on the job)? Which ones (such as anxiety, anger, and guilt) hinder your ability to function as a helper?

3. *Sensation:* Are there any negative sensations, such as tension, butterflies in your stomach, muscle tightness, light-headedness, blushing, rapid eye blinking, or tapping, that you experience when you are in the helper role?

4. *Imagery:* What pictures or images come to mind when you are helping? Do they bother you? Help you?

5. *Cognition:* What ideas, values, opinions, and attitudes get in the way of your helping? What do you find yourself saying? You may refer to Ellis's list of irrational ideas to see which negative self-statements seem familiar.

6. *Interpersonal relationships:* Write down concerns you have about working with others, your teacher, your classmates, or your supervisor. In class exercises, do you have any problems with the classmates with whom you role-play? When your

teacher observes you, does that inhibit you? Are you more, or less, comfortable as helper, helpee, or observer? Discuss.

7. *Diet/drugs:* Write down any health habits or illness or effects of medication that interfere with your ability to help, such as hangovers or skipping dinner.

What do you learn about yourself as you review what you have written?

EXERCISE 7.30 ■ In small groups, discuss or role-play the following scenarios to determine (1) targets for change and (2) possible action strategies for achieving those changes. (See our comments at the end of the chapter.)

1. A European American graduate student comes to you because she is distressed at her family's rage about her romantic involvement with an African American student. She also feels that other students in the dorm are talking about her behind her back and that she is being shunned by both white and black students.

2. An Asian female worker bursts into tears whenever her boss reprimands her. He is known for being insensitive and harshly demanding. The helpee is experiencing agitation and distress, which increases the likelihood of her making mistakes. One of her peers sent her to you for help. She is uncomfortable talking about her problems with a stranger.

3. An African American parent whose youngster is bussed to school in a predominantly white suburb is upset by the way one of the teachers "talks down" to her. She's conflicted: she wants her child to get a good education, but she feels increasing resentment about incidents she perceives as racist.

4. A middle school teacher comes to you for advice about how to manage one of her classes. A young boy is being scapegoated by all the other kids, who taunt him about being a "queer." The teacher does not know the boy's sexual orientation, but she is anxious about his classroom antics, which elicit these responses and which she finds disruptive. She wonders if she'll ever learn classroom management.

5. An employee in middle management comes to see you because he has been told by his manager that if he doesn't accept a night shift assignment, he may lose his job. This helpee, a loyal, effective employee, has assumed child-care responsibilities in the evenings while his wife goes to her night shift nursing job. His wife cannot change her shift, and he is terrified of angering her and his boss.

The following exercise serves as a review of the criteria on which to base your choice of approach. Remember, the more strategies you can learn to use effectively, the wider the variety of problem situations you can help with.

EXERCISE 7.31 ■ Based on your understanding of this chapter, circle the letter of the strategy(ies) or technique(s) you would consider most appropriate for each of the following cases. Then, in small groups, discuss the reasons for your selections.

Remember, there are no hard-and-fast rules, except for some very specific cases, and even then more than one strategy or technique can be applied. Possible answers are discussed at the end of the chapter.

1. Lisa, age 18, is deathly afraid of flying. She is unable to identify the source of this fear, but she is concerned because her fiancé has accepted an out-of-town job, and she is expected to fly in to see him once a month for the next year.
   a. person-centered therapy
   b. rational-emotive behavior therapy
   c. systematic desensitization
   d. reality therapy
   e. Gestalt therapy
   f. ecological/systems therapy

2. Ms. Rubenstein is feeling anxious because her supervisor has unexpectedly left and the new supervisor hasn't arrived yet. She was very close to her old supervisor and doesn't know anything about the new one. Her work is suffering, and she is scared.
   a. person-centered therapy
   b. rational-emotive behavior therapy
   c. assertiveness training
   d. reality therapy
   e. Gestalt therapy
   f. systems therapy

3. Mr. Delgado, age 45, married with three children, has just been told he'll have to take a 20 percent salary cut in order to keep his job. The firm for which he works has been having difficulty for several months. Because Mr. Delgado's living costs have risen considerably due to inflation, he does not think he can manage on this reduced salary.
   a. person-centered therapy
   b. rational-emotive behavior therapy
   c. decision-making therapy
   d. reality therapy
   e. Gestalt therapy
   f. systematic desensitization

4. Letitia, age 13, is causing her mother great distress because of her low marks and sassy conduct at school and at home. Her mother has come for help because she is "at the end of her rope" and doesn't know what to do.
   a. person-centered therapy
   b. cognitive-behavioral therapy
   c. contract therapy (behavioral)
   d. reality therapy
   e. Gestalt therapy
   f. ecological/systems therapy

5. Phyllis, a 34-year-old divorcée, is unable to pay child-care costs for her son on her salary. However, if she quits work, she won't have any income, because her

ex-husband is out of work and can't help out at all. She doesn't know what to do, and she is very depressed.

a. person-centered therapy
b. rational-emotive behavior therapy
c. assertiveness training
d. reality therapy
e. Gestalt therapy
f. ecological/systems therapy

6. Edward's family has told him he is welcome to come home for Christmas, but his boyfriend, Manuel, is not welcome. This will be the first Christmas that Edward will not be with his family if he decides not to go, and while he prefers to go to Manuel's family, he is feeling hurt and confused by his family's rejection of him as he truly is. Edward's family does not mind seeing Edward with Manuel as "roommates," but they do not want anyone in their extended family to see them together.

a. person-centered therapy
b. cognitive-behavioral therapy
c. assertiveness training
d. reality therapy
e. Gestalt therapy
f. ecological/systems therapy

7. Mr. Agostino feels that his boss is constantly criticizing him in front of others in the office. He works in a small office, can't really get out of sight of his boss, and has become increasingly nervous and distraught.

a. person-centered therapy
b. rational-emotive behavior therapy
c. assertiveness training
d. Gestalt therapy
e. reality therapy
f. cognitive-behavioral modification

8. Martha, age 15, is very angry with her mother. She says her mother is unfair, too punitive, and not at all understanding. Martha's marks in school have dropped considerably this year, and she is much moodier than previously.

a. psychoanalysis
b. person-centered therapy
c. rational-emotive behavior therapy
d. assertiveness training
e. reality therapy
f. Gestalt therapy

9. Tom, age 14, comes for help because he is scared. Several of his friends were involved in a house break-in over the weekend, and although he didn't go into the house, he was outside waiting for his friends to come out. Everybody in town is talking about the vandalism this gang did in the house, and Tom is afraid he'll be implicated sooner or later.

a. psychoanalysis
b. reality therapy

c. rational-emotive behavior therapy

d. person-centered therapy

e. Gestalt therapy

f. cognitive-behavioral therapy

10. Mayda, age 23, is distressed because another love affair has just ended. She feels very sorry for herself and resents this always happening to her. "Every time I get close to or begin to get close to someone, he leaves me."

a. psychoanalysis

b. rational-emotive behavior therapy

c. modeling

d. cognitive-behavioral therapy

e. Gestalt therapy

f. person-centered therapy

11. Larry, age 22, is very angry and bitter because he did not get into graduate school. He feels he had to settle for second best in college, too. Larry says, "I never get what I want. I always end up with second best."

a. psychoanalysis

b. rational-emotive behavior therapy

c. reality therapy

d. person-centered therapy

e. ecological/systems therapy

f. assertiveness training

12. Marianne, age 32, is severely depressed and has not eaten or slept more than a few hours in days. She has a long history of illnesses and a high incidence of absenteeism from work. She doesn't know what's bothering her and just wants to be left alone.

a. psychoanalysis

b. person-centered therapy

c. reality therapy

d. systematic desensitization

e. Gestalt therapy

f. ecological/systems therapy

13. Max, age 18, has been accepted by the four colleges to which he applied. Although he is overjoyed, he is baffled by the need to choose a college and has become increasingly nervous and irritable as the deadline approaches.

a. reality therapy

b. decision-making therapy

c. person-centered therapy

d. rational-emotive behavior therapy

e. assertiveness training

f. Gestalt therapy

14. Ms. Wolfe is the divorced mother of three young children. She's come for help because she can't manage her children and is always losing her temper and slapping them. She feels that 100 percent of her time and energy are devoted to motherhood and that she has no time for herself.

   a. behavioral contracting
   b. rational-emotive behavior therapy
   c. psychoanalysis
   d. systematic desensitization
   e. ecological/systems therapy
   f. person-centered therapy

15. Mr. Esposito has recently been released from a mental hospital. He is having trou-
    ble finding work. He is very nervous and always lets others get ahead of him in
    employment lines.
    a. rational-emotive behavior therapy
    b. assertiveness training
    c. psychoanalysis
    d. cognitive-behavioral modification
    e. person-centered therapy
    f. Gestalt therapy

EXERCISE 7.32 ■ Now go back over these 15 cases and see which of the modalities
from the BASIC ID model you would emphasize as priorities in each case.

SUMMARY

This chapter's brief overview suggests the skills and some criteria necessary
for selection of strategies. We presented examples and exercises to provide an
initial exposure to representative strategies emanating from the helping theories discussed in Chapters 5 and 6. Helpers modify and adjust various com-
binations of effective strategies and techniques according to their own
personalities and preferences, as well as the needs of helpees. The strategies
and techniques discussed in this chapter range from commonsensical (such
as decision making) to complex and powerful, from individual to interpersonal to ecological and systemic. *All* interventions require training, supervision, and experience to be used effectively. Again, it cannot be stressed
enough that there is no one strategy or technique to fit any particular problem. For example, in Exercise 7.31 some interventions appeared to be more
effective than others for each of the situations presented, but a skillful helper
could have effectively adopted many of the possible strategies and techniques for any one problem. The best guidelines are to learn from your own
and others' experiences and to work with whatever seems right to you at the
particular moment.

   The model on which the categorization of strategies in this chapter is based
is the affective-cognitive-behavioral continuum. The helper identifies which
domain is the primary context for the problem and which holds most promise
for its resolution. Everyone's ultimate goal is to function effectively in all three
domains in multiple contexts.

EXERCISE ANSWERS

Exercise 7.18 Numbers 2 and 4, the second part of 6, and numbers 11, 13, and 15 are behavioral statements. The others express subjective conclusions, attitudes, and evaluations.

Exercise 7.24 1. a, 2. c, 3. b, 4. c, 5. b, 6. c, 7. a, 8. b, 9. c, 10. b

Exercise 7.30

1. Possible targets for change might be the graduate student's understanding of white and black racial identity development, her family's attitudes, and her peer group's attitudes. Strategies might include psychoeducation, checking things out with peers, biracial couple support groups, family sessions, small groups in her dorm, and so on.

2. Possible targets of change would be the female worker's feelings of shame regarding seeking help, attitudes in her department, and strategies for dealing with job pressures. Strategies might include empathic validation of her cultural worldview, involving the peer who referred her in change-agent strategies, proposing cultural sensitivity training within the organization, and coaching her about talking to her supervisor.

3. Possible targets are the teacher and other school personnel to become more aware of the impact of their behaviors on parents who already feel "outside"; the perceptions and inferences of the mother; and policies and implementation of the bussing program. Strategies might involve meeting with the teacher and school administrators, joining with the program administrator; becoming more involved with parents' groups, and seeking community supports.

4. Possible targets are the curriculum, the teacher's classroom management, and the students in small groups. Strategies might involve curriculum development and implementation about diversity; bringing in consultants to help the teacher understand her fears and insecurities and suggest better management techniques; and sensitivity training with students.

5. The principal target might be the organization's assignment policies and human resource policies. The major strategy would be to empower the employee to determine his rights and options.

Exercise 7.31   Possible answers are as follows:

1. Systematic desensitization has been proven to be effective with phobias. One can use person-centered therapy at the same time.

2. We would opt for person-centered therapy here, involving the client in a relationship that would reduce her anxiety.

3. Some decision-making and/or reality therapy would be helpful here, examining all the options and values involved so that Mr. Delgado can accept responsibility for taking the cut or looking for a new job.

4. Teaching the mother how to use behavioral contracts may clear up some of the hassling that is occurring at home. We don't know enough to know what the problem is or whose problem it is, but if Letitia becomes the client, reality therapy may be helpful, and if the mother remains the client, cognitive-behavioral techniques can be useful in helping her to clarify her expectations.

5. Except for assertiveness training, any of the strategies could be appropriate in this case. Person-centered therapy could help her feel better about herself, rational-emotive behavior therapy could get her in touch with her irrational ideas, reality therapy could help her with choosing responsible behavior, and Gestalt could enhance her emotional and intellectual awareness. Ecological/systems theories might enable her to locate resources and options.

6. Assertiveness training could help Edward deal with his family; cognitive-behavioral therapy could help him examine his belief systems about families, individualism, authority, relationships, sexual orientation, and so forth. Ecological/systems strategies could help him change the ways he reacts to his family system and not only empower him to feel more comfortable with himself and his decisions but also teach him strategies to find ways to help his family come to terms with who he is.

7. Assertiveness training along with some rational-emotive behavior therapy could be effective here. Cognitive-behavioral modification could reduce his stress by teaching him new verbal self-instructions.

8. In cases such as this, we have found a combination of person-centered therapy and Gestalt therapy to increase insight and self-concept.

9. Reality therapy, person-centered therapy, and/or cognitive-behavioral therapy can be helpful here: the first to help Tom evaluate his own behavior, person-centered to help him feel better about himself, and the last to help him challenge his catastrophizing thoughts.

10. Psychoanalysis or cognitive-behavioral therapy could be helpful here to enable Mayda to gain some insight into patterns of relating and help her to change her thinking about herself, others, and relationships.

11. Again, psychoanalysis or cognitive-behavioral therapy could be helpful here. We'd opt for the cognitive-behavioral therapy, because it sounds as if Larry has made an early decision never to be successful based on faulty assumptions.

12. Psychoanalysis could be helpful here if this has been going on for a long time. Reality therapy could be effective, too, in forcing Marianne to assume some responsibility for her behaviors. Ecological/systems strategies could teach her new interactional patterns.

13. Decision-making therapy is the obvious choice here. Gestalt techniques might supplement this therapy by incorporating affective material into the cognitive elements of decision making.

14. Some rational-emotive behavior therapy or cognitive-behavioral therapy might help here. It sounds as if Ms. Wolfe has some unreasonable ideas about motherhood. Some contracting principles could help her with child management. Ecological/systems strategies might empower her to locate support systems and enable her to broaden her perspectives.

15. Some person-centered therapy could help him gain self-confidence. Assertiveness training would also be useful.

These answers are only suggestions and are open to discussion.

REFERENCES AND FURTHER READING

General

Corey, G. (2005). *Case approach to counseling and psychotherapy* (4th ed.). Belmont, CA: Brooks/Cole.

Corsini, R. J., & Wedding, D. (Eds.). (2005). *Current psychotherapies* (7th ed.). Belmont, CA: Wadsworth.

Okun, B. F. (1990). *Seeking connections in psychotherapy.* San Francisco: Jossey-Bass.

Affective-Cognitive Strategies

Cashdan, S. (1988). *Object relations therapy.* New York: Norton.

Freud, S. (1943). *A general introduction to psychoanalysis.* Garden City, NY: Doubleday.

Freud, S. (1949). *An outline of psychoanalysis.* New York: Norton.

Gabbard, G. (2000). *Psychodynamic psychiatry in clinical practice* (3rd ed.). Washington, DC: American Psychiatric Press.

St. Clair, M., & Wigren, J. (2004). *Object relations and self psychology: An introduction* (4th ed.). Belmont, CA: Brooks/Cole.

Watkins, C. H., Jr. (1983). Transference phenomena in the counseling situation. *Personnel and Guidance Journal, 62,* 206–210.

Affective Strategies

Person-Centered

Carkhuff, R., & Truax, C. (1967). *Toward counseling and psychotherapy: Training and practice.* Chicago: Aldine.

Combs, A. W. (1989). *A theory of therapy: Guidelines for counseling practice.* Newbury Park, CA: Sage.

Farber, B. A., Brink, D. C., & Raskin, P. M. (Eds.). (1996). *The psychotherapy of Carl Rogers: Cases and commentary.* New York: Guilford Press.

Rogers, C. (1951). *Client centered therapy.* Boston: Houghton Mifflin.

Rogers, C. (Ed.). (1967). *The therapeutic relationship and its impact.* Madison: University of Wisconsin Press.

Gestalt

Fagan, J., & Shepherd, I. (Eds.). (1970). *Gestalt therapy now.* Palo Alto, CA: Science and Behavior Books.

Levitsky, A., & Perls, F. (1970). The rules and games of Gestalt therapy. In J. Fagan & I. Shepherd (Eds.), *Gestalt therapy now* (pp. 140–150). Palo Alto, CA: Science and Behavior Books.

Passons, W. (1975). *Gestalt approaches in counseling.* New York: Holt, Rinehart & Winston.

Perls, F. (1969). *Gestalt therapy verbatim.* Moah, UT: Real People Press.

Perls, F. (1973). *The Gestalt approach and eye witness to therapy.* Palo Alto, CA: Science and Behavior Books.

Polster, I., & Polster, M. (1973). *Gestalt therapy integrated.* New York: Brunner/Mazel.

Yontef, G. M. (1993). *Awareness, dialogue and process: Essays on Gestalt therapy.* Highland, NY: Gestalt Journal Press.

Yontef, G. M. (1998). Dialogic Gestalt theory. In L. S. Greenberg, J. C. Watson, & G. Litaer (Eds.), *Handbook of experiential psychotherapy* (pp. 82–102). New York: Guilford Press.

Zinker, J. (1991). Creative process in Gestalt therapy: The therapist as artist. *The Gestalt Journal, 14,* 71–88.

Cognitive and Cognitive-Behavioral Strategies

Alford, B. A., & Beck, A. T. (1997). *The integrative power of cognitive therapy.* New York: Guilford Press.

Barlow, D. H. (Ed.). (2001). *Clinical handbook of psychological disorders: A step-by-step treatment manual* (3rd ed.). New York: Guilford Press.

Beck, A. T. (1976). *Cognitive therapy and emotional disorders.* New York: New American Library.

Beck, J. S. (1995). *Cognitive therapy: Basics and beyond.* New York: Guilford Press.

Ellis, A. (1962). *Reason and emotion in psychotherapy.* New York: Lyle Stuart.

Ellis, A. (1998). *Rational emotive behavior therapy: A therapist's guide.* San Jose, CA: Impact.

Ellis, A. (2005). *Myth of self esteem: How REBT can change your life forever.* Essex, UK: Prometheus Books.

Ellis, A., & Dryden, W. (1987). *The practice of rational-emotive therapy.* Secaucus, NJ: Lyle Stuart.

Ellis, A., & Grieger, R. (1986). *Handbook of rational-emotive therapy* (Vol. 2). New York: Springer.

Ellis, A., & Harper, R. A. (1997). *A guide to rational living* (3rd ed.). North Hollywood, CA: Wilshire Books.

Ellis, A., & Whiteley, J. (Eds.). (1979). *Theoretical and empirical foundations of rational-emotive therapy.* Pacific Grove, CA: Brooks/Cole.

Freeman, A., & Dattilio, F. M. (1992). *Comprehensive casebook of cognitive therapy.* New York: Plenum Press.

Glasser, N. (Ed.). (1989). *Control theory in the practice of reality therapy: Case studies.* New York: Harper & Row.

Glasser, W. (1986). *The control theory–reality therapy workbook.* Canoga Park, CA: Institute for Reality Therapy.

Glasser, W. (1998). *Choice theory: A new psychology of personal freedom.* New York: Harper & Row.

Glasser, W. (2000). *Counseling with choice theory: The new reality therapy.* New York: HarperCollins.

Glasser, W. (2004). *Warning: Psychiatry can be hazardous to your mental health.* New York: HarperCollins.

Maultsby, M. C. (1984). *Rational behavior therapy.* Englewood Cliffs, NJ: Prentice-Hall.

Meichenbaum, D. (1977). *Cognitive behavior modification: An integrative approach.* New York: Plenum Press.

Meichenbaum, D. (1993). Stress inoculation training: A 20 year update. In P. M. Lehre & R. L. Woolfolk (Eds.), *Principles and practice of stress management* (pp. 373–406). New York: Guilford Press.

Meichenbaum, D. (2000). Letter writing, audiotaping and videotaping as therapist tools: Use of healing metaphors. In M. J. Scott & S. Palmer (Eds.), *Trauma and post traumatic stress disorder* (pp. 96–102). Newbury Park, CA: Sage.

Meichenbaum, D., & Goodman, R. (1971). Training impulsive children to talk to themselves: A means of developing self-control. *Journal of Abnormal Psychology, 77,* 115–126.

Persons, J. B., Davidson, J., & Tompkins, M. A. (2000). *Essential components of cognitive-behavior therapy for depression.* Washington, DC: American Psychological Association.

Wubbolding, R. E. (2000). *Reality therapy for the 21st century.* Muncie, IN: Accelerated Development (Taylor & Francis).

Behavioral Strategies

Alberti, R., & Emmons, M. (2001). *Your perfect right: A guide to assertive action* (8th ed.). Atascadero, CA: Impact.

Homme, L. (1970). *Use of contingency contracting in the classroom.* Champaign, IL: Research Press.

Kanfer, F. H., & Goldstein, A. P. (Eds.). (1986). *Helping people change: A textbook of methods.* New York: Pergamon Press.

Kazdin, A. E. (2001). *Behavior modification in applied settings* (6th ed.). Belmont, CA: Wadsworth.

Spiegler, M. D., & Guevremont, D. C. (2003). *Contemporary behavior therapy* (4th ed.). Pacific Grove, CA: Brooks/Cole.

Sulzer-Azaroff, B., & Mayer, G. (1977). *Applying behavior analysis procedures with children and youth.* New York: Holt, Rinehart & Winston.

Watson, D. L., & Tharp, R. G. (2002). *Self-directed behavior: Self-modification for personal adjustment* (8th ed.). Pacific Grove, CA: Brooks/Cole.

Wolpe, J. (1990). *The practice of behavior therapy* (4th ed.). New York: Pergamon Press.

Strategies That Cut Across Domains
Eclectic and Multimodal Strategies

Corey, G. (2001). *The art of integrative counseling.* Pacific Grove, CA: Brooks/Cole.

Ivey, A. E. (1991). *Developmental strategies for helpers: Individual, family, and network interventions.* Pacific Grove, CA: Brooks/Cole.

Lazarus, A. (1976). *Multimodal behavior therapy.* New York: Springer-Verlag.

Lazarus, A. (1989). *The practice of multimodal therapy.* Baltimore: Johns Hopkins University Press.

Lazarus, A. (1997). *Brief but comprehensive psychotherapy: The multimodal way.* New York: Springer.

Ecological and Systems Strategies

Haley, J. (1976). *Problem-solving therapy.* San Francisco: Jossey-Bass.

Madanes, C. (1984). *Strategic family therapy.* San Francisco: Jossey-Bass.

Minuchin, S., & Fishman, H. C. (1981). *Techniques of family therapy.* Cambridge, MA: Harvard University Press.

Norcross, J. C., & Goldfried, I. R. (Eds.). (1992). *Handbook of psychotherapy integration.* New York: Basic Books.

Prochaska, J. O., & Norcross, J. C. (2003). *Systems of psychotherapy: A transtheoretical analysis* (5th ed.). Pacific Grove: Brooks/Cole.

Satir, V. (1967). *Conjoint family therapy* (2nd ed.). Palo Alto, CA: Science and Behavior Books.

Steenbarger, B. N. (1993). A multicontextual model of counseling: Bridging brevity and diversity. *Journal of Counseling and Development, 72,* 8–15.

Sue, D. W., & Sue, D. (2003). *Counseling the culturally diverse: Theory and practice* (4th ed.). New York: Wiley.

Wachtel, E. F., & Wachtel, P. L. (1986). *Family dynamics in individual therapy: A guide to clinical strategies.* New York: Guilford Press.

Wachtel, P. L. (1997). *Psychoanalysis, behavior therapy and the relational world.* Washington, DC: American Psychological Association.

Visit the book companion site at www.thomsonedu.com to access tutorial quizzes.

8

Stage 2:
Applying Strategies

The boundary line between the first (relationship) and second (strategy) stages of the helping relationship is not distinct. You will know when you are at the point of crossing the boundary when you are able to focus on identifiable problems, when you find yourself thinking "OK, now that we know what the trouble is, what can we do about it?" Remember that you do not want to rush into the strategy stage until you have clearly ascertained and clarified the helpee's problem and until you have agreement from the helpee that he or she wants to do something about it.

In this chapter, we will examine the six steps in applying strategies during the second, strategy stage of the helping relationship. These six steps are (1) mutual acceptance of defined goals and objectives, (2) planning of strategies, (3) use of strategies, (4) evaluation of strategies, (5) termination, and (6) follow-up. At the end of the chapter, we'll examine some case studies that will take you through the steps of both the relationship stage and the strategy stage. We will integrate the theories we have studied with the strategies.

STEP 1: MUTUAL ACCEPTANCE OF
DEFINED GOALS AND OBJECTIVES

The helping relationship must focus on areas of concern to the helpee, not on concerns that the helper thinks the helpee ought to work on. This necessity may become a serious issue in some organizational settings where a conflict may exist between organizational policies, which you as the helper may represent, and the needs of the helpee. For example, if you are working in a correctional institution and are sent an inmate who is causing some disruption and is seen as a "troublemaker who must be changed," you may find that you and this inmate have different objectives. Yours may be, of institutional necessity, to help the inmate conform to the system, whereas the inmate's objectives may be to disrupt and get whatever attention results from the disruption. No one can tell you how to handle this kind of conflict, but you really have to think it out and come to a decision with which you are comfortable.

If the client is limited by managed care to a specified number of sessions and you both think that you cannot meet the agreed-upon objectives within that time period, you need to decide among (1) redefining your objectives, (2) making arrangements for meeting privately beyond the number of reimbursable sessions, (3) seeking authorization for further sessions from the managed care company, or (4) making a referral. Some managed care contracts preclude private sessions.

It is important to have a theoretical rationale for your understanding of the client's problem and definition of goals and objectives. This theoretical framework will help lead you to a specific choice of strategies. Your theoretical framework can be inclusive rather than exclusive. By that, we mean you can have an understanding of a client's individual problems within the affective, cognitive, and/or behavioral domains, along with an understanding of person/environment difficulties. You can integrate individual strategies with ecological/systems strategies. Also remember that in order to be of help you must have a strong helping relationship, and that building this relationship involves identifying goals and objectives that are accepted by all involved parties. Strategies and techniques will not be as effective if a strong helping relationship does not exist.

The following examples illustrate negative outcomes when this first step is not taken into consideration.

> Mary and Tom entered counseling with an accredited marriage counselor for intensive sex therapy. Their objective was to improve their sexual relationship. The counselor felt that he needed to explore the dynamics of their marital relationship, because he believed the underlying problems in the marital relationship were maintaining the sexual dysfunction. When Mary and Tom achieved success through some behavioral sex therapy, they wished to terminate the therapy. They became upset when the counselor suggested they remain in treatment for more intensive marriage counseling. The point is that the helper and the helpees had not clarified the nature and extent of the problem and treatment. Thus, what began as an effective helping relationship ended with confusion and misunderstanding on both sides.

> Lisa, age 25, was admitted to a state rehabilitation counseling program for job training after her release from a state hospital psychiatric unit. Her understanding was that this program consisted of coursework and job counseling as well as placement advice. When the six-week group human

relations course was completed, Lisa expected to receive some résumé and job-seeking skill counseling. The counselor told her to look at the ads in the newspaper every day and that he would check in with her by phone once a week. After several weeks of no contact from the counselor and no job possibilities, Lisa's symptoms of suicidal depression began to reappear. Investigation by the welfare worker indicated that the printed information about this program, the verbal promises of the counselor, and the actual circumstances were incongruent. Again, the lack of clearly specified goals and objectives resulted in pain and illness rather than growth and health.

John went to a vocational counselor for tests, to help him make a career decision. He was very disturbed when the counselor tried to get him to talk about his personal feelings and lifestyle instead of presenting him with factual results of his interest and aptitude tests. After the third session, he quit and decided to go elsewhere. This is another example in which the counselor's approach and focus were not consistent with the client's understanding of what the sessions would involve.

Ms. Escadero agreed to have her daughter, Christina (age 8), work with a volunteer aide for individualized help. Ms. Escadero thought that Christina would receive some academic skills help in reading and arithmetic. The aide was told by the classroom teacher that her objective was to "develop a relationship with Christina to improve her self-concept." The aide played games with Christina and took her for walks. Christina's social skills improved and she seemed happier in her class, but her mother became angry when she found out that academic tutoring was not occurring and insisted that the relationship terminate. This case is still another example of what may happen when objectives of a helping relationship are not clarified.

EXERCISE 8.1 ■ Discuss in small groups how you could handle the preceding four cases in a different manner. Act out different approaches, and share your feelings and reactions. How can you be sure that the helpee really accepts the goals and objectives and is not just trying to please you?

Here is another example of the importance of the first step of the strategy stage.

Lauren was referred to a counselor in May of her senior year in high school. The presenting problems were promiscuity and possible pregnancy. (However, it turned out that Lauren was not pregnant.) In the first three sessions, the counselor discovered that Lauren had a very low self-concept; received little, if any, positive feeling from her parents (who were divorced); had no close girlfriends despite her popularity; and was, in fact, quite the opposite of her outward image of a beautiful, talented, bright, "model" teenager. Lauren has just expressed some concerns about going away to college in the fall.

Counselor: You're wondering if you're going to be able to find the kinds of friends and relationships you want there without getting into trouble.

Lauren: I'm not sure I'll be able to handle difficult situations when they come up. I always get messed up.

Counselor: You really don't think much of yourself.

Lauren: (*laughs nervously*) I know . . . it's just that sometimes I try to think so much, I get awfully confused.

Counselor: Well, we have eight weeks left before you leave, and we've agreed to meet weekly. How about if we focus on talking about your concerns and situations as they come up, and see if we can help you to feel better about yourself before you go away?

Lauren: I'm already feeling better since I've been coming in here. I do want to make it on my own next year.

In this case, the counselor and Lauren decide that the major goal will be to increase Lauren's self-confidence and to afford her the opportunity to receive empathy and support from the counselor.

STEP 2: PLANNING OF STRATEGIES

The second step of the strategy stage is similar to the decision-making process; in both instances, we think of all the possible options and then select the most effective strategy or combination of strategies. We try to determine which strategy is best for *this* individual at *this* time, given our understanding of the client, his or her problem, our theoretical orientation, and the treatment context. The client's participation in this decision making increases the possibilities for successful outcomes. We carefully explain to the helpee the approaches we are considering, their rationale, possible consequences, time and activities involved, and any other pertinent information. If the helpee seems to be resistant to some interventions, we discuss the resistance and then decide together whether to hold off or tentatively try them out. Some strategies and techniques may seem threatening at first but become less so as the helping relationship develops. For example, we often use Gestalt techniques. Unless the relationship is well established and the client trusts us and our professional ability, a common response to the suggestion that we engage in a particular Gestalt dialogue or role play is "That's silly; I can't do that." Sometimes, if strategies have not been adequately explained, helpees get scared away because they do not understand what is going on. If the helper describes techniques in a tentative way, the helpee can refuse without losing dignity or self-respect.

Timing and manner of introducing alternative approaches are important factors in planning strategies, as illustrated in the following example.

Helper: We seem to agree that one of the immediate goals you want to work toward is to be able to say "no" to people, to see if we can find some other ways for you to feel good about yourself so you won't always have to buy friendship.

Client: Yeah. My way certainly hasn't worked either.

Helper: Evelyn, I wonder if we can do some role playing and practice what you might say to Benny the next time he calls you.

Client: Sure. What do you mean?

Helper: Well, I'll be Benny, and I've called you to have you come up for the weekend. Now what do you really want to say to me?

Here the helper has given the helpee an outlet. The relationship is such that the helpee knows she will not be rejected if she does not go along, but because she believes that the helper knows what she is doing, she is willing to go along and try something new.

Another example of strategy planning can be drawn from the case of Lauren.

Counselor: Lauren, in addition to our talking about you and what's happening in your life in the session, I'd like to ask you to keep a diary. If each night you'll write down all the things that happened that day to help you feel good about yourself, it will be helpful.

Lauren: I don't know if there'll be any, but I'm willing to try.

Counselor: We can go over your list when you come in. It might help us both to find out what pleases you. To get started, I'd like you to draw up a list of all the things you like about yourself. You don't have to show it to anyone, and you can bring it in next week.

Lauren: OK.

The purpose of this "homework assignment" is to help Lauren focus on her strengths. It also provides some continuity between sessions.

EXERCISE 8.2 ■ How would you plan strategies for the helpees in the preceding two examples? Role-play the scenes, and then create your own cases that you can act out. Discuss in small groups the criteria and reasons for your selections. Remember that there is not just one intervention for any one problem. There are times when helpers try something that both parties agree to and find it doesn't work very well. However, if the relationship is effective, this does not need to be viewed as a failure. In fact, gains can be made by talking about what did not work, and then the strategy-planning step can be repeated.

STEP 3: USE OF STRATEGIES

A particular strategy or combination of strategies may be used for short-term or long-term goals. The helper may spontaneously decide to change strategies, and this is fine, as long as the helpee knows what is going on and agrees to the change. Often, the helper's intuition sparks appropriate selection of techniques midway through this step. For example, several years ago I (BFO) was using systematic desensitization with a college physical education student who had a phobic reaction to balloons and who found that she needed to be able to tolerate being in the same room with balloons during some school affairs. She was an excellent candidate for systematic desensitization and responded beautifully. One day after a successful session, while she was still relaxed, I asked her to engage in some Gestalt dialogues with balloons. She was equally responsive to this technique, and we both learned some important information about her aversion to balloons. I also learned that relaxation facilitates Gestalt dialoguing.

As you gain experience as a helper, your self-confidence in the use of strategies will increase and you will feel more comfortable trying out new techniques. However, do not be afraid to let the helpee know if you are trying something you have not used before. You can say something like "I have a new idea that we can try, but I'm not sure how it will work. Let's try it out and see if it works." It is important to arrange for some supervision or consultation from someone more experienced with a particular strategy. Pretending to be an expert when you're not can backfire, and even if it doesn't, it is ethically questionable. However, if you restrict yourself to the familiar and comfortable, you won't be able to extend your capabilities. In any case, for both your benefit and the helpee's, any significant use of new strategies should be accomplished carefully and under the guidance or supervision of someone who is qualified in that particular area. If you reach a point in counseling where you believe the client would benefit from a strategy you do not know well or a modality, such as group therapy, that you are not offering, it may be appropriate to refer.

It is impossible to say how much of the entire helping relationship will be devoted to using strategies—it may be a little; it may be a lot. The amount of time available for each session, as well as for the entire relationship, affects the use of strategies. The nature of the problem and the setting in which you work have a major impact. Some strategies can be used in a shorter time span than others: behavioral strategies are relatively short term, whereas psychoanalytic and client-centered strategies can last indefinitely. It seems that those strategies that lean toward the behavioral domain are more specifically evaluated and easier to limit to a particular time frame; strategies that lean toward the affective domain take a longer time for application.

Strategies facilitate learning. Coupled with a strong helping relationship, they can expedite the helpee's emotional, cognitive, or behavioral changes.

EXERCISE 8.3 ▪ The purpose of this exercise is to give you some experience in planning and using strategies. In triads, rotate the roles of helper, helpee, and observer. You can choose your settings and circumstances, but assume that both helper and helpee have agreed to one of the following goals for the helping relationship. After selecting an objective, role-play it as far as you can. Assume that you already have an effective helping relationship. What strategies would you want to use? How would you want to use them? Discuss your choice and use of strategies in small groups. Here are the goals:

1. To learn how to make friends of the opposite sex

2. To get to work on time

3. To get homework assignments in on time

4. To learn how to get along better with the boss

5. To decide whether to tell your parents that you are seriously involved with a romantic partner of another race

6. To decide whether to have a baby

7. To try to control anger when things don't go your way

STEP 4: EVALUATION
OF STRATEGIES

Evaluation (assessing the effectiveness) of strategies is ongoing from the beginning of their use. If at any time both helper and helpee feel that the strategies are not effective, it is necessary to review and reassess the situation. However, it sometimes takes a while for something to work, and a sensitive helper knows when to apply evaluation criteria.

Evaluation of counseling effectiveness has always been difficult because counseling strategies (except for behavioral strategies) do not always produce observable changes. Actual behavior changes provide the best criteria for evaluating strategies. These behavior changes can be reflections of emotional and cognitive changes. Self-report alone can be deceptive; we may be fooled by some people who say they feel good because they want to please us. Increasingly, third-party payers are requiring documentation that counseling outcomes have been attained. Written records measuring behavior changes can satisfy this requirement. We can almost always tell if something has been effective by observing behavior.

Behavioral change is not limited to the helping relationship; it can generalize to other situations in the helpee's life. The helpee may report change or the helper may hear about it from significant others, such as a supervisor, parent, spouse, or teacher. The helper and helpee can seek objective criteria for evaluating change and can validate these criteria rather than take effectiveness for granted. The timing of evaluation is important because realistically some ups and downs are to be expected during the course of a helping relationship, and new behaviors, attitudes, and thoughts take time to become stable.

The results of an evaluation may prompt the helper to decide to use another strategy, work on some other objectives and goals, or terminate the helping relationship. The helpee participates in the selection of one of those outcomes.

The following example illustrates the strategy evaluation step.

Dr. Jovanovic is a 52-year-old dentist who came for help when his 22-year-old son dropped out of everything he had previously been involved with and joined a religious cult. Terribly distressed, Dr. Jovanovic didn't understand what had gone wrong and how this could have happened to his family. The counselor has been using rational-emotive techniques and assigning homework to Dr. Jovanovic to dispute his irrational ideas. This excerpt is from the ninth session.

Helper: I'm wondering how things are going at home for you now.

Client: They're beginning to change. Every time I start to think or say that my wife or one of the kids *should* be or do something, I catch myself and shudder at that awful word "should."

Helper: And what happens?

Client: I don't get so angry anymore. I keep telling myself that everyone doesn't have to be perfect all the time and neither do I. Also, things don't always have to go my way. I'm beginning to believe it.

Helper: (*laughs*) You're learning.

Client: Well, my wife says things are much pleasanter, and we don't have so much quarreling at the dinner table.

In this case, the helper is evaluating the effectiveness of some strategies and, in addition to learning whether the strategy is working, gaining some insights into future directions of this helping relationship.

EXERCISE 8.4 ■ The purpose of this exercise is to familiarize you with evaluative criteria. For the following objectives of helping relationships, pick out what you think would be appropriate evaluative criteria. More than one answer is acceptable. Suggested answers are at the end of the chapter. Discuss your answers and reasons for them in small groups.

1. Objective: Learning to get along better with coworkers
    Criteria: a. Fewer complaints from supervisor
        b. Positive report from helpee
        c. Your observation of friendlier relationships in department
        d. Your observation of helpee in cafeteria engaged in friendly relations with coworkers

2. Objective: Feeling less depressed
    Criteria: a. Client improves appearance
        b. Client reports feeling better
        c. Client reports more involvement in activities
        d. Client doesn't cry as much

3. Objective: Increasing self-understanding
    Criteria: a. Client reports feeling better
        b. Client wants to continue sessions

        c. Client talks in sessions with more assurance and confidence

        d. Client reports better interpersonal relationships

4.   Objective: Learning to make friends of opposite sex

     Criteria: a. Client talks about going to singles' bars

             b. Client reports making a date for tonight

             c. Client asks if your receptionist is single

             d. Client says he has struck up a conversation with a girl in his class

5.   Objective: Improving marital happiness

     Criteria: a. Client says spouse doesn't nag so much anymore

             b. Clients report they spend more time together

             c. Clients say during counseling sessions that their communication is good outside of sessions

             d. Clients report they try but never complete homework exercises

STEP 5: TERMINATION

Termination is an important part of the helping relationship; some believe that all of therapy, from the first session, should be viewed as preparing for termination. If termination is not acknowledged and handled appropriately, helpees may end up with more distress and unresolved issues than when they entered the helping relationship.

Termination of Session

It has been said that one can tell how counselors and clients will handle the final termination process by how they handle the end of each session. Several minutes before the end of the session, it is important for the helper to communicate nonverbally or verbally to the helpee that the allotted time is almost up. This allows for summarization of what has occurred during the session, to be sure that both parties are clearly in accord, and for assigning between-session tasks or planning for future sessions. In sessions that have been particularly "heavy" or emotional, both helper and helpee need time to regain composure so as to comfortably make the transition back to the outside world.

    Helpers may have to set clear limits with the ending time, so that clients do not have their "hand on the doorknob" and continue to talk after the session is formally over. Helpers may need to process with certain clients their tendency to stop talking several minutes before the end or with other clients their pattern of bringing up difficult issues moments before the end of each session.

Termination of the Helping Relationship

Evaluation of the results or progress of the application of strategies may lead to termination of the helping relationship. Termination can occur in one of four ways.

1. Both helper and helpee feel that all objectives have been reached. This is a positive, mutual termination, albeit one involving sadness because of the loss of a meaningful relationship. Sad feelings usually occur in both helper and helpee, and both may experience some anxiety about the impending loss of a significant other and the uncertainty of the future. These feelings should be explored and shared so that both can leave each other feeling the sense of growth and satisfaction that comes from the achievement of objectives. It is important for both parties to know when the last meeting will occur and to leave enough time to discuss their feelings.

2. The helper initiates termination before the objectives have been achieved. This happens often in schools when a term ends or an internship concludes or in settings where the personnel changes frequently and rapidly. In these cases, it is essential that the helper inform the helpee as soon as possible of the impending termination and that they both fully explore the feelings aroused by this necessity. The helpee often feels angry and rejected, and the helper often feels guilty and uncomfortable. It is useful to review what gains the helpee has made in the relationship and what can be anticipated in a new helping relationship. Ideally, the helper arranges for a referral before termination occurs. If the helper has had an effective relationship with the helpee, it will be that much easier for the helpee to work effectively with someone else.

3. Termination is necessitated and determined by a third party to the helping process. For example, a health care plan allows one or two sessions for evaluation. The helper and the helpee agree on the nature, goals, and objectives of the helping relationship, and the health plan administrator informs the helper and the helpee how many sessions will be allowed. In this type of situation, the number of sessions may be known in advance of the strategy phase so that adjustments may be made in the selection and implementation of strategies or anytime during the strategy phase. Though the termination may be in the best economic interests of the health care plan, it is not necessarily in the best interests of the helpee or in accordance with the helper's professional judgment. Another version of this type of termination is when the helpee switches health insurance and the helper is no longer on the panel. While some insurance plans will allow the helper to continue, most give only a few sessions, if any, to plan for termination. Even if the helper offers a sliding scale fee, many clients cannot afford these out-of-pocket costs and will decide to go to a new therapist who is covered by their insurance. It is important that the frustration and anger that the helper and helpee may feel in these situations not interfere with the processing of the work and relationship that have been achieved.

4. The helpee terminates the relationship prematurely. In this case, the helpee may be escaping from a threatening situation, leaving the helper feeling useless and inadequate. If premature termination seems likely, the helper must try to determine whose problem this premature termination is; it

might be the helpee's problem if he or she refuses to work anymore and chooses avoidance over approach. On the other hand, it might be the helper's problem in that he or she has been unable to develop an effective helping relationship or has selected an inappropriate strategy.

In any of these kinds of termination, helpers can provide positive support to the helpee and communicate interest in being of assistance should the need for help arise in the future.

For the first two types of termination, Ward (1984) has conceptualized four steps that can facilitate and strengthen outcomes of the helping relationship.

1. *Evaluation of goal attainment* is a mutually shared process in which helper and helpee specifically check to see whether the presenting problems or symptoms have been reduced or eliminated. The helpee is encouraged to list specific behavioral changes made during the helping process and to discuss his or her thoughts and feelings about those changes. Helpees may be asked to refer to previous assignments, such as a written journal or audio- or videotapes, or to check out changes with significant others. The next part of this assessment process can be to talk about how resolution of the presenting problems has affected the helpee's self-esteem, relationships with others, work or school functioning, and ability to plan the next steps in life. This step may take several sessions, particularly for helpees working on growing up, individuation/separation, and dependency/independence issues.

2. *Closure of relationship issues* requires talking about the helpee's feelings about the helper and the helping relationship. These feelings can probably be related to other relationships, separations, and losses in the helpee's life experience and may arouse powerful emotions. When appropriate, the helper can disclose his or her feelings about the helpee and impending termination. This is a step that requires much discussion and contributes to achieving the ability to express and experience an appropriate and meaningful good-bye to a significant person.

3. *Preparation for self-reliance and transfer of learning* includes specific planning for the future. How is the helpee going to take his or her new learning to the outside world? What kinds of supportive relationships can the helpee develop and maintain? A number of our clients have told us that they have internal dialogues with us whenever they get into a bind. Other clients contract with themselves or others. We often ask clients to imagine future problems and deal with them through imagery in a session. We leave open the possibility that at some point in the future they might decide to contact us, letting them know that it will not be perceived as a "failure" if they decide to come back.

4. *The final session* is the culmination of the preparation and often includes lighter, more social discussion. Often, I (BFO) give the client a memento, such as a poster, that is significant as a reminder of the work we've done together. We specifically plan for follow-up evaluation and discuss whether there is a possibility of follow-up telephone or session contact.

Some helpers extend terminations over several weeks. For example, they may lengthen the time between sessions by reducing weekly sessions to biweekly sessions, then to monthly sessions, then to one session every three months. Extending termination has the effect of reducing anxiety and providing follow-up and evaluation while maintaining necessary support. However, helpers must be aware of the possibility that the helpee's dependency needs may be prolonging the helping relationship. Helpers may need to set some limits in order to avoid reinforcing those dependency needs.

The same conditions necessary for the success of the initial contact in a helping relationship (encouragement, warmth, focusing on the helpee's needs) are necessary for the final contact. It is all right for you to share your true feelings with helpees and let them know that you will miss them, too.

The following is an excerpt from the end of the final session with Lauren.

Counselor: You've come a long way this summer.
Lauren: I feel so good about myself, and I'm looking forward to college. Did I tell you I found out the name of my roommate?
Counselor: No, but that does make it more real. You're looking forward to making new friends and a new life.
Lauren: I think everything's going to be fine. If I need to, can I come see you?
Counselor: Of course, you know how to reach me. Listen, you've worked through some tough situations this summer. We both know you can do it.
Lauren: Yes, that's true. I'm going to miss you.
Counselor: I'm going to miss you, too. Let me know how you're doing, OK?
Lauren: Sure thing.

The counselor leaves the door open so Lauren may come back at any time, and the counselor feels free to express sadness at the end of the relationship.

If the client abruptly ends the relationship by not showing up for an appointment and not contacting the counselor, the counselor may attempt contact by phone or letter to see if the client was testing his or her concern and interest or needed reassurance for some other reason; it may be possible to schedule at least one more session to work through unresolved issues, make a referral, or at the very least gain some understanding of the reasons for termination.

EXERCISE 8.5 ■ Pick as a partner someone you feel particularly close to, someone with whom you have shared information about yourself. Find a place where you can spend some time together and role-play helper and helpee roles, with each of you having the opportunity to play each role. Pretend this is the last time you will meet together, and see how effectively you can share your feelings and concerns. Does this exercise remind you of other experiences in your life? How do you usually cope with separation anxiety? Discuss your reactions to this exercise with other people in your group.

EXERCISE 8.6 ▪ This is a Gestalt exercise to put you in touch with feelings of separation anxiety. Take something out of your purse or pocket that is very necessary to you (your wallet, your car or house keys). Put that article under your chair, lean back, and close your eyes. Now imagine that you are not going to retrieve that article and that you need it. Let yourself get in touch with the panicky feelings that emerge, and try to experience these feelings for several minutes. Then discuss the exercise with others.

EXERCISE 8.7 ▪ With a partner, identify 5 to 10 interactions you have had in the last week. Describe how they ended. Who or what ended them? What kinds of feelings did you have? These interactions may have been over the telephone, in person, or even by letter. For the coming week, try to become more aware of how you end telephone and personal contacts.

EXERCISE 8.8 ▪ How have you handled good-byes? Think back to friends who have moved away or have gone to different schools. Have you ever gotten into an argument as a way of dealing with the loss? Have you tried to deny that someone was leaving, perhaps by getting so busy you did not make time to say good-bye in person? When you do say good-bye in a direct way with someone you might not see again, what do you talk about with that person? Select a partner and share what you have learned about how you handle termination.

STEP 6: FOLLOW-UP

Follow-up involves checking to see how the helpee is doing, with respect to whatever the problem was, some time after termination has occurred. This is a step that many helpers do not take. However, some work settings require formal follow-up by mail or telephone. And in other work settings where follow-up is not required, many helpers informally do their own by dropping in on former helpees to say hello and see how everything is, dropping them a note, or giving them a call.

Here again, the helper must distinguish between genuine follow-up and extension of a helpee's or helper's possible dependency. The purpose of follow-up is to evaluate long-term effects of helping strategies and the effectiveness of the helper. Occasionally, follow-up will result in additional helping; in most cases, however, it simply serves as an evaluation of both helper and helpee. It is a form of recognition that both parties can appreciate, in that it can communicate genuine caring and interest.

We generally telephone former clients six months to a year after termination to let them know we've been thinking of them and are wondering how they are. We allow enough time for them to fill us in on developments in their lives, and we check to see if they have been able to use what they learned from the helping relationship in other aspects of their lives.

Now that we've briefly discussed each of the six steps of the strategy stage of the helping relationship, we'll do an exercise that reviews all six of them.

EXERCISE 8.9 ■ The purpose of this exercise is to help you recognize the different steps of the strategy stage. Which step do you think each of the following numbered excerpts represents? The answers are at the end of the chapter.

1. **Helper:** Hello, Mr. Witkins. This is Mr. _____ calling. How are you?

    Client: Oh! . . . I'm fine, thank you. How are you?

    Helper: I guess you're surprised to hear from me. I've been thinking about you and wondering how everything is going.

    Client: Well, everything is real OK. I've been working since March, and I really like it . . . in the accounting office of _____ Associates. The hours and pay are better than the last job, and I'm home to help out more after supper with the kids.

    Helper: Are you and your wife getting out together more now?

    Client: Oh, yes. We make a point of going out alone once a week. And we're beginning to have company in now, too. Things really have been better since I found the new job. And I have to thank you for seeing me through that rough period.

    Helper: Well, I'm glad I called. Hope things continue to go well for you. Give my regards to your wife.

    Client: Thanks. Appreciate your calling.

2. **Client:** I'm really in a bind. There's no place for the old man to go. We can't afford a home, and Jim's brother is out of the country, and I'm just stuck, that's all.

    Helper: Let's focus on what we can do to make this situation tolerable for you and your family. Since, as you say, your father-in-law's residing with you is a given . . .

    Client: Yes, I need to learn not to react so much, not to get so upset every time he says or does anything. I know it's not good for Jim and the children, but I just can't help myself.

    Helper: OK. We'll focus on the home situation before we talk about your idea of getting a job.

3. **Helper:** How'd you do on your last math test?

    Client: I passed it! And my homework assignments are OK.

    Helper: Do you feel you're meeting the terms of the contract?

    Client: There was one day I didn't do my work. I just went without watching TV. I didn't like that, though, because the next day my friend Jeff told me I missed a great game.

    Helper: What are you going to do about that?

    Client: I'm not going to miss any more.

4. **Helper:** It sounds to me like somebody once told you when you were a kid that it's not OK to cry.

   Client: I never cry. Yes, I remember something happened when I was very little, around 4 or maybe even 3.

   Helper: I'd like to try a role-play with you that may get us in touch with that early decision. OK?

   Client: Sure.

   Helper: Now be that little girl and tell me what happened.

   Client: I left my doll carriage on the driveway, and my dad ran over it when he came home that night.

   Helper: Go on.

   Client: I cried . . . and he came up to me and hit me . . . and he said I'll show you what happens to little girls who leave their doll carriage on the driveway and cry. And he took the doll off the driveway—it was a raggedy type of doll—and he tore her apart and threw her away.

   Helper: And you decided never to cry again.

   Client: (*crying*) Poor little girl.

   Helper: (*throwing her a large cushion*) This is your dad. Be that little girl and tell him what you want to tell him.

5. **Helper:** We have only two more sessions together. I'm wondering how you feel about that.

   Client: Well, in a way I'm glad, and in a way I'm not sure. I think I'm doing much better. I don't get stoned anymore. But every now and then, I get scared . . . and lonely. I think I'll take your suggestion and join that group you were telling me about.

   Helper: We can use the next two sessions to talk more about that, if you'd like.

6. **Helper:** What often works in cases like yours is what we call systematic desensitization. Have you ever heard of it?

   Client: No.

   Helper: It's a form of counterconditioning. I teach you how to relax each of your muscle groups, and when you're able to master that, we begin to imagine all aspects of flying while you're relaxed. It's impossible to be anxious and relaxed at the same time, and this is a technique that can be used whenever you're anxious. I have a paper you can read about it.

   Client: How long does it take?

   Helper: It usually takes about three sessions for relaxation, and then somewhere between 10 and 15 sessions for desensitization. I often use other techniques along with desensitization, but we can see as we go along.

   Client: I'm willing to try.

EXERCISE 8.10 ■ Select a partner with whom you have already established some degree of trust. One of you will be the helper and the other the helpee. Work through the following steps; then reverse roles and start the steps again.

1. Helpee suggests a problem to work on.

2. Using responsive listening, the helper explores and clarifies the problem with the helpee.

3. The helper restates the problem in terms that are clear, goal directed, and acceptable to the helpee.

4. The helper and helpee proceed to break down this problem into a specific goal statement.

5. Next, the helper aids the helpee in identifying the psychological needs of both parties in this helping relationship (for example, the need to be liked, the need to be successful, the need to control).

6. The helper suggests at least three different helping strategies that will meet the previously identified psychological needs of the helpee.

7. Next, the helper suggests at least three different helping strategies that will meet the previously identified psychological needs of the helper.

8. Then the helper, in collaboration with the helpee, determines whether any strategies have been suggested that will meet the needs of both helpee and helper. If possible, the helper selects the one strategy that will best meet the needs of both parties in the helping relationship.

9. Once a strategy has been selected, determine who is going to do what, and when and where he or she is going to do it. Determine what the terms of the relationship and the interventions will be and how you will know if and when the problem is resolved.

The purpose of the preceding exercise is to show you that the needs of both parties in the helping relationship must be taken into account when selecting strategies. For example, a helper who has a need to be liked and to refrain from expressing emotion might not select a Gestalt strategy even if that strategy is likely to be most effective for this particular helpee at this particular time. The more one is in touch with one's own values and needs, the more aware one is of the reasons for choosing particular helping strategies.

CASE STUDIES

Five brief case studies will now be presented to show how counseling progresses through the relationship and strategy stages. These five case studies have been selected to illustrate the steps in building a relationship and applying strategies. You will note that the steps flow freely into one another and often you go back one or two steps and then return. The names and identifying information in these case studies have been changed to protect the clients' identities.

The Case of Ms. Souza

Ms. Souza, age 48, was referred to this counselor by her counselor at the outpatient clinic of a state hospital because her counselor was leaving the state. Ms. Souza had been in and out of treatment for 10 years, although she had never been hospitalized. She was diagnosed as being depressed with phobic reactions. For 10 years she had refused to leave her home except with her husband, a truck driver for a large baking firm. Thus, all her marketing, shopping, and other errands were done with her husband, who worked an early shift and was home by 4 P.M. Ms. Souza lived in a lower-middle-class neighborhood with her mother (age 82), her husband (age 52), and her 22-year-old son who has developmental disabilities. At this particular time, a crisis had arisen because Mr. Souza was being transferred to another route, which would involve him in work all day and not leave time for marketing at Ms. Souza's favorite small markets.

Session 1 Mr. Souza drove Ms. Souza to the session and arrived a few minutes late. He waited outside in the car. Ms. Souza apologized for being late, took a while to get comfortable, and then sat primly with her hands folded on her lap. Because she seemed to expect to be questioned and because I (BFO) already had background information, I asked her to tell me about what she had been doing all day. (*initiation/entry*) Very slowly, she told me about her sewing, her cleaning, and the time her son and mother took. Her great joy and pride in life was her cooking, and she was very fussy about the foods she bought and what she cooked. She refused to shop in supermarkets; she had known the vendors where she marketed for years and could depend on them for fresh, high-quality produce, cheeses, and meats. On Sundays the highlight of the week occurred: her daughter and son came for dinner with their families.

(Counselor's comments: "Ms. Souza is neat, nicely groomed, and pleasant to talk with. She does not express much animation, and she talks very slowly and carefully. It took about an hour to get the preceding data.")

Session 2 Ms. Souza continued to talk about her family and cooking. She described in great detail the past Sunday: the food and the sayings of her grandchildren, who were quite young. (*clarification of problem*) Toward the middle of this session we began to talk about her fear of leaving the house. She could not remember the onset of this fear, and she could not clarify what she was afraid of. She seemed to think it happened gradually and that it was nothing to get upset about. However, when I reminded her that her husband was starting a new route in a few days, she became agitated (her fingers started to play with each other and she licked her lips a lot). She then explained that she lived about eight blocks, less than a mile, from the markets and that if her husband came straight home from work and there was no traffic, maybe they could still make it. I asked her if she thought she would be physically able to walk that distance, and she replied that sometimes on spring and fall weekends she took walks longer than that with her husband and their son.

Session 3 (*Structure/contract*) After a few minutes of being caught up on Ms. Souza's household chores, I asked her if she would be interested in learning to be able to walk to the markets alone to get her food. (*exploration of problem*) She said she didn't think she would be able to do that, and we spent the entire session talking about the pros and cons. (*possible goals*) I suggested that we take no more than 10 sessions to try it out and see if we could together enable her to overcome her fear. We went over and over the consequences of her not being able to market where she wanted to, of her husband's new route, of maintaining the status quo. Toward the end of the session we returned to less anxiety-provoking events, and she proceeded to tell me about some outfits she was making for her granddaughter.

Session 4 This session began with some more relationship discussion about my perceptions of and feelings toward her and resulted in her expressing pleasure at our meetings. (*mutual acceptance of goals*) We then talked about her agreeing to focus on the behaviors of being able to go out of the house alone and walk to the market, shop, and return home. (*planning of strategies*) She agreed to give "my way" a chance, and I described a step-by-step behavioral procedure to her whereby I would come to her house each day for the next 12 days; if she was able to meet the directives for the day, I would take her marketing and/or take her to her daughter's house for a visit. When she agreed, we asked Mr. Souza to come into the office, explained the procedure to him, and asked him not, under any circumstances, to market for Ms. Souza or take her marketing. He agreed and Ms. Souza agreed (but with reservations).

Intervention Period The following 12-day period consisted of graduated steps. A summary of these steps follows.

> *Day 1:* (*Use of strategies*) Ms. Souza put on hat and coat and came to front door and walked downstairs. I said that she did not have to go any farther than that, and I asked her if she wanted to go marketing with me. She said no, she was too nervous; but she was pleased when I offered to go to the bakery for her and get her some of her favorite pastries (which Mr. Souza had told me about).
>
> *Day 2:* Ms. Souza was able to walk to the curb with me. During this walk, I talked calmly to her, urged her to take long, deep breaths. When we got to the curb, we returned to the house, and I went to the butcher for her and picked up her order.
>
> *Day 3:* The goal was to walk down the block to where my car was parked. When we got to the next house, Ms. Souza said she was dizzy and wanted to return home. We did so. No reinforcement. I left immediately, not wanting to reinforce her with my company.

Day 4: Ms. Souza expressed concern about letting me down yesterday. As I reassured her, we left the house, and we were halfway down the block before she realized where we were. She was pleased and surprised and, as we were by my car, she agreed to be driven to the market. She said she was out of produce and she had been "worried sick" about how she would manage.

Days 5–8: Each day, Ms. Souza was waiting for my arrival with her hat and coat on, and each day we extended our walk until day 8, when together we reached the market, filled the cart with groceries, and walked home together. This called for a celebration, and we called Ms. Souza's daughter, who came over for a visit, bringing a favorite grandchild. Ms. Souza reported that she was so busy talking that she had not been nervous or afraid, even when crossing the streets.

Day 9: (*Evaluation of strategies*) I waited for Ms. Souza halfway to the market. She arrived at the appointed time, and we proceeded to the market together. She had a longer list today, as it was her son-in-law's birthday.

Day 10: Ms. Souza was able to come alone to the market, where I met her. We returned home together, and her daughter joined us for lunch. We agreed to add two more days to this period.

Day 11: Following a weekend, I phoned Ms. Souza and told her that I would be at her home waiting for her when she returned from the market. She was about ten minutes later than I, and she explained that the produce trucks were slow in being unloaded. She was out of breath, but in good spirits and very busy bustling about the kitchen.

Day 12: Repeat of day 11.

Sessions 5 and 6 (*Evaluation*) These were short sessions held in Ms. Souza's home (her husband was no longer able to drive her to my office). We discussed what had happened and her feelings. It was very hard for her to talk about her feelings, but she appeared to be OK and had much to report about her family and cooking.

Sessions 7 and 8 (*Evaluation/termination*) These sessions occurred at two-week intervals and consisted of checking things out and discussing forth-coming termination. Ms. Souza was continuing to do her own marketing, although she did not leave the house for any other reason, except with her husband.

Session 9 (*Termination*) This session occurred three weeks after session 8. We talked about what we had accomplished, and I asked Ms. Souza whether she thought she might want to go out alone for purposes other than marketing. She wasn't sure about that and seemed reluctant to discuss it. As we had fulfilled our contract with each other, I did not pursue the matter.

Session 10 (*Follow-up*) This session occurred six weeks after session 9. Ms. Souza was still totally involved in her family, household, and culinary efforts. She accepted her husband's changed route now that she could market herself, but she had not made any attempts at or expressed any interest in expanding her independence out of doors.

The objective of being able to leave the house to market was accomplished. At the time of follow-up, there was no generalization of this to other situations, but it could be that there was no reason or motivation for Ms. Souza to go other places alone, since her family readily came to visit her, as did neighbors and friends. No attempt was made to resolve depression or underlying causes of phobic behavior.

The Case of Rory

Rory, age 17, was referred to a community counselor by the school drug counselor after he was expelled from his senior year of high school because of drug use. Rory had not been in trouble before high school, although he had been placed in a special program for behavior problems and slow learners after one year in high school. He was such an appealing person that teachers and parents found it easy to forgive his misbehaviors and "give him another chance." His behavior problems before the drug usage were more passive than active—he would not hand in assignments, would be unresponsive to adults who made demands of him, and would engage in foolish activities with other kids that would disrupt the class. Finally, when found dealing drugs to other students, he was put on probation by the courts and ordered to seek therapy.

Rory's school record indicated average intelligence and no specific learning disabilities. His personal appearance was attractive and friendly. He had a cute smile and a twinkle in his eye, and he was easy to talk with. Rory was the youngest by five years of eight sons in an Irish American family; his parents were retired and in their late 60s at the time of this referral. Mr. O'Malley had been a mail carrier, and Mrs. O'Malley had worked in a nursing home as an aide. Two of Rory's brothers had attended college, four were married, and all were self-supporting. Several of his older brothers had had drinking problems while in high school and were viewed retrospectively by their parents as "tough kids."

Session 1 Rory and his parents attended the first session together. Rory talked about how boring school was, how much his parents nagged him to be like his brothers and "make something of himself," and how the only fun he had was going out with his friends. Mr. O'Malley expressed his frustration about not being able to get Rory to do anything—when he was younger and physically stronger, he was able to "make his boys behave," and he would not have tolerated Rory's sassing back and making his mother so unhappy. Rory never helped around the house and didn't talk to his folks at all. He was moody and sullen. Mrs. O'Malley expressed dismay at her failure to keep peace in the family (Rory and his dad were always arguing) and said she was very worried about her dying mother. Both parents described their physical ailments at great length—they were worried about their health and worn out by their parenting responsibilities. The counselor noticed that while they were talking, Rory tuned out. He stared at the ceiling with an impassive expression on his face. All three family members agreed that Rory came and went as he pleased no matter what restrictions his folks tried to impose, and that they were at an impasse. The counselor commented that while there was a lot of frustration in this family, there was no anger and rage, but rather a great deal of caring and concern. (*initiation/entry/joining*) Perhaps each person's frustration and depression came from so much caring. At the end of this session, it was agreed that Mr. O'Malley would bring Rory to an individual session (part of Rory's probation included the lifting of his driver's license). In the interim, the counselor agreed to look into community-based programs for Rory's drug rehabilitation and schooling, and the parents and Rory were directed to look into the school's own alternative program.

Session 2 The counselor met with Rory alone to develop a relationship and make some immediate drug rehabilitation and educational plans to deal with these entry problems. During this session, Rory talked more openly about how hard it was to be the only kid in the house, how all his friends had younger parents, how his brothers were also on his back because they heard from his folks about how bad he was, and how only his friends understood him. He acknowledged that he smoked pot every day, usually before, during, and after school. He did not seem upset that he had been caught and thrown out of school. He did seem to be interested in getting help, but he seemed to be puzzled about taking any kind of responsibility for himself. His behavior appeared apathetic and depressed. The counselor pursued Rory's thinking and past patterns of helping himself when he got into trouble (*clarification of problems*) and helped him to talk more about his feelings about his family and his wanting to be liked and supported. At this stage, Rory did not seem to take responsibility for himself or his problems and seemed content to let the drugs and others make him feel better.

Sessions 3–5 (*Deepening relationship, exploration of problems and possible goals*) The focus of these sessions was to engage Rory in the helping relationship so that he would become more actively involved in making his own life decisions. During this time, he and his parents visited several possible program sites and a family contract was developed regarding his going out and his use of daytime hours since he was not in school.

Rory agreed to attend Narcotics Anonymous meetings (also a term of his probation) as well as to keep his appointments with various resource people. He reported less arguing at home and by the end of session 5 (*structure/contract*) had worked out some objectives with the counselor: (1) to regularly attend NA meetings, (2) to attend the alternative school program if he was admitted, and (3) to regularly meet with the counselor. He was intrigued by the counselor's suggestion that all of the brothers who lived in the area attend one meeting with him without the parents, and he even offered to make the arrangements.

(*planning of strategies*) This was the first time he had really actively engaged in the helping process. Other strategies suggested were the use of limited behavioral contracts, Gestalt dialogues, cognitive restructuring, and reality therapy questioning. For example, Rory was directed to stop before smoking and ask himself two basic questions: (1) Do I know what I am doing? (2) Is this what is best for me?

Session 6 This session was another planning session as the counselor worked with Rory to prepare his application materials for the alternative program and helped him rehearse for the interview by role playing. At the end of the session, Mr. O'Malley, who would wait in the car during the sessions, was asked to come in to share his perceptions of how things were going at home. He reported that the fights were fewer and that while he was worried at how much time Rory was spending lying on his bed listening to his tape player with his earphones, he was able to keep his worries to himself. He still talked about how worried "the missus" was. Rory had told him about the forthcoming session with his brothers and Mr. O'Malley thought it was a fine idea and did not seem to be upset that he and his wife were not invited.

Session 7 (*Implementation of strategies*) This was a critical session in that four of Rory's older brothers came to the session. At first, Rory sat as far away as possible and seemed to be very wary of what was going to happen. As the counselor encouraged each brother to share with Rory what it was like for him growing up in this family and how he worked out his problems, Rory became more alert and interested and joined in the conversation. This one-and-one-half-hour, very emotional session ended in a group hug with the brothers openly expressing their concern and their availability to Rory. Rory left this session with a grin and looking happier than ever. The purpose of this session was twofold: (1) to assess Rory's difficulties within a larger family system context, and (2) to obtain support and modeling for Rory.

Sessions 8–30 (*Use of strategies*) Rory was admitted to the alternative program and was able to abide by the contract (daily attendance, no drug use, compliance with assignments) with the program administrator. This was a small, structured, individually designed program on a local university campus several miles from the high school where Rory had gotten into so much trouble. At first, he would try to return to the high school after hours, but he was directed by his probation officer to stay away from the high school. Gradually, he was weaned away from some of the kids at the high school who had not been a good influence on him. While his drug usage did not disappear, he did curtail it so that it did not interfere with his school attendance. During these sessions, Rory developed a greater attachment to the counselor and would bring in his schoolwork to show her as well as talk about his friends and his family with much more understanding. Person-centered and cognitive-behavioral strategies predominated, although occasionally Gestalt dialogues were used to heighten Rory's self-awareness. He became involved with a new girlfriend in the alternative school program and they helped each other to abide by the program contract. He had more contact with his brothers, and he was able to become more caring to his parents about their health and family concerns. A great deal of time in these sessions was devoted to planning for his graduation from high school and post–high school life. When his girlfriend became pregnant and decided to have and keep the baby, he responded responsibly and spent a lot of time asking the counselor for information and resources. He read books about pregnancy, took his girlfriend to the prenatal clinic, and sought an after-school job in a warehouse so as to save some money. Occasional family sessions indicated that while Mr. and Mrs. O'Malley were upset about the pregnancy, they were supportive of Rory's responsible behavior and included his girlfriend in their family. His brothers followed through more on their agreement to be available to Rory, and Rory learned to initiate contact with them and not just wait for them to make the first move.

Many of the helping strategies used involved decision making—brainstorming options, collecting information, and planning what to do. When Rory realized in April of his senior year that he would graduate, he decided to enlist in the marines. Because of his drug record, he was unable to do so, but he was able to get into the army. Luckily, he had a very supportive and encouraging recruiting officer who helped him over some of the rough application hurdles.

Sessions 31–40 (*Evaluation/termination*) These sessions took place between Rory's high school graduation and his induction into the army. Rory was saving money, hoping to be able to return from basic training for the birth of his baby, and looking forward to the structure of the army and opportunities for finding a vocation. He was able to talk about his anxieties and how it would feel going away from home for the first time. In preparation for the army, he had stopped smoking pot and gotten himself into better physical shape. His whole self-image had changed, and he and the counselor talked about and role-played saying good-bye, both in the counseling and with family and friends. Rory felt very good about himself and his progress and said that he realized that he had to think more for himself and not be so easily influenced by others. He understood his parents better and was looking forward to taking care of his girlfriend and baby. The actual termination session was emotional and sad for both Rory and the counselor. It included a review of decision-making and problem-solving steps and of specific ways that Rory could help himself feel better about himself.

Three-Month Follow-Up Follow-up at three months occurred by telephone when Rory returned for the birth of his child. He reported that he was doing very well in the army and that he had remained drug-free and had made good friends, but was primarily focused on his girlfriend and the baby, so most of his free time was spent writing letters home. He had been homesick but was kept so busy, it wasn't as bad as he had feared. He hoped to save enough money to get married within a year.

Two-Year Follow-Up Before being sent to the war in the Persian Gulf, Rory returned home and requested a session with the counselor to thank her for "standing by him" but, more important, to ask her if his wife could come see her while he was out of the country. Rory reported that he wanted to remain in the military. He liked the structure and opportunities, and he felt more successful and energetic than he ever had. He no longer felt as if he was "just going along."

This case involved both individual and family counseling sessions. The systems perspective enabled the helper to understand Rory's need for structure and support in his family and at school and to help Rory change the way he related to his family so that they could simultaneously change their ways of relating to him. The steady, continuous support and practical skill building that Rory received during the counseling helped him achieve the primary objectives of (1) completing his high school education and (2) freeing himself from his drug dependency. This was a positive experience for Rory because he was lucky to have a family with the capacity to be caring and supportive and because he lived in a community with available resources. It was also a positive experience for the counselor in that Rory and his family were so open.

The Case of Martha

Martha, age 30, entered counseling to find out whether she wanted to have a baby. She'd been married for eight years and reported a relatively happy marriage. She was an elementary school teacher with many activities and interests, and Bill, her husband, was a middle-level research scientist in an industrial laboratory. They had never tried to have a baby; what precipitated this entrance into counseling was a chance remark by Martha's physician during her annual checkup to the effect that if Martha and Bill were going to have children, they ought to think about getting started.

Session 1 Martha arrived early for her appointment and was eager to talk about herself. (*initiation/entry*) She told the counselor that she was the second of two daughters from a traditional Jewish middle-class background. She recalled a relatively placid, happy childhood, although she remembered a lot of squabbling with her sister. Her lingering impression was of an all-female, matriarchal home. Her father seemed almost nonexistent, and Martha was vague in her references to him. Martha was an above-average student, although not as academically gifted as her sister. She was easygoing, anxious to please, and easily led by others.

Her sister went to a prestigious college, but Martha attended the state university, where she maintained a B– average and dated moderately. She met Bill during her senior year, and they were married right after graduation. She had been teaching fourth grade ever since and said she liked teaching and maintained a well-organized, well-run classroom. She did express disdain for parents and teachers who didn't know how to "control and discipline" children. Martha had supported Bill while he studied for his master's degree. They now lived in a two-bedroom apartment in a suburb. When they got married, they had not discussed having children because they had decided that was a long way off.

Martha described Bill as quiet, introverted, and a loner. They didn't see too much of each other because she had her women's group, her art class, and her card group during the week. However, on Saturday nights they either had company or went out. Sundays were for visiting their families, who lived nearby.

Martha had been "shocked" by her doctor's comment. She'd had no idea she'd have to start thinking about children. A friend suggested she come for counseling, and she eagerly accepted that suggestion.

(Counselor's comments: "Martha is attractive, bright, and very outspoken. She is eager to talk and speaks rapidly and egocentrically—practically every statement begins with 'I.' Near the end of the session, when asked about Bill, she seemed genuinely startled. Does not know how Bill feels about having children, but has decided that she needs to figure out how she feels first before she discusses it with him. She definitely does not want him to come to counseling with her but has agreed to come by herself.")

Session 2 Martha arrived early again, but she seemed a little subdued, her rate of speech was slower, and she was more reflective. (*clarification of problem*) She described her eight years of marriage as if she were relating an article from a women's magazine, with little affect. She talked about their different interests— she liked to keep busy, always doing things and doing them as perfectly as possible, liked to be with people and go to cultural events. Bill's idea of fun was reading a mystery novel or watching TV. In the evening, when they were both home, he tended to watch TV, and she usually read and corrected papers. She had high expectations of her students and wrote long comments on their papers.

The counselor and she discussed her feelings about children: no one she knew was happy with his or her children; they're too much work; she'd be trapped and tied down; she'd hate to give up teaching, yet she wouldn't dream of working while her children were young; it seemed like such a burden. The only positive reason she could think of for having children was that "it's the thing to do" and that "it would please our parents." She said that Bill didn't really care—"He wants what will make me happy."

The session concluded with Martha agreeing to keep a diary containing all the thoughts, feelings, and observations she had or made about having children during the week.

(Counselor's comments: "The fact that she's come for counseling is the only behavioral evidence that there is a positive side to her feelings about having children. There seems to be some anger and fear underneath the bright exterior.")

Session 3 Martha produced her diary for the week, which elaborated her ambivalences. (*clarification*) On the one hand, she was afraid that if she decided not to have children she would regret it when it was too late, and on the other hand, she had many "shoulds" in her head that she was afraid of, such as "I should have children because it is expected of me"; "If I have children, they should be perfect"; "If I have children, I should stop teaching and stay home and be the perfect mother." The counselor and she spent much time talking about these beliefs and what they meant to Martha—the feelings behind them. She had great difficulty experiencing her own feelings. She could talk about, but not experience, them.

(*Structure/contract*) The counselor and Martha decided to set up seven more sessions, one per week, to see where they could go. Martha agreed to continue her diary and to read some books that the counselor had selected for her.

(Counselor's comments: "Slowly but surely, she's becoming a little less guarded and more relaxed. She's not trying to impress me as much. Less talk about all her activities and achievements, and today she expressed some genuine feeling [compassion] for one of her students.")

Session 4 (*Exploration*) They talked about where Martha got some of her beliefs and what kinds of things occurred in her childhood to reinforce them. As she talked about her mother expecting her to live up to her older sister and to keep on trying harder, she began to get in touch with some anger. (*use of strategies*) Using some Gestalt strategies, the counselor encouraged her to experience the anger, and she did remarkably well for the first attempt. Martha briefly mentioned that she had begun to read one of the books suggested by the counselor.

Sessions 5 and 6 (*Exploration and possible goals*) They decided to focus on Martha's feelings about herself and her self-understanding, rather than on the decision making about children. (*mutual acceptance of goals*) It became apparent that there was much material to work through before a decision could be made. Martha decided that she really didn't like herself very much and that she hid behind lots of activities and fast talk.

(Counselor's comments: "She seems somewhat relieved, although anxious, that she doesn't have to play 'perfect' games anymore and that she can say and do what she feels like here.")

Sessions 7–10 (*Planning of strategies*) In these sessions, the counselor explained how they could use some rational-emotive and Gestalt techniques to help Martha get in touch with and understand her feelings and beliefs. She agreed and easily got into dialoguing, developing fantasies, and so forth.

Martha came into the ninth session disturbed by the anger she was feeling toward her family. She found now she was feeling angry every time she spoke to or thought of them. (*use of strategies*) The counselor emphasized that it was OK to be angry and that she would be able to work it through once she allowed herself to feel the anger. During a dialogue session with her imagined mother, some anger spilled over to her father and Bill, both of whom she saw as "passive," "almost not there." They spent the rest of the ninth and all of the tenth sessions dealing with her anger toward men. (*recontracting*) At the end of the tenth session, they agreed to meet for five more sessions.

Sessions 11–14 They continued intense exploration and working-through of anger and the early script decision wherein Martha had vowed always to try harder.

(*Use of strategies*) Each session ended with a behavioral contract for the interval between sessions, such as talking to Bill about a particular feeling or doing something fun and enjoyable. The contract after session 13 was to tell both families that Martha and Bill would not visit that Sunday because they were going to spend the day together alone. Session 14, Martha came in glowing: she had had a wonderful day with Bill, and they had really talked for the first time in years. (*evaluation*) She said that Bill was saying and doing things she had never noticed before, such as being concerned and caring and telling her that he wanted her to stop running around and to pay more attention to him.

Session 15 This was the final session of the contract. (*termination*) Martha said that she was ready to be on her own and that she believed that over the next few months she and Bill would be able to decide about having children. She felt good knowing that whatever they decided would be fine for them, and she agreed that she was now able to balance the scales a bit by seeing and looking for people who enjoyed having children.

Three-Month Follow-Up Martha reported over the telephone that although they still had not made a final decision with regard to children, they were getting there. She reported that she was able to continue to refute her "silly" beliefs and that she was able to relax and to enjoy Bill's company more. She laughed as she told the counselor about how funny her students had been in a recent classroom activity. She ended the call by saying that she thought Bill and she would both want to come in for some counseling together at some point in the future, as she knew there were still some marital issues.

You will note the use of bibliotherapy (the assigning of pertinent reading material) and weekly homework assignments. These behavioral strategies go hand in hand with the more experiential strategies used in sessions. In this case, it was important not to rush into decision making but to take the time to explore the underlying dynamics of the presenting concerns.

The Case of Ms. Stewart

Ms. Stewart, age 39, was referred to a counselor by her children's school counselor. Married, and the mother of two elementary school children, Ms. Stewart was frightened and anxious about her children's behavioral problems at school. Limited to five sessions by her health insurer, Ms. Stewart agreed to complete a background form (see Appendix C) prior to the initial session. The counselor spoke to the referring school counselor, who reported that the children were talking about their father's "hitting Mommy" and "Mommy being bad for wanting to break up the family."

Session 1 (*Initiation/entry and clarification of problem*) Ms. Stewart came to the session neatly dressed, nervously twisting her fingers and tapping her foot. Her husband had been laid off from his teaching job six months earlier and was collecting unemployment insurance. He spent most of his time moping around the house, finding things to complain about. She worked part-time as an art instructor. She described herself as being "scatterbrained and artistic" and her husband as being "short-tempered and rigid." Their fights centered on her housekeeping and parenting. He did not think she was strict enough with the children, and he considered her a "slob." He had taken away the telephone, refused to give her money, and insisted she turn over her earnings from her part-time job. When asked about physical violence, Ms. Stewart acknowledged that it did occur, but felt that she probably brought it on by displeasing him.

The counselor asked Ms. Stewart what she wanted to get out of the counseling, and Ms. Stewart replied that she wanted "to get her head straight." Further exploration led to her stating that she wanted to find a way to leave her husband without harming the children. Whenever she told him she wanted to leave, he told her that it would be "over his dead body" and that he would get the kids. As the counselor explored Ms. Stewart's fear and intimidation, certain information was revealed: Ms. Stewart came from a nonsupportive family, where she was ridiculed as being "crazy," and her husband was holding her previous extramarital affair over her head.

The counselor was able to conclude at the end of the first session that Ms. Stewart had no family, friends, or community support except for the school counselor, who was very sympathetic and supportive. Therefore, the counselor's first goal was to empower Ms. Stewart to locate support resources. (*goal setting*) She proposed a list of resources that Ms. Stewart could contact prior to the next session: a battered women's shelter for a safety net; a legal aid consultant; and a women's support group at the community center. (*structure/contract*) They also discussed the importance of calling the local police if she ever felt in imminent danger.

Session 2 Ms. Stewart indicated her motivation to confront her problem and take action by coming to the second session with information from each of her contacts. She reported several arguments with her husband and noted how he brought the children, particularly the older, 7-year-old boy into these arguments. As she outlined the sequence of these fights, the counselor suggested role plays of more effective ways of managing conflict with her husband and handling the children. (*planning and use of strategies*) Cognitive restructuring and cognitive-behavioral modification along with empowerment and psychoeducation were the major strategies utilized.

Ms. Stewart had been advised by the legal consultant to prepare to take the children to the shelter at the next incidence of physical abuse. She and the counselor talked about how she could prepare the children for this possibility and the steps she could take to get support from the school and other community resources. A written plan was drawn up. Ms. Stewart wanted to bring the children to the next counseling session, but her legal consultant had warned her that she could not do this without her husband's consent. It was agreed that Ms. Stewart would ask her husband and would notify the counselor prior to the next session.

Session 3 Prior to the session, Ms. Stewart called to say her husband wanted to come in with Ms. Stewart and the children. Thus, the third session turned out to be a family session. (*exploration of problem and use of strategies*) The counselor asked each of the family members what they would like to change in their family. The son replied that he wanted his folks to stop fighting and his mom to stop trying to break up the family. The 5-year-old daughter agreed with her brother. Mr. Stewart said he agreed too, and Ms. Stewart said she wanted to end the marriage. At this point, Mr. Stewart turned to his children and said "See? I told you she is no good." He boasted proudly that he was honest with his children and shared everything with them. The counselor intervened, first explaining to the children how it takes two people to both make and break a marriage and that their parents' difficulties were separate from the parents' relationship with the children. She then calmly asked Mr. Stewart what his reasons were for wanting to maintain the marriage since he obviously did not care for his wife. His reply was that the Bible dictated retaining the marriage no matter what, and he wanted the children to know that he was keeping the marriage even though their mother was an "evil bitch." At this point, the children were excused from the session and the counselor confronted both parents with the deleterious effects of these kinds of exchanges on the children. Mr. Stewart was chastened by this confrontation, and both parents agreed to refrain from airing their dirty linen in front of the children. A specific contract of "do's" and "don'ts" was written up for all participants. (*reiteration of structure/contract*)

Session 4 Prior to Session 4, the counselor conferred with the school counselor, who reported that the son had come to talk to her about Dad's having a "girlfriend." Ms. Stewart came to Session 4 alone. She and the counselor constructed a decision-making tree, listing all the pros and cons of leaving the marriage, the practical realities and possible consequences. Ms. Stewart appeared to be stronger and more in control of her life. She had attended several group sessions at the battered women's shelter, had met with the lawyer to draw up separation papers, and felt that she was responding differently to her husband by not engaging in his attempts to fight. She reported that the children felt better after the family session and that she did not think their father was "filling them with lies and distortions" anymore. In fact, she found her husband to be more conciliatory than ever. The counselor continued to utilize psychoeducation, empowerment, and cognitive restructuring strategies so that Ms. Stewart could feel supported and encouraged to continue her active pursuit of resources.

Session 5 Prior to this session, Mr. Stewart phoned the counselor to complain about a restraining order Ms. Stewart had obtained. He was now living at his parents' house (they were away for the winter), and he wanted the counselor to know how "irrational" this was. He could not believe his wife had done this and insisted that it was all her fault. He wanted the counselor to know what was being done to him. The counselor responded empathetically and offered Mr. Stewart the opportunity to come in and talk. He declined but said he might call again. When Ms. Stewart came in for the fifth and final session (*evaluation*), she reported that the precipitating event for obtaining the restraining order was that her husband had taken her car keys away and tried to keep her from leaving the house. She was filing for divorce, and she was feeling tremendous relief that she was able to follow through on her decision. Through her new women's group and the school counselor, she had located counseling groups for the children, and she was feeling better and stronger than ever. In the final moments of the session, Ms. Stewart said that she had begun feeling stronger after the first session, when she felt the counselor's validation, support, and empowerment. She had been "stuck" and had not known what to do or with whom to talk. She now feels connected to other people and is amazed that there are so many supportive people.

Follow-Up   The counselor followed up by telephone monthly for the next six months with the school counselor and Ms. Stewart. She learned that Mr. Stewart did not contest the divorce or custody decisions and was keeping pretty well to the agreed-upon visitation arrangements. The children did not seem to be so divided in their loyalties, and the school reported fewer classroom behavioral problems. The school counselor felt that the children were functioning better than ever and that Ms. Stewart was much more relaxed and self-confident. Ms. Stewart was preparing to take a full-time teaching job the following year and was actively involved in single-parent groups.

Note that the counselor did not deal with the problems that underlay Ms. Stewart's fearfulness and isolation. The focus was on the presenting problem, on resolution and establishment of other supportive systems.

Although these cognitive-behavioral and ecological/systems approaches worked extremely well in this particular situation, one cannot assume that will always be the case. Some clients may not be as ready to take action as was Ms. Stewart, who had passed a threshold of anxiety tolerance.

The Case of Ellen

Ellen, age 31, lives on a military base with her two children, ages 9 and 12. Her soldier husband, Reed, has been in Iraq for 18 months. Prior to his deployment, the couple had been fighting and were considering divorce. Reed refused to attend couples counseling, stating that he did not believe in "that kind of crap." The conflict centered around Reed's temper, occasional "hitting," and refusal to allow Ellen to visit her family or relatives off base. He believed that Ellen did not keep the house clean enough and that she spent too much time away from home. After Reed left, Ellen was relieved to be living without the continuous bickering and feelings of resentment. She visited family and friends and became "friendly" with a former high school boyfriend. Her sister suggested she go to the counseling center on base.

Session 1 (*Entry, relationship*) Ellen arrived on time for her first session, casually dressed and appearing nervous. The counselor told her she was entitled to eight visits and reviewed confidentiality and informed consent. Ellen explained that she was pretty sure that she wanted to leave Reed but she was afraid he would gain full custody of the children and leave her penniless (he had threatened this prior to his leaving). She believed Reed was intelligent and powerful, and was apparently intimidated by him and unsure of her self-worth. During the first session, the counselor drew her out about the stories of her upbringing and her marriage. Listening carefully to Ellen's story, with a few probing comments, he learned that Ellen had been raised in an alcoholic family and that her father had been verbally abusive to the children and physically abusive to her mother. After graduating from high school, Ellen went to work as a clerk in a small store and continued to live at home. She was 19 when she met Reed at a dance in town and was attracted to his intelligence, independence, and "strength." They married two months after meeting, and Ellen became pregnant shortly thereafter. She reported that once, during her first pregnancy, Reed hit her hard enough that she fell to the floor. Her face struck the corner of the kitchen table, and she needed stitches by her eye. Over the years, he has hit her several times, with no discernable injury, but he has often threatened to hurt her. At the end of the session, the counselor recommended that they meet the next week to determine what goals they could achieve within the seven remaining sessions. As a homework assignment, he suggested that Ellen visit the Base Legal Clinic to learn about her rights should she decide to leave her husband.

Session 2 (*Continued relationship development and clarification of goals*) Ellen arrived early and smiled as she greeted her counselor. She reported learning that state law favored joint custody arrangements unless one parent was shown to be unfit. She had also learned there was a formula for distribution of assets. She was more relaxed with the counselor and thanked him for encouraging her to obtain this information. The counselor asked her if she saw any similarities between her current family and the family in which she had grown up. Ellen replied that she was afraid of her husband, just as she had been of her father, that she experienced the same feelings of worthlessness when around these two men, and that she always tried to avoid conflict. They talked about her fear of anger, including her own, and decided that the foremost goal of these sessions would be to teach her to become more assertive and to find "her own voice." The next priority would be to understand her marriage, as well as fantasies about a former boyfriend, so that she could make an informed decision about her marriage. (*setting goals*) The counselor assigned homework using cognitive-behavioral strategies. He asked Ellen to read material he provided about women's development and to attend Al-Anon meetings on the base, so that she could begin to understand the dynamics of intimidation and avoidance. (*homework and empowerment*) Furthermore, he gave her worksheets on which she could write three things she felt good about each day, practice saying "no" in an assertive way, and begin to think in terms of making statements such as "I feel angry (feeling) when you _____ (behavior) because _____."

Session 3 (*Further assessment and use of strategies*) Ellen came in tense and agitated. She had just received word that Reed would be coming home in two months for a one-month leave. She was frightened and resentful but also felt guilty about her lack of patriotism and support for her soldier husband. The counselor encouraged her to express her feelings and empathized with her. He taught her relaxation exercises (*behavioral strategy*) to reduce tension and anxiety. He reviewed her homework assignments, noticing that her voice and nonverbal language became more confident as she relayed the positive achievements of the week. He asked her about her "friendship" with her high school boyfriend. It became clear that this relationship was more Ellen's fantasy than a reality. He was supportive as he provided psychoeducation about the realities of divorce and assigned her the task of writing down the pros and cons of staying in the marriage and the pros and cons of leaving the marriage (*cognitive*).

Session 4 (*Continued use of cognitive-behavioral, feminist, and constructivist strategies*) In discussing the pros and cons of staying in or leaving her marriage, Ellen began to express her opinion that she and the children would be better off without Reed. She told the counselor that she had shared feelings about her marriage and husband with family and selected friends on and off the base and learned that they believed Reed treated her "poorly" in public and at family functions. This feedback was surprising to her as she had never allowed herself to share her personal pain before and had convinced herself that everyone thought she had a great relationship. She told the counselor that participating in therapy seemed to have given her permission to share her true thoughts and feelings with others as well as with him. She also acknowledged that while Reed is not an alcoholic, she found the Al-Anon meetings helpful in thinking about her upbringing and she learned that other families had similar difficulties to hers. Her homework assignment was to draft a letter to Reed telling him about her thoughts and feelings. They agreed that this letter would be used only in the counseling sessions and she could decide later if she wanted to send it.

Session 5 Ellen came in to the session announcing that she had struggled with the letter assignment but had completed it. The counselor suggested she read the letter to Reed in an "empty chair" and then reply as Reed (*Gestalt intervention*). After several minutes of changing seats, she edited her own letter to make it clearer but also softer. She and the counselor spent the rest of the session talking about her decision-making process and what kinds of plans she would need to make. Her assignment was to create a plan of action for staying in the marriage and one for leaving.

Session 6 Ellen came in with a well-developed plan for leaving the marriage. She reported that she was unable to imagine a plan for staying. She said the children had been so much happier and more relaxed while Reed was gone that she just could not stay in the marriage. Her plan was to write her husband before he came home for his furlough. Before he arrived, she was going to talk to an attorney about a divorce and figure out how she could live and find a job near her hometown, 20 miles from the base. She expressed concern about the effects of divorce on her children and asked the counselor for some resources. Together, the counselor and Ellen decided that the next session, the next to last one, would be devoted to fine-tuning her plan and to evaluating what strides she had made so far. To assess the gains she had made in assertiveness and self-esteem, he asked her to complete a worksheet.

Session 7   Ellen was very excited because she had talked to the manager of a department store at a nearby mall who suggested she consider their training program. She had never thought her previous sales experience would count for anything! She had already written Reed once, but did not expect to hear from him as he rarely wrote or called. She and the counselor went over her plan step by step and did not have time to review the homework sheets she had filled out. They discussed the fact that the next session was the last.

Session 8   (*Evaluation*) Ellen and the counselor reviewed their sessions and what they had accomplished. They were able to discuss the worksheets Ellen had previously completed, and Ellen said she was nervous about ending these sessions. The counselor said that, due to the circumstances, his director had approved three more sessions, to be used after Reed came home, and Ellen could come alone or with Reed. They then used role plays to practice how Ellen could respond to Reed without provoking him and how she could detach herself when he tried to provoke a fight. They also created a safety plan should things get out of hand: Ellen had two friends she would call if anything threatening occurred, and she arranged to leave the children with a cousin off base the second night of Reed's return. She had the phone number for the base's 24-hour help line, as well as the military chaplain who knew her husband well. A counseling session was scheduled for the end of Reed's first week home.

Follow-Up   Ellen came to this session alone. To her surprise, Reed did not seem to care about her decision and was not at all attentive to the children. He spent most of his time playing basketball with his buddies. He could not wait to go back to Iraq—he told her that his unit needed him and he felt accepted. His anger was directed toward the insurgents, and it became clear that he, too, had gone on to another life and was satisfied with it.

Three-Month Follow-Up   The counselor called Ellen at her new phone number. She reported that the legal work for the divorce was progressing smoothly since Reed was not opposing it, and that the kids seemed happy in their new rented house and school. Ellen had completed two months in the training program and was now an assistant manager in the housewares department. She hoped to begin night classes the next semester at the local community college. She said that she was more relaxed and happier than she had ever been. She was making new friends but was not yet interested in dating. She was not seeing her old boyfriend anymore. She said that she was thinking more about what she wanted for herself and her children and she had more confidence that she could achieve her goals.

SUMMARY

In this chapter, we have discussed the six steps of the strategy stage: mutual acceptance of defined goals and objectives; planning of strategies; use of strategies; evaluation of strategies; termination; and follow-up. We stressed the importance of a theoretical framework within which helpee problems are defined. The goals and objectives of the helping process are derived from this problem definition, and the helper's theoretical framework helps in the selection and application of strategies.

Examples and exercises were presented to help you understand the steps. We particularly emphasized the termination and follow-up steps, as they are too often neglected in favor of the relationship development steps. We presented five case studies to illustrate the steps of the human relations counseling model. Remember that these steps are not necessarily distinct and discrete. Each case is different, and flexibility and modifications are encouraged. Further, the effectiveness of the strategy stage depends on the quality of the relationship stage, as demonstrated in the case studies. Thus, the steps in applying strategies can be viewed only within the context of an empathic helping relationship.

EXERCISE ANSWERS

Exercise 8.4 1. c and d; 2. a, c, d; 3. c, d; 4. b, d; 5. a, b. The correct answers are based on observable behaviors rather than subjective feelings.

Exercise 8.9 1. follow-up; 2. mutual acceptance of objectives; 3. evaluation; 4. use of strategies; 5. termination; 6. planning of strategies

REFERENCES AND
FURTHER READING

Breunlin, D. (1980). Multimodal behavioral treatment of a child's eliminative disturbance. *Psychotherapy: Theory, Research and Practice, 17,* 17–23.

Corey, G. (2005). *Case approach to counseling and psychotherapy* (6th ed.). Belmont, CA: Brooks/Cole.

Corsini, R. J. (Ed.). (2001). *Handbook of innovative therapy* (2nd ed.). New York: Wiley.

Mirkin, M. P., Suyemoto, K. L., & Okun, B. F. (Eds.). (2005). *Psychotherapy with women: Exploring diverse contexts and identities.* New York: Guilford Press.

Okun, B. F. (1990). *Seeking connections in psychotherapy.* San Francisco: Jossey-Bass.

Ward, D. W. (1984). Termination of individual counseling: Concepts and strategies. *Journal of Counseling and Development, 63,* 21–26.

Wedding, D., & Corsini, R. J. (Eds.). (2005). *Case studies in psychotherapy* (4th ed.). Belmont, CA: Brooks/Cole.

Visit the book companion site at www.thomsonedu.com to access tutorial quizzes.

9

Crisis Theory
and Intervention

More and more frequently, helpers are working with people who are experiencing some type of crisis; in other words, helpers are *intervening* in crises. Crisis intervention is an approach to helping relationships that is usually distinct from the counseling model developed previously in this text. However, it requires the same communication skills for establishing a relationship and clarifying and understanding the crisis, and it can use many of the problem-solving strategies of the human relations counseling model.

Crisis intervention is active, direct, and brief and occurs shortly or immediately after the crisis becomes evident. It involves the short-term use of specific skills and strategies, ranging from provision of immediate contact and support to referral for intensive therapy; its goal is to help people cope with the turmoil resulting from specific emergencies. It may focus on one or several victims and may involve conventional one-to-one helping. Over the years, crisis theory has been broadened to include disaster or trauma theory. Disaster or trauma intervention requires coordinated team efforts to deliver services to large groups of sufferers and the use of multiple modalities of helping. In reality, there is much overlap in what is considered a crisis situation or a disaster and in the types of services provided.

An understanding of current trauma and resilience literature and studies on evidence-based early interventions is a requirement for crisis and disaster mental health workers. It is also imperative that these helpers realize that both crisis/disaster survivors and helpers are vulnerable to **compassion fatigue** or **secondary traumatization** (Watson & Shalev, 2005).

The purpose of this chapter is to familiarize you with basic crisis and disaster theories and with the application of helping strategies in basic intervention. The chapter is an overview; more training is required before a helper is adequately prepared to perform many aspects of crisis and disaster work.

WHAT IS A CRISIS?

A crisis is a state that exists when a person is thrown completely off balance emotionally by an unexpected and potentially harmful event or a difficult developmental transition. Crises are not usually predictable or expected, and it is this unexpectedness that can intensify the reaction to crisis situations. When we talk about crises, we are referring to people's emotional reactions to a situation, *not* the situation itself. Therefore, crisis intervention helpers work with a person's perceptions and judgments of the crisis, not with the event itself.

When we are in crisis, we feel powerless and overwhelmed, often experiencing a loss of control over ourselves and the course of our lives. Common terms used to describe the personal experience of crisis are *disequilibrium, disorientation,* and *disruption.* Common feeling responses to crisis situations include apathy, depression, guilt, and loss of self-esteem. People in crisis find that the ways they solved problems and coped with difficulties in the past no longer work, and they become more and more upset and frightened.

If a person comes to you in crisis because of an accident, you deal with that person's feelings and thoughts about the accident, not with the accident as an isolated event. How one responds and reacts to crisis depends on one's past learning and experiences (how one has reacted to meeting previous crises), one's lifestyle and social support, and one's life philosophy, as well as the duration and intensity of the crisis situation. Sociocultural variables affect one's meaning-making and reactions to crises. Disaster studies have found that ethnic minorities are more vulnerable to mental health consequences than European Americans (Norris & Alegria, 2005). Minority groups do not have as much access to services as do mainstream groups, language may be an obstacle, and cultural expectations differ. But even within homogeneous groupings, there is variability. For example, a volunteer rape counselor reported that two married women in their 40s with similar educational, sociocultural, and socioeconomic backgrounds came to her for crisis counseling on the same night. The situations were so alike that the police suspected that both women were assaulted by the same person. One victim collapsed hysterically and required intensive care and counseling, missing work for two weeks. The other victim required factual information about police and court procedures before driving herself home (20 miles), having a drink with her husband while she related the details of her assault, going to bed, and reporting for work the next morning. Neither reaction is "better" or "more normal" than the other. These two women had different histories, philosophies, and coping and defense mechanisms. They needed different amounts of time and types of help in working through their feelings about their crisis.

EXERCISE 9.1 ■ Close your eyes and reflect on the last loss you experienced. It may have been the loss of a job, a loved one, a pet, a wallet, or whatever. Focus on the feelings you experienced as a result of that loss, not on the loss itself. Remember where you were, with whom, and what everything looked, sounded, and felt like. How did your distress show itself? See if you can remember all of your feelings, their physical expressions (for example, tight stomach, clenched fists, palpitations), and the thoughts you had about the event and your feelings. Were those feelings familiar to you? How long did you feel the acute pain from loss? What coping strategies do you remember using to work through this state? After you have remembered these details, pick a partner and share your findings. See what you can learn about your own way of dealing with loss and how it may differ from someone else's way. What are the similarities and differences related to the type of loss experienced?

KINDS OF CRISES

There are six generally accepted classes of emotional crises:

1. *Dispositional crises:* These crises can ensue from a lack of information, such as not knowing which job to take, what type of medical referral to seek for a particular symptom, what one's options are about living arrangements, and whom to ask for what.

2. *Anticipated life transitions:* These are normative, developmental crises that are fairly common in our society. They may result from midlife career changes, getting married, becoming a parent, divorce, the onset of chronic or terminal illness, or changing schools.

3. *Traumatic stress:* These crises result from externally imposed stress situations that are unexpected, uncontrolled, and emotionally overwhelming. Examples are 9/11, rape, assault, sudden death of a loved one, sudden loss of job or status, sudden onset of illness, accident, war, hurricane, or earthquake.

4. *Maturational/developmental crises:* Most of us experience these general crises as we pass through our life stages. They may reflect issues of dependency, value conflicts, and sexual identity, or our capacity for emotional intimacy, our response to authority, or our level of self-discipline. Usually, these crises surface in relationship patterns or at crucial transition points in our development. Examples are the repeated loss of jobs because of an inability to get along with supervisors, the intense homesickness or depression of college students away from home for the first time, and midlife crises.

5. *Psychopathological crises:* These are emotional crises precipitated by preexisting psychopathology. In other words, one's psychopathology significantly impairs or complicates the way one deals with a situation, inflating it to crisis proportions. For example, a teenager diagnosed with bipolar disorder becomes so emotional and upset whenever she menstruates that she throws objects and is unable to attend school.

6. *Psychiatric emergencies:* These are crisis situations in which one's general functioning is severely impaired and one is rendered incompetent or unable to maintain responsibility for oneself; in other words, one is dangerous to oneself, to others, or both.

As we look at this classification scheme, we see that crises fall into one of two major categories: they are either developmental, in that they have to do with growth and passing through various life stages; or they are situational, in that they are the result of internal stresses, external stresses, or both. In addition to helping us understand the nature of crises, the classification scheme helps us to put crises in perspective so that we can determine the best means of immediate intervention.

EXERCISE 9.2 ■ Using the preceding classification scheme, place the following crisis situations where you think they belong. When you have finished, compare your answers with those of your classmates and discuss the reasons for your answers.

Bad drug trip

Alcoholic binge

Suicide attempt

Acute bereavement over loss of a parent

Loss of job

Discovery of unwanted pregnancy

Discovery that spouse is involved in extramarital affair

Severe marital fight

Abandonment by spouse

Car stolen

Transferring to new high school midyear

Emergency appendectomy in foreign country

Seeing pet run over by hit-and-run driver

Being rejected by college of choice

Being beaten by spouse

Discovering that child is mentally retarded

Finding home vandalized and burglarized

WHAT IS A DISASTER?

A disaster is a traumatic stress that involves a group of people and organizations. Disasters are classified as natural or human-made and range in size and duration. Generally, disasters are defined by levels of financial impact and scope of response required (Hamilton, 2005). The Oklahoma City bombing,

9/11, a plane crash, school shootings, war and "ethnic cleansing," a major hurricane (such as Katrina in 2005), and the tsunami in December 2004 are all examples of disasters. As a result of news media and rapid communication, the consequences of a disaster may reach across the world; the effects have no defined limits.

One important feature of a disaster is that it is a shared experience with shared meaning and influence on group activities, roles, and relationships. Thus, immediate societal support is usually available to survivors of disasters, which can help validate their perceptions and experiences. This is in contrast to the confusion, isolation, and alienation that many victims of individual crisis (such as any type of abuse) experience as they struggle with whether the abuse actually occurred and whether they have a right to their feelings and claims of victimization. Researchers (Norris & Alegria, 2005) claim that feelings of belonging and being cared for are crucial to disaster recovery and resilience. Early prevention and intervention are becoming the focus of regional and national planning for natural and human-made disasters (Boscarino, Adams, & Figley, 2004; Herman, 2005; Watson & Shalev, 2005).

We now recognize **acute** and **posttraumatic stress disorders** (including symptoms such as feelings of intense guilt, anxiety, and/or depression resulting from repeated intrusive thoughts related to the trauma) as possible immediate or later responses to both individual crisis and disaster trauma. These disorders can develop in victims and helpers (secondary traumatization), as well as television viewers around the world who become so identified with the disaster experience TV provides that they develop symptoms. We are attempting to learn more about these disorders, to discover why some people recover from the acute event and others experience either the delay of stress symptoms or cyclical or continued chronic symptoms. Such factors as genetics, temperament, the biological or physiological response to stress, an individual's subjective response to stress, and the impact of early experience prior to the stress are being studied. Epidemiological studies conducted following traumatic events have shown that most trauma survivors are resilient and that only 9% of trauma victims will develop chronic posttraumatic stress disorder (Gray & Litz, 2005), thus challenging the myth that all who experience crisis or disaster will be affected for life.

WHO DEALS WITH CRISES AND DISASTERS?

We can see that different levels of helping may be required in different types of crises and disasters. Certainly professional medical help is necessary in psychiatric emergencies, and professional psychological help is necessary in crises involving psychopathology. However, any one of us can help with dispositional crises, and many of us can help with anticipated life transitions, traumatic stress, and maturational/developmental crises.

Police, friends, pastors, family, or physicians are usually the first to be alerted to a crisis. They, in turn, usually call in the counselor or human services worker to help in direct problem solving and working through the feelings associated with the crisis. With regard to disasters, a variety of lay, generalist human services, and professional helpers are involved. The International Red Cross trains and supervises disaster relief helpers around the world. The American Psychological Association Disaster Response Network (DRN) collaborates with local, national, and international Red Cross divisions.

EXERCISE 9.3 ▪ Choose a partner for a role play between helper and helpee. The helpee should pick one of the crisis situations from Exercise 9.2 and act it out. The helper is to draw out the helpee's feelings and thoughts about this crisis. See if together you can decide how to resolve it. After you have finished, process your thoughts and feelings. What stereotypes and value conflicts did you encounter? How comfortable were you talking about this crisis situation? How well do you think you could deal with others' intense emotion in similar situations? What would you want to do differently the next time around?

CRISIS THEORY

Crisis theory is based on the pioneering work of Eric Lindemann, who studied the reactions of bereaved families of victims who died in the Coconut Grove nightclub fire in Boston. Lindemann (1944) discovered that crisis usually involves some type of loss that necessitates a grieving (bereavement) period. Part of this grieving includes the expression of emotions and intense distress. This distress may take various forms, such as tightness in the throat, choking, shortened breath, sighing, exhaustion, lack of strength, digestive problems, insomnia, altered sensitivity, preoccupation with guilt, and disturbed interpersonal relationships. These expressions of grief are acute, have an identifiable onset, and last for a relatively brief time (about six weeks).

Together with Gerald Caplan, Lindemann began a community mental health program based on his discoveries. Lindemann and Caplan believed that people in crisis choose adaptive or maladaptive ways of coping with problems and that the nature of their problem solving will affect their later adjustment and ability to cope. They believed that people can be helped to identify, understand, and master the psychological tasks involved in grieving and posed by crises.

In developing this crisis theory, Caplan described four phases of a crisis reaction:

Phase 1: In the initial phase, one experiences the beginning of tension and attempts to use habitual kinds of problem solving to restore one's emotional equilibrium.

Phase 2: This phase is characterized by an increase in tension, leading to upset and ineffectual functioning when one's habitual problem-solving strategies fail; at this phase, one attempts trial-and-error strategies to resolve the problem.

Phase 3: This phase is characterized by increased tension, requiring additional helping resources such as emergency and novel problem-solving strategies; if one is successful at this phase, one is able to redefine the problem and resign oneself to it or resolve it.

Phase 4: This phase occurs when the problem has not been resolved in the previous phases and may result in major personality disorganization and an emotional breakdown.

From Lindemann and Caplan's crisis intervention work, we learn that a person in crisis can be receptive to major change in a brief period of time and can be influenced and helped by others during that period. Relationships with significant others (helper, family, friends) are an important part of crisis intervention. A person in crisis needs as much support and help as possible from whoever is available to give it. Lindemann and Caplan found that adaptive crisis resolution *can* result in enduring positive change.

Current crisis theory suggests that unresolved bereavement from earlier losses (of a person, a relationship, security, capacity, a dream) that may or may not be associated with crisis or trauma affects not only one's later day-to-day functioning, but also one's reactions to subsequent crises. Thus, it is important for helpers to learn about the victim's past experiences with abuse and loss so that helping strategies can be planned that enhance the person's style of coping.

Although crisis theory is indeed distinct from helping theory, it is consistent with and influenced by the models of helping discussed in this text. For example, the influence of the psychodynamic model on crisis theory is shown by the extensive research on suicide, which examines the connection between the current crisis and earlier experiences, as well as birth trauma, birth order, and familial and other interpersonal relationships. The influence of phenomenological theory is evident in the existential approach of crisis intervention, which emphasizes the here and now and the positive growth potential of crisis. Learning to cope effectively with a crisis will facilitate problem solving during future difficulties. The use in crisis intervention of supportive relationships with significant others and with an empathic helper, allowing the helpee to express intense feelings without interfering with his or her functioning, also demonstrates the influence of phenomenological helping theory.

The cognitive helping models are represented in crisis intervention theory in that helpers focus on improving the helpee's cognitive appraisal of the crisis and correcting his or her faulty or irrational thoughts. The cognitive-behavioral approaches contribute an understanding of reinforcement and problem-solving theory. The ecological/systems theories enable us to understand the crisis event in the context of the person's significant relationships and systems, focusing on both the contributing sources and available helpful resources. Multicultural theories remind us that understanding the influence of variables such as race, culture, class, religion, age, and sexual orientation can facilitate the accurate assessment of culturally appropriate services for people in crisis.

The major difference between helping strategies and crisis intervention strategies is the latter's focus on immediate, time-limited reactions to a specific source of stress. In the next section, we'll examine in more detail how helping strategies are an integral part of crisis and disaster intervention.

CRISIS AND DISASTER INTERVENTION

The major goal of short-term crisis and disaster intervention is to provide as much support and assistance as possible to individuals, their families, and victim groups in order to enable helpees to regain their psychological equilibrium as quickly as possible. From the crisis and disaster theory we have discussed, we can derive six major components of intervention.

1. The focus of crisis and disaster intervention is on specific and time-limited treatment goals. Attention is directed toward reduction of tension and adaptive problem solving. The time limits can enhance and maintain client motivation to achieve the specified goals.

2. Intervention involves clarification and accurate assessment of the source of stress and the meaning of the stress to the helpee, and it entails active, directive cognitive restructuring.

3. Intervention helps clients develop adaptive problem-solving mechanisms so that they can return to the level at which they were functioning before the crisis.

4. Intervention is reality oriented and focuses on clarifying cognitive perceptions, confronting denial and distortions, and providing emotional support rather than false reassurance.

5. Whenever possible, crisis and disaster intervention uses existing helpee relationship and survivor networks to provide support and help determine and implement effective coping strategies.

6. Intervention may serve as a prelude to further treatment. When the intensity of the feelings lessens and one is able to tolerate, not repress, these feelings, talking to someone about them can lead to working through or understanding and coming to terms with them.

Lazarus's BASIC ID model (see Chapter 6) may be useful as a comprehensive assessment scheme for crisis intervention helpers. One can quickly elicit information about the impact of the crisis event in the seven modalities—behavior, affect, sensation, imagery, cognition, interpersonal relationships, and diet/drugs—to determine which modality requires immediate attention and to determine which strategies best fit the particular client in the particular circumstances.

EXERCISE 9.4 ▪ Social networks can be useful in a variety of helping situations. This exercise is designed to help you articulate your own support systems. Draw an ecogram, or social network inventory, to see who actually comprises your current support network. List in columns on a sheet of paper your immediate family, extended family, neighbors, intimate friends, lover(s), casual friends, work associates, school associates, recreational friends, formal helpers (such as doctors, teachers, clergy), and other community members. After you have completed your list, place the appropriate number(s) from the following list next to each name. What can you conclude about your social support network? How would you like it to change? For the purposes of this exercise, contact includes in-person, telephone, or e-mail.

1. Close contact, at least once per week

2. No contact within past year

3. Casual, infrequent contact—only a few times per year

4. Have actually experienced support from this person in the past

5. Know I can *always* depend on this person for help

6. Not sure whether I can depend on this person

7. Know I *cannot* depend on this person

8. Would feel uncomfortable receiving support from this person

Stages and Steps of Intervention

Although there are many different models for intervention, our human relations counseling model can be modified and used to delineate commonly accepted crisis intervention stages and steps.

Stage 1: Relationship

Step 1: Initiation/entry

a. Assess cognitive, affective, and behavioral reactions to crisis and disaster incident(s) and how its meaning impacts helpee's identity as a victim.

b. Explore significant relationship systems (family, work, peer, neighborhood).

c. Create ongoing opportunities for helpee to express and ventilate intense feelings (for example, anger, fear, anxiety, sadness).

Step 2: Clarification of problem being presented/assessment of crisis and disaster

a. Assess major environmental variables (such as where and how one can receive social, physical, economic, and emotional support).

b. Determine helpee's perceptions of personal strengths/weaknesses.

c. Determine precipitating events (particularly those of the past 24 hours) resulting in psychological crisis—that is, significant change or loss.

d. Determine reason helpee is seeking help at this time.

e. Determine kinds of problem solving and coping strategies helpee has attempted in dealing with crisis/disaster (approach, avoidance, immobility).

f. Assess phase and classification of crisis/disaster: Is helpee dangerous to self, to others?

Step 3: Structure/contract for helping relationship

Inform helpee of what you can and cannot do within a limited time period to help him or her regain self-esteem, self-confidence, and efficacy.

Step 4: Intensive exploration of crisis/disaster situation and reactions

Step 5: Discussion of possible goals and objectives as well as time limits of intervention

a. Reiterate problem focus.

b. Reaffirm time limits.

c. Determine how other people and resources can be used.

d. Clarify who is responsible for what (for example, for drugs, referral).

Stage 2: Strategies

Step 1: Mutual acceptance of defined goals and objectives of intervention

Step 2: Planning of strategies

Consider utilization of support groups and other resources.

Step 3: Use of strategies

a. Cognitive restructuring

b. Referral

c. Supportive, empathic, responsive listening

d. Assertiveness training

e. Behavioral contract

f. Ventilation of feelings

g. Decision making

h. Systematic desensitization

i. Gestalt experiments

j. Social and political advocacy

Step 4: Evaluation of strategies

Step 5: Termination when crisis has been resolved or when referral is made

a. Formulate realistic plan for immediate future, which may include longer term treatment.

b. Verify that helpee is detached from intense emotional reaction.

c. Confirm that helpee has accurate cognitive appraisal of crisis event and appropriate management of affect.

d. Ensure that helpee is willing to seek and accept help from others when appropriate.

e. Confirm that helpee understands how present experience can help him or her cope with future events.

Step 6: Follow-up

Depending on context of intervention, determine whether resolution has been maintained.

The strategies listed under stage 2, step 3, are taken from Chapters 7 and 8 and are merely suggestions of strategies that can be used for crisis/disaster intervention. The point is that any strategy that works for a particular helpee quickly and effectively is valid for crisis/disaster intervention.

Brief Therapy

Brief therapy is a solution-focused form of therapy limited to 10 or fewer sessions. While there are many approaches, techniques, and philosophies of brief therapy, the four-step helping model developed by Watzlawick, Weakland, and Fisch (1974) is useful in some types of crisis intervention.

1. Describe the problem (or crisis) in concrete behavioral terms: frequency, duration, consequences, situational variables; try to understand the function of the problem and what the payoffs and purposes are.

2. Investigate previous attempts at problem resolution. "What have you done about this in the past?" "How?" "What happened when you tried something?"

3. Obtain a clear definition of the change to be achieved. What needs to happen for the helpee to feel better about this? How much change is the helpee willing to accept in order to be satisfied?

4. Formulate and implement a plan to produce the change. What will happen if the change actually takes place? How will the helpee deal with the consequences of change? What may happen to prevent change from occurring?

The focus of brief therapy is on solutions not problems, on what works for helpees rather than on what has not worked, on helpees' strengths rather than weaknesses. The approach is direct, active, and present/future oriented. A favorable helping relationship and problem definition must be established in the first meeting.

Consider the following case.

Ms. M., age 35, called the counselor sobbing about her husband's latest episode of coming home drunk and beating their only child, 11-year-old Tina. The counselor arranged to see the distraught mother that same day.

In describing her problem, Ms. M. reported that Mr. M. came home drunk about once every three or four weeks, usually after receiving his paycheck. When this happened, he immediately picked on Tina, using whatever excuse he could find, like her coat being out of place or her books being on the kitchen table. He yelled more than he hit, but this time he had really gone out of control and persisted in his hitting. After most altercations, Tina went to her bedroom crying and Mr. M. fell asleep on the couch. Ms. M.'s usual practice was to go into Tina's bedroom to comfort her. Until today she had been successful in convincing Tina to placate her father; by the next morning, things usually would have calmed down and everyone would act as if nothing untoward had occurred. Ms. M. was afraid of her husband and had never mentioned his drinking or treatment of Tina to him. What distinguished this incident was the severity of physical abuse and Tina's refusal the next day to talk to her father, who was acting hurt and bewildered.

In most states and in most agencies, the helper would have a duty to report child abuse to the authorities. In fact, most helpers review the limits of confidentiality in their initial sessions with clients. In this case, with the guidance of the supervisor or director of the agency, the helper would need to inform Ms. M. about this law as soon as the abuse is discussed. This is always a difficult task for the helper, as it will affect and perhaps even destroy the helping relationship. Yet without making this disclosure, the helper is failing to meet his/her ethical obligations to protect endangered children. In many cases, clients like Ms. M. are relieved by the disclosure and, though angry at first, go on to form good relationships with the helper. Most centers and agencies have clear guidelines and policies to follow and, hopefully, there is support and guidance for the helper from peers and supervisors.

It took two sessions before Ms. M. could verbalize the change that she wanted: for her husband to cease picking on Tina when he came home drunk and for Tina to resume friendly relations with her father. After much discussion, Ms. M. was able to see that if Tina were no longer the target of her father's drunken bouts, Ms. M. might be, and that she would have to learn assertive behavior to protect Tina and confront her husband.

Cognitive restructuring and assertiveness-training techniques were used. In addition, the helper and Ms. M. created a safety plan so that if she felt in danger she would know where she could go for help and what essential documents she should take with her. By the sixth session Ms. M. felt that the situation had changed: she reported meeting her husband at the door the next time he came home drunk and dealing with him directly—and she felt more in control of the situation. Although Mr. M. refused to come in for counseling, Ms. M. was amenable to attending some Al-Anon meetings and learning more about alcoholism.

Forms of Crisis Intervention

There are two main forms of crisis intervention: (1) hot lines, drop-in centers, and crisis clinics where victims can come in person or telephone 24 hours a day; and (2) outreach counseling, in which helpers go to the victims to provide immediate support and comfort as soon as they are notified of the crisis. Crisis intervention settings are often staffed by volunteers who undergo intensive, short-term, on-the-job training. They may or may not be supervised by professional helpers. In addition to developing crisis intervention centers, many schools and communities are working on crisis prevention programs.

Hot Lines, Drop-In Centers, and Crisis Clinics

Helpers working through hot lines, drop-in centers, and crisis clinics deal with suicide, drug, runaway, rape, alcoholic, and abortion crises, to name just a few. Helpers receive specialized training about hot line work and they are taught specialized knowledge about the issues involved in different kinds of crises. For example, a drug counselor knows the names of commonly used drugs, the effects of those drugs and their duration, and how to help a user on a bad trip. The suicide counselor knows how to recognize suicide threats, has studied the facts and statistics (not the myths) about suicide, and is aware of different kinds of intervention, such as providing a network of supporters for the victim during the crisis, helping the victim and his or her family change behaviors to alleviate the crisis, and helping the victim gain a different perspective on the crisis and the situation precipitating a suicide attempt.

In these settings, helpers must focus on immediate concerns. Sometimes they get only one or two chances to work with the victim. Therefore, they must be skillful at establishing empathic relations and providing accurate information and alternative options to the victims, all within a short period of time. Personal contact is important—whether over the telephone or in person. This contact may involve helpers working overtime, continuing a conversation by telephone, or arranging immediate referrals. Hot lines are often more accessible than face-to-face counseling and afford anonymity to the caller. But there is a lack of continuity due to the transitory nature of the hot line encounter, and there is little or no feedback to the helper and no follow-up. Also, some helpers find the lack of visual cues disquieting.

The following is an example of a late-night hot line call to a university crisis center.

Caller: Hello? Are you there?

Helper: This is the _____. May I help you?

Caller: I just need to talk to someone . . . I'm worried about my friend. I think he may be thinking about taking pills.

Helper: You're worried what can happen if someone overdoses on—what kind of pills?

Caller: Well, I dunno. Maybe Tylenol . . . he said that's what he'd take.

Helper: It's depressing and scary when someone is all alone, worrying. Taking too many pills may seem a way to get out of it.

Caller: Yeah. I wouldn't do that, of course, but he might.

Helper: Sounds like your friend needs to talk to someone about how bad he's feeling.

Caller: Well, he called some friends but they weren't home and his folks don't ever give a damn (*lots of anger in voice*).

Helper: So he's feeling lonely and rejected.

Caller: Yes, I guess so . . . actually, it's not my friend, it's me—and sometimes I feel like there's no one who cares enough to listen to me.

In this case, the helper spent about 35 minutes on the phone and then referred the helpee to the university counseling center. During this interview, the helper did a thorough suicide assessment. This included asking whether the caller had access to means to hurt himself, whether he had a specific plan for how and when he would hurt himself, whether he had ever tried to hurt or kill himself before and whether he had engaged in any behavior, such as giving away favorite possessions, that might signal an intent to follow through with his suicidal feelings and thoughts. Follow-up indicated that the helpee did report to the counseling center the next morning.

Telephone skills necessary for this type of work include the ability to use responsive listening to establish quick rapport and the patience to nondirectively follow the helpee's messages to assess the nature and severity of the problem. In the preceding example, if the helper had pushed the helpee to acknowledge that the problem was his rather than his friend's, the helpee might have hung up before help could be obtained. Patience, calm, and the courage to hang in there are necessary attributes for hot line workers.

Outreach Counseling

Sometimes helpers must go to the crisis victim rather than wait for the victim to come to them. This is a relatively new concept in human services and is based on the "visiting nurse" concept, in which primary care is taken to the client in the client's own setting. The advantage is that the helper is able to see the victim in context and to draw on immediately available resources such as family and neighbors. In addition, the helper is able to provide direct assistance in immediate problem solving (for example, finding a sitter for the children in the case of a parental accident, talking down a drug victim on a bad trip in a familiar setting, or arranging for immediate medical care). Outreach counseling usually involves more time and cost than other types of counseling, which may be why it is relatively rare. The time the outreach worker spends traveling to and from clients is time not used for helping and so is typically not reimbursable.

The outreach counselor feels comfortable in different settings and is not limited by the clock or the site. Some are on 24-hour call and think nothing of accompanying clients to the welfare or employment office or helping them obtain legal, educational, and health care. They engage in recreational and leisure-time activities with clients, know how to break up fights and deal with implosive violence, and have learned to establish trusting relationships in the most suspicious climates. Research, though limited, has shown that the best outreach counselors are those recruited from and trained within the communities where they will work. They are in touch with the customs and lifestyles of their neighbors and can overcome distrust and establish and maintain relationships more easily than an outsider could.

Outreach counseling requires unlimited patience and dedication. Crisis intervention is only one part of outreach counseling, which occurs throughout the community—on the streets, in bars, in houses and schools, in social centers, and on playgrounds.

Disaster Relief

Although the two forms of crisis intervention can apply to disaster survivors, the main form of disaster relief involves teams that work directly on site and in the community with victims, survivors, and others associated with major catastrophes. The teams may be composed of professionals, generalist human services workers, and volunteers in several areas, such as firefighters, police, health care personnel, mental health workers, and military personnel.

Disaster relief is a crucial response to disasters, such as airplane crashes, earthquakes, terrorist attacks, or war. Effective disaster response requires coordinated teamwork. Immediate attention is provided to the victims, the bereaved (the family or friends of victims), service and support providers (other people in contact with the victims such as the police, firefighters, or mechanics), and those who just happen to be in the immediate environment. Because of the immediacy of a disaster to media viewers, help is often even necessary for those peripheral to the actual event. For example, during the events of 9/11, some television viewers suffered symptoms of distress as severe as those experienced by those actually involved in the destruction. While most cities have medical disaster plans, only recently have mental health disaster plans been developed. Organized mental health disaster plans will speed the delivery of services and allow for better coordination and quality of help, thereby reducing the chaos that naturally follows a disaster.

The first step in disaster intervention is **triage,** the quick assessment of severity and scope of need. When a catastrophe occurs, the intervention team may organize into small groups for informational and assessment purposes. The use of teams facilitates information exchange among individuals, small groups, and rescue workers and allows for emotional venting and **critical incident stress debriefing** of reactions to the event within hours of the catastrophe. Concerns have been raised about using this type of intervention, questioning whether emotional venting can contribute to retraumatization.

Helper observations, feedback from others on site, and direct interactions facilitate decisions about what type of help is needed first. In some disasters, the pressing need is for food, water, and physical safety and deciding who is in need of what kinds of immediate services, who can wait, and who can be enlisted as a helping resource. Over the next few days, team members meet with families and other affected members of the community. The objectives of meeting with family and community members are to distribute information, provide an opportunity to express feelings, and enable family and community members to achieve mastery by getting and giving support.

Many communities and professional organizations have disaster relief teams that include mental health workers. They respond rapidly to school shootings, bomb scares, and other such incidents in their local communities. These teams have mobility and are trained to work with local resources and coordinate after-care services. The teams are organized, and leaders, supervisors, and role assignments are in place.

Prevention

Many educational programs have arisen on college campuses and in communities to help people avoid certain kinds of crises and cope with some of the developmental crises that are inevitable. For example, it is routine today for college first-year orientation programs to include rape prevention classes, sex education classes, drug education classes, and so on. In fact, some of these classes are now part of the regular curriculum in secondary and elementary schools. Crisis intervention workers often contribute directly or indirectly to these educational programs; needless to say, their experience provides them with invaluable knowledge and information.

Community agencies are often instrumental in producing and disseminating literature about potential crises, such as pamphlets on how to avoid assault, on neighborhood watch programs, and on first aid procedures. Local, regional, state, federal, and international agencies are developing prevention and intervention plans, such as evacuation plans for natural disasters, alertness to warnings of terrorism, and vaccinations for large-scale health disasters such as Avian flu.

EXERCISE 9.5 ■ In pairs, role-play a helpee and helper during a crisis intake interview. After approximately 30 minutes, each helper should write down (1) treatment goals and (2) favored crisis/disaster intervention strategies. Switch roles. Then everyone in the group should compare and discuss his or her evaluations. Possible crisis situations to role-play are a bad drug trip, date rape, discovery of an unwanted pregnancy, loss of necessary financial aid in the last year of school, or having survived a hurricane that destroyed one's house. Try out different forms of helpee reactions to the crisis situation, such as extensive crying, shock and numbness, anger, or suicidal thoughts.

EXERCISE 9.6 ■ In pairs, sit back to back and role-play a hot line situation. The helpee can select any type of crisis situation. Remember, as the helper, you have just this one time to talk to the helpee. Continue your dialogue as long as is natural. When you have finished, discuss your experience together and then share your reactions with the rest of the class. How did it feel not to have visual stimuli? What kinds of pressure did you experience?

Skills for Intervention

In crises and disasters, helpers' abilities to remain calm in an emergency, to use common sense, and to project self-confidence are important. Helpers rely greatly on their responsive listening communication skills, both to get at the nature of the crisis and its stressful ramifications and to communicate comfort, support, and respect to the helpee. In addition to responsive listening, in some cases physical gestures such as holding hands and putting an arm around the helpee's shoulders may communicate caring and concern.

Generally, it is important to differentiate between empathy and sympathy, as the latter can impede recovery from a crisis by fostering prolonged dependence. One way to avoid fostering dependence is to focus on what can be done about the personal crisis rather than repeating over and over again the details of the actual crisis or disaster situation. In other words, after the initial ventilation period, during which the victim describes in great detail the actual event, focusing on future action rather than on what happened is more conducive to recovery. Focusing on the helpee's past and current strengths and positive experiences emphasizes the positive rather than the negative and builds the helpee's faith in his or her capacity to recover.

In the beginning steps of intervention, the helper may judiciously pose some questions to the helpee in order to determine which intervention strategy to follow. In addition to asking questions about the actual event, the helper may ask the following kinds of questions:

What changes have occurred in your life recently, particularly in the past few days?

Have you had any particular difficulties with people who are important to you, like a family member, boss, valued friend?

What kinds of things have you already tried to do about this?

Have you ever experienced these kinds of feelings before? If so, when, and what did you do about them?

What do you think you need to have happen in order to get through this?

Who in your life do you think might be most helpful to you at this time?

You can see that the purpose of these questions, in addition to eliciting information quickly, is to engage the helpee in the process of understanding his/her emotional, cognitive, and behavioral reactions and in the development of adaptive strategies.

At the same time that helpers are providing respectful comfort and support to survivors, they may need to take some kind of direct action. They may have to physically prevent someone from hurting himself or herself or others; seek medical help; actively recruit networks of family, friends, or neighbors to stay with the helpee until the crisis has passed; arrange for some kind of immediate placement (for example, in a hospital or shelter); talk to others to understand the cause of stress for the victim; or arrange for burial rites and insurance benefits. Crisis or disaster victims are often unable to take these actions themselves and need to feel they can depend on others for a short while.

The dependency of a crisis/disaster survivor on the helper is accepted by the helper until such time as the survivor is ready for a referral or to take over for himself or herself. The counselor may need to keep in contact and share information with others involved with the helpee in order to reach this stage of readiness and have other people provide support for the survivor.

Reactions to crises and disasters involving loss, such as divorce and death, may have distinct stages, as noted by Kübler-Ross (1969). The initial reaction is one of shock and denial. The feeling is "this can happen to others, but not to *me.*" Helpers provide empathic support during this stage. As the denial fades, anger emerges, and helpers and those close to the helpee often receive the brunt of this anger. Acceptance and then coping occur when the helpee can remobilize coping strengths and resources and begin to plan and implement action leading to recovery.

Another skill used by crisis workers in certain kinds of situations is confrontation, in which the helper shows the helpee discrepancies in or ramifications of the crisis situation in order to stimulate immediate action. An example is a helper saying to a remorseful alcoholic who has beaten his wife while on a binge, "It's hard for you to control your temper when you drink. Now your wife is in the hospital, and she is thinking about pressing charges. In any case, she says she'll take the children and leave this time. It seems to me that you have to decide what you want to do about your drinking. If you want to keep your family, you'll have to deal with it. Let's go over the options you have." In a sense, this helper is telling the helpee to "shape up or ship out." Often this kind of "shock treatment" confrontation is necessary to get someone off dead center and moving in some direction.

In crisis and disaster situations, time is often a crucial variable; helpers do not have the luxury of building up long-term helping relationships before attempting problem solving. Therefore, confrontation often occurs earlier in crisis/disaster intervention than in other forms of helping. However, it is possible to be empathic and confrontational at the same time; the helper's tone of voice, body posture, and facial expression can make the difference between hostile and constructive confrontation. Constructive confrontation is not negative: it includes acknowledgment of the helpee's strengths and ability to choose a course of action. When using confrontation, it is vital that you do so for the helpee's benefit, not to let off steam, prove your superiority, or impose your will. In other words, the confrontation should be assertive rather than aggressive, and can be in line with your helping objectives.

In addition to the knowledge required for specific types of disasters and crises (for example, drugs, alcohol, child abuse, suicide), human services workers involved in intervention programs need to become thoroughly familiar with the sociological, economic, and cultural characteristics of the community in which they are working and the resources available within the community. Such knowledge is needed to make good referrals, especially when time is of the essence.

Following are four examples of crisis intervention.

Cecilia, a 19-year-old university student, came to see me (BFO) unexpectedly. I had met her once, when she accompanied her roommate to my office, but I had had no direct contact with her. She was in obvious distress and incoherently blurted out that she had some pills and was seriously thinking about taking them because she "didn't want to live anymore." I immediately notified my secretary to hold all calls and appointments and spent the next couple of hours talking with her. She told me that her fiancé and brother had been killed in an automobile accident six weeks before and that she just couldn't get over it. She didn't feel she had anything to live for. She cried . . . I held her . . . we went over her loss and her anger at being left alone, over and over again. Finally, when she was completely exhausted, I asked her if she thought we could work together to find some meaning in her life. When she tearfully agreed, I pushed for some commitment: Would she give me the pills and promise not to do anything to herself until I could see her the next day at 3:30? I asked her to look me in the eye and promise that much. It took some time for her to be able to do that. I then suggested that it might be helpful for her to have some friends with her. She said that she had friends here, including her roommate, but that she had tried to keep her grief from them. I secured her permission to telephone her roommate and to arrange for constant companionship until our next appointment. This was arranged to everyone's satisfaction. The next day, Cecilia felt that the immediate crisis was over and that we could begin to meet regularly to work her problem through without fear of suicide. Whether Cecilia's threats were legitimate is not important. I would never ignore such a threat nor discount it, and I do not leave clients until I have secured a commitment that they will not harm themselves.

Ari, 24, who worked at a beauty salon, phoned his employer to tell him that he was "sick" and could not come into work. He sounded very agitated and upset, and Robert, his boss and a hot line volunteer in his spare time, sensed that something was very wrong. Robert went over to Ari's house and found him disheveled, wild-eyed, and disoriented. Ari talked about dying and seemed incoherent. Knowing that Ari's family lived in the Middle East and that war had broken out, Robert thought that was the cause for this upset and tried to calm Ari down by talking quietly. It turned out that the precipitating crisis for Ari had occurred at work the previous day when Ari had overheard other workers and some customers making racist comments about him. Ari had worked in this shop for 10 years and was devastated by the abrupt loss of what he had experienced as safety and security. This had pierced his defense of keeping busy to avoid feeling and thinking about the war. Robert communicated empathy and demonstrated calm, supportive behavior. He encouraged Ari to return to the shop with him, and he was able to soothe and reduce tensions among his staff by his manner and actions. After work that day, Robert took Ari to a community center where he could receive some group support from other Arab Americans awaiting word about their families and friends in the Middle East. In this case, Robert's supportive communication skills as well as his active strategy of locating a resource to provide group support enabled him to help Ari emerge from his terror and deal more effectively with his situation.

Lieutenant Vinsen, a National Guard nurse, came for help because she was waking up in the middle of the night with tremors, gasping for breath. She had spent 10 days in New York City after the attack on the World Trade Center as part of a disaster relief team and had been cited for exemplary service. A school nurse in civilian life, she did not experience any symptoms until several months after returning from New York. During the initial session, the helper asked her if she had ever experienced the death of anyone close to her. It took Lieutenant Vinsen a while to volunteer that her younger sister had been killed at the age of 6 in a school bus crash. (The lieutenant was 8 at the time.) She surprised herself by commenting that she had "almost forgotten." Witnessing the brutal deaths of so many and tending to their surviving families in New York rekindled intense feelings of anger, helplessness, and sadness for Lieutenant Vinsen. Coming from a culture that did not allow emotional expressiveness within the family, she had always prided herself on being stoical and not feeling "sadness" or "weakness." In the two allotted crisis intervention sessions, Lieutenant Vinsen was encouraged to remember and talk about her sister's death and its impact on her and her family. Rather quickly, she began to see how it related to what she had experienced in New York. Crying, as well as acknowledging and talking about her pain, provided the therapeutic relief and release she required. She was then able to regain her feelings of mastery and self-esteem.

Suzanne, a mental health professional, was sent to Louisiana after Hurricane Katrina as part of a disaster response team. Although she was ready to assess the dazed evacuees, to ask them how they were doing emotionally, and to offer counseling, she quickly learned that her most important task in the first few days was to help the cooks in the kitchen and to participate in the distribution of clothes and toilet articles. As she performed these responsibilities, she made a point of warmly acknowledging and greeting staff and incoming evacuees. Within a few days, she was so accepted as a community member that people began to approach her to discuss their emotional concerns. A colleague of mine (REK) recently returned from volunteering at a post–Hurricane Katrina shelter. He said that the mental health workers were referred to as "paper clips" because they held everything together at the shelter.

EXERCISE 9.7 ■ Reenact the hot line role-play in Exercise 9.6, using the following situation. A woman calls you on the hot line and hysterically says, "Hello, my 22-year-old son tried to kill me. He actually went at me with a knife. I can't believe it. He's acting like he's crazy. I don't know what to do. I'm calling from the corner phone. I'm scared to go home, but I can't call the cops. He's my son. I love him. Help me. What should I do?" Compare your reactions to this exercise with your classmates' reactions, and discuss what critical information you would need to find out and what crisis intervention strategies you would use.

EXERCISE 9.8 ■ Which of the following statements do you believe to be true, and which are myths? Compare your answers with other students' and discuss your differences and agreements.

1. Nice girls don't get raped.
2. It is better to give a robber what he wants rather than resist.
3. Divorce is always harmful to children.
4. It is not really rape if you did not resist.
5. People who lose their jobs are obviously partially responsible.
6. Strong people do not crack up in crises.
7. Alcoholics go on binges because people drive them to it.
8. A man has the right to rape a woman who dresses seductively or accepts rides.
9. People who have sudden financial reverses must have brought them on by poor planning.
10. People who threaten to commit suicide are not really likely to do it.
11. People who undergo natural disasters are in more distress than those who undergo human-made trauma (such as abuse, assault, torture).
12. First responders (police and fire personnel, EMTs) have been trained to handle disasters and thus do not suffer any symptoms of distress.
13. It is important to encourage survivors of trauma and disaster to emotionally vent as quickly as possible after the event.

EXERCISE 9.9 ■ Imagine that you have been working with a student, Peg, for several months about her difficult relationships with family members. Peg just learned that her brother was killed in a suicide bombing in Iraq. She is distraught and tells you that she plans to drop out of school immediately. Role-play the therapist and client.

EXERCISE 9.10 ■ You have been assigned to go to Otis Air Force Base in Massachusetts to work with a Hurricane Katrina evacuee family from Mississippi.

They have enrolled their children in the public schools, and the father has been able to find a restaurant job. The mother wants to go back to Mississippi, even though they have no housing or jobs there. The father wants to remain in Massachusetts, at least until the end of the school year. Role-play the mother, the father, and the helper.

SUMMARY

This chapter presented an overview of crisis and disaster theories, their relation to helping theory, and the practice of crisis and disaster intervention. The extension of crisis intervention theory to disaster and trauma was discussed. We formulated six classes of emotional crises, in order to differentiate between developmental transitions and situational traumas. We highlighted the intervention phases of crisis and disaster theories. Many people—nonprofessionals, generalist human services workers, and professionals—deal with crises and disasters through face-to-face contact, over the telephone, or through various outreach programs and disaster response networks.

Our review of crisis and disaster theory indicates that short-term intervention can be effective and that identifying and using available support networks are critical components of intervention. It is interesting to note that people in crisis can be very open to change; thus, mental health interventions can lead to positive results, such as further counseling, recognition of personal strengths, and the ability to cope better with problems in the future.

Although crisis/disaster intervention sometimes demands a helping approach different from that of the counseling model developed in this book, it still requires good communication skills and the development of effective helping relationships. The helping strategies discussed in Chapters 7 and 8 can be modified and applied to crisis/disaster intervention. In addition, we presented a synopsis of brief therapy as a viable form of crisis/disaster intervention because of its active focus on problem solving.

This chapter also included a review of the stages and steps of crisis/disaster intervention and the skills needed to practice it.

REFERENCES AND
FURTHER READING

Aguilera, D. C. (1998). *Crisis intervention: Theory and methodology* (8th ed.). St. Louis, MO: Mosby.

Ashinger, P. (1985). Using social networks in counseling. *Journal of Counseling and Development, 63,* 519–521.

Barry, K. L. (1999). *Brief intervention and brief therapies for substance abuse.* Rockville, MD: U.S. Department of Health and Human Services.

Bell, J. L. (1995). Traumatic event debriefing: Service delivery designs and the role of social work. *Social Work, 40*(1), 36–43.

Boscarino, J. A., Adams, R. E., & Figley, C. R. (2004). Mental health service use 1 year after the World Trade Center disaster: Implications for mental health. *General Hospital Psychiatry, 26,* 346–358.

Budman, S. H., & Gurman, A. S. (1988). *Theory and practice of brief therapy.* New York: Guilford Press.

Caplan, G. (1961). *An approach to community mental health.* New York: Grune & Stratton.

Caplan, G. (1964). *Principles of preventive psychiatry.* New York: Basic Books.

Farber, M. (1968). *A theory of suicide.* New York: Funk & Wagnalls.

Farberow, N. L., & Schneidman, E. S. (Eds.). (1965). *The cry for help.* New York: McGraw-Hill.

Fiefel, H. (1959). *The meaning of death.* New York: McGraw-Hill.

Figley, C. R. (Ed.). (1985). *Trauma and its wake.* New York: Brunner/Mazel.

Fisch, R., Weakland, J., & Segal, L. (1982). *The tactics of change: Doing therapy briefly.* San Francisco: Jossey-Bass.

Gerber, S. K. (1999). *Enhancing counselor intervention strategies: An integrational viewpoint.* Philadelphia: Accelerated Development.

Gist, R., & Lubin, B. (Eds.). (1989). *Psychosocial aspects of disaster.* New York: Wiley.

Gray, H. J., & Litz, B. (2005). Behavioral intervention for recent trauma: Empirically informed practice guidelines. *Behavior Modification, 29,* 189–210.

Hamilton, S. (2005). Disaster/psychology. *Register Report, 31,* 28–32.

Herman, J. L. (2005). Early intervention for trauma and traumatic loss. *American Journal of Psychiatry, 162*(5). 1036–1037.

Horowitz, M. J. (1986). *Stress response syndromes* (2nd ed.). Northvale, NJ: Jason Aronson.

Kavel, K. (1999). *A guide to crisis intervention.* Pacific Grove, CA: Brooks/Cole.

Kübler-Ross, E. (1969). *On death and dying.* New York: Macmillan.

Lindemann, E. (1944). Symptomatology and management of acute grief. *American Journal of Psychiatry, 10,* 141–148.

Lystad, M. L. (Ed.). (1988). *Health response to mass emergencies.* New York: Brunner/Mazel.

Menninger, W. C. (1978). *Psychiatry in a troubled world.* New York: Macmillan.

Myer, R. A., Williams, R. C., Ottens, A. J., & Schmidt, A. E. (1992). Crisis assessment: A three-dimensional model for triage. *Journal of Mental Health Counseling, 14*(2), 137–148.

Norris, F. H., & Alegria, M. (2005). Mental health care for ethnic minority individuals and communities in the aftermath of disasters and mass violence. *CNS Spectrum, 10*(2), 132–140.

Osterweis, M., Solomon, F., & Green, M. (Eds.). (1984). *Bereavement.* Washington, DC: National Academy Press.

Parad, H. J., & Parad, L. G. (Eds.). (1999). *Crisis intervention: Book 2. The practitioner's sourcebook for brief therapy.* Hertsfordshire, UK: Manticore.

Richman, J. (1986). *Family therapy for suicidal people.* New York: Springer.

Satcher, D. (1999). *The surgeon general's call to action to prevent suicide.* Washington, DC: U.S. Public Health Services.

Sederer, L., & Rothschild, A. (Eds.). (1997). *Acute care psychiatry: Diagnosis and treatment.* Baltimore: Williams & Wilkins.

Slaikeu, K. A. (1990). *Crisis intervention: A handbook for practice and research* (2nd ed.). Boston: Allyn & Bacon.

VandenBos, G. R., & Bryant, B. K. (Eds.). (1986). *Cataclysms, crises, and catastrophes: Psychology in action.* Washington, DC: American Psychological Association.

Watson, P. J., & Shalev, A. Y. (2005). Assessment and treatment of adult acute responses to traumatic stress following mass traumatic events. *CNS Spectrum, 10*(2), 123–131.

Watzlawick, P., Weakland, J., & Fisch, R. (1974). *Change: Principles, problem formation, and problem resolution.* New York: Norton.

Wright, K. M., Ursano, R. J., Bartone, P. T., & Ingraham, L. H. (1990). The shared experience of catastrophe: An expanded classification of the disaster community. *American Journal of Orthopsychiatry, 60,* 35–43.

Visit the book companion site at www.thomsonedu.com to access tutorial quizzes.

10

Issues Affecting Helping

U nderstanding the first two dimensions of the human relations counseling model—stages and strategies—will not, by itself, allow us to completely understand the helping process. Given the complexities of both the readership of this book and the client populations of today's world, we need to continuously reassess, adapt, and modify our attitudes and beliefs associated with the third dimension of the model—issues. Unexamined values and beliefs can seriously hamper our usefulness as helpers. We must learn to respect individuality, as well as develop an appreciation that every life is shaped by institutions—family, school, work, community, church, government, culture—and that gender, class, race, age, sexual orientation, and ethnicity are among the powerful influences on our ever-developing self-identity, as well as on our views of others and the world.

Most of us choose friends with whom we can relate easily, share similar value systems, and feel comfortable revealing our true feelings and beliefs. This may restrict our understanding and appreciation of the plurality and diversity of people's lives outside our social network. As helpers, we are not always able to choose who will come to us for help or with whom we will work. Most helpers are willing to work with diverse clients and work continuously to increase self-awareness, so that their values, beliefs, and ideology do not have a deleterious effect on helping relationships. Helpers who are willing to work only with those who are similar to themselves must acknowledge this to prospective employers because they are unlikely to develop effective helping relationships with helpees who do not share their worldviews.

Many personal, societal, professional, and ethical issues affect helping relationships. It is not the intent of this chapter to explore all of these issues in depth but to make you aware of some of them. Consciousness-raising exercises and the reading list at the end of the chapter will enable you to study these issues further.

PERSONAL VALUES

The traditional models of helping maintained that if helping relationships were objective, distant, and neutral, the helper's values and beliefs would not contaminate the relationships. However, in recent years we have recognized that in any interpersonal relationship, whether a helping relationship or not, values are transmitted either directly or indirectly between the participants. The more self-aware helpers are, the less likely they are to hinder the helping relationship by imposing their own values on the client.

We cannot assume that our personal beliefs and values are universal. Since they are shaped by sociocultural variables, and we live in a multicultural society, multiple perspectives are inevitable. As we learn to respect differences, we can help our clients become more comfortable with differing views.

Discussion of values can enhance the helping relationship if both people are genuine and empathic. For example, one helper recalls her first counseling session with a lesbian. When she informed the helpee that she did not know, other than from reading, much about gay and lesbian issues, but that she wanted to learn, the helpee replied that she also was learning and that they could learn together. In another similar situation, the helpee responded that she wasn't coming for help in order to be the teacher and she would prefer to work with a "straight" counselor who had clinical experience with lesbian issues. (This particular helpee's reason for preferring a heterosexual helper was that she was struggling with her lesbian identity and she was concerned that she might risk persuasion from a lesbian helper.) Trying to change another person's value system is fraught with dangers, but helpers can at least help clients become aware of their own values in order to increase their self-understanding and ability to make effective choices.

Clarification of Values

Discussion of values is a form of teaching that provides information and alternative viewpoints; it differs from the imposition of values, which insists that there is a "right" view to adopt.

Values clarification is a systematic, seven-step approach developed by Simon, Howe, and Kirschenbaum (1972) that helps people process their values through structured exercises. Throughout the 1970s, these exercises were incorporated into school curricula and other organizational programming. Glaser and Kirschenbaum (1980) present examples of questions in the seven-step values clarification process that can be used in the helping relationship.

1. Prizing and cherishing one's beliefs and behaviors
   a. "Is that something that is important to you?"
   b. "Are you proud of how you handled that?"
2. Publicly affirming, when appropriate, one's beliefs and behaviors
   a. "Is this something that you'd like to share with others?"
   b. "Who would you be willing to tell that to?"
3. Choosing one's beliefs and behaviors from alternatives
   a. "Have you considered any alternatives to that?"
   b. "How long did you look around before you decided?"
4. Choosing one's beliefs and behaviors from alternatives after consideration of consequences
   a. "What is the thing you like most about that idea?"
   b. "What would happen if everyone held your belief?
5. Choosing one's beliefs and behaviors freely
   a. "Is that really your own choice?"
   b. "Where do you suppose you first got that idea?"
6. Acting on one's beliefs
   a. "Is that something you'd be willing to try?"
   b. "What would your next step be if you chose to follow that direction?"
7. Acting on one's beliefs with a pattern, consistency, and repetition
   a. "Is this typical of you?"
   b. "Will you do it again?"

Obviously, it is important for the helper to know when to question and when to listen, when to elicit feelings and when to reflect back the feelings expressed by the helpee.

As discussed in Chapter 1, one's personal values are intertwined with one's beliefs about such matters as gender, family, money, politics, religion, work, race, authority, and culture, as well as with one's personal taste and lifestyle. Values confusion usually results in interpersonal difficulties, the major reason that many people seek help from agencies and institutions. If helpers are uneasy about their values in any one of the previously mentioned areas, they may deliberately and subtly avoid those areas in helping relationships. For example, if you find that you never seem to get around to talking about sexuality with helpees who are involved in sexual relationships, you might ask yourself what's going on and why. You may find that you are the one who is uneasy about discussing sexuality, not the helpee.

Respect for Different Values

For helpers to create the necessary empathic conditions for effective helping relationships, they must be able to understand and accept people with different value systems. This necessity can create quite a dilemma for you as a helper. How can you be both genuine and nonjudgmental with someone whose values you dislike? How can you acknowledge the dignity and worth of an individual whose actions, attitudes, and ideology are unacceptable to you?

Accepting people means that you respect them as dignified, worthy individuals. It means that you recognize that they have as much integrity and right to be alive as any other human being. This does not mean you have to accept their behavior or concur with their values. Neither does it mean you cannot feel and express anger and disagreement when the timing is appropriate. It does mean that you can tolerate differences, ambiguity, and uncertainty, that you can accept that what is an acceptable choice or good for one person may not be an acceptable choice or good for another. It also means that you are sensitive to multicultural worldviews and the values they engender.

Responsive listening and sending "I" messages (for example, "I feel angry when you . . ." rather than "You are mean and nasty when you . . .") can help you communicate not only respect for the helpee as a worthwhile human being but also your genuine feelings and reactions along with your personal values and views, without imposing them on the helpee. In this way, the helper aids helpees in learning to acknowledge and evaluate their own values. By sharing our values at carefully chosen times, based on the needs of the helpee and the formation of the helping relationship, we may be adding options and alternative values for helpees to consider. By the same token, we may gain insight into our own value systems. Research by Enns and Hackett (1990, 1993) concludes that explicit helper value statements provide useful information, help clients and counselors define reciprocal roles, and promote an atmosphere of equality, respect, and trust.

An example of values sharing occurred in my (BFO's) office when a couple came in for marriage counseling.

Counselor: Can you try to tell me what you see as the problems in this marriage?

Husband: Yes. She's not a good wife. She won't have sex with me, and she's always going out with friends after work, and she's not a good mother either—our boys don't listen to her. I make four times as much money as she—I give her a nice house, everything, and she won't even let me touch her.

Wife: You're always criticizing me, telling me what to do, and when I say "no" to the kids, you say "yes." I'm fed up with this. I'm not your slave, and I won't follow your orders. You make me sick.

Counselor: (*to husband*) It's important to you that your wife do things for you the way you want them to be done because then you would know she cares for you.

Husband: That's right! That's her job. Without me, she'd have nothing. Her job pays peanuts. I'm a self-made man; I work very hard, and I give her everything.

Counselor: (*to husband*) You're angry and disappointed because you feel your wife is not meeting her obligations to you.

Wife: (*interrupting*) He always wants more and more. He's angry because finally I have my own friends and my own life. I don't care that I don't make much money. I like what I do and having some freedom now that the boys are in high school.

Counselor: (*to husband*) I'm having a hard time with your concept of a wife's obligations. However, I do see that, in your view, she is rocking the boat and that it's hard for you to understand or look at it any way other than as a sign that she is disloyal and uncaring.

In the preceding excerpt, I (BFO) expressed my views without deriding or punishing the husband. This seemed to help both husband and wife begin to acknowledge and evaluate some of their different values and beliefs about sex roles and marriage.

Another example of values sharing is provided by the following example of a 19-year-old college student who was talking about flunking out.

Client: My dad's going to be very angry about losing all this money. I'm going to see if I can get my tuition back.

Counselor: You're really afraid of your dad's reaction to your flunking out again.

Client: I'm going to tell them I was sick. I think I'll tell them I had an operation and that's why I couldn't attend classes. Don't you think they'll give me my money back? They did it for my girlfriend. She had her appendix out.

Counselor: It seems to you that you can ease your dad's reaction and anger at you if you can at least get some money back for him . . . the money will make it all right.

Client: Yes . . . that's what I'll do. Do you think they'll give me my money back? It's so much money . . . twenty thousand dollars.

Counselor: I'm uncomfortable with claiming illness as the reason for not going to classes.

Client: Really? Why?

Counselor: To me, that would be lying. You must think I'm pretty square, but I want you to know how I feel.

Client: Um-m. It's always worked before.

Counselor: Sometimes the ends seem to justify the means for you.

Client: M-mmm. I never thought of it like that.

The session then focused on the client's need to defend herself against her father's reactions. She became aware of the manipulative devices that had worked for her in the past. The counselor's statement of values did not inhibit the relationship. Two weeks later, the client reported that she had received a 75 percent rebate and that it had not been necessary for her to lie to get it.

Helpers who have strong ideologies are often dismayed by the philosophy that they should not impose their values on helpees. But imposition of values and beliefs rarely results in growth and independence. Rather, it results in submission to or withdrawal from the counselor. Helpers can share their ideologies and offer them as options for consideration, but it is important for all choices and decisions to be the helpee's, not the helper's.

An example of withdrawal occurred in a counseling session in which the counselor was working with a couple. The wife was concerned about having children because she did not want to give up her career; her husband felt it was important for children to be with their mothers full-time for the first five years and that, since his job was more important than his wife's, she would have to be the full-time parent. This couple was in their late 30s, and because most physicians believe it becomes riskier to have children as middle age approaches, it was important that they resolve this issue before too many years passed. Thus, they went to a community agency for counseling. They were assigned to a female counselor who identified strongly with the wife and immediately proceeded to berate the husband for being a "selfish male chauvinist." By so strongly interjecting her value system, this counselor completely alienated both husband and wife by the end of the first session, and the couple chose not to return. The wife commented afterward that despite her anger at her husband, and even though she agreed with the counselor's values, she so resented the attack on her husband that she became protective of him. If the counselor had used responsive listening and had spent time developing a relationship with the couple and drawing them out, rather than reacting to their struggle, she would have been able to suggest some alternatives reflecting her values for their consideration. Thus, she would have had a better opportunity to expose them to different values and perhaps to help them.

Rogers (1967) suggests that if you continue to have negative feelings about a client, you should first do some "homework" about those feelings to determine where they are coming from and whether they relate to some of your own concerns. You can then check them out with the client by focusing on the areas causing the negative feelings, and if they continue to persist, you can finally confront the client, using "I" statements. Examples of this kind of confrontation are "I find myself feeling angry whenever I hear you talk about your husband in such a deprecating way, such as when you said that 'all men are really babies and Joe is no exception.' I'd like to talk about this with you because my angry feelings are getting in the way"; or "I'm having a hard time listening to you talk about spending money on buying a new TV when you know that Jamie needs to see a dentist. I know that for me a kid's health care is more important than TV. I don't want my values to get in the way, and I want to try to understand. Can we talk about this some more?"

There *are* going to be situations in which you find it difficult to be genuine and nonjudgmental at the same time. It would be irrational to believe you can like and work well with all people. If, after you have tried talking it out with the helpee and you are still unable to feel genuine positive regard for him or her as a person, you have certain options to consider: (1) locating another helper, (2) seeking consultation (from a supervisor or colleague) in working the problem through with the client, or (3) limiting your relationship to the accomplishment of specific, immediate, concrete goals, such as obtaining food stamps, processing papers, or providing factual information.

The following exercises will help you become more aware of how you react in uncomfortable situations.

EXERCISE 10.1 ▪ In small groups, role-play the roles of helper and helpee in the following situations and then discuss your feelings and reactions to see if different people role-play in similar or different manners. The purpose of this exercise is to help you become more aware of the effect of your values on your helping. Some controversial topics that will get you in touch with your values and others' are the following:

1. A 12-year-old comes to see you because she is pregnant and wants to keep her baby.

2. A nurse's aide comes to see you because she is in conflict about the issue of euthanasia with regard to a terminally ill 37-year-old woman in great pain, who keeps pleading for an overdose of drugs.

3. A 16-year-old boy tells you he is having a homosexual affair with his 17-year old cousin.

4. A couple is considering an interracial marriage.

5. A 17-year-old girl comes to you to talk about whether or not she should tell her mother that her father is having an affair with his secretary.

6. A 48-year-old woman tells you that her husband is physically abusing her but she does not want to leave the relationship.

Now let's do an exercise that will help you clarify some of your own values in relation to helping.

EXERCISE 10.2 ▪ Write your immediate reaction to the following situations. Identify your personal values and beliefs. See whether you can determine which sociocultural values and beliefs influence your feelings—including gender, race, class, ethnicity, community, religion, and sexual orientation. How would you hope to work with the client(s) in these circumstances? Discuss your answers in small groups.

1. An interracial couple comes to you because they are fighting about the minority parent's desire to spend extended time with his child and his parents without his dominant-culture wife.

2. Parents come to you because they suspect their 40-year-old son is gay and they don't know whether to let him know that they know. They love him and are willing to accept him, whatever his orientation. Now repeat the example and imagine that they love him but tell you they are not willing to accept him if he is gay.

3. An 18-year-old college freshman wants to sell one of her eggs to a fertility clinic for $50,000, and her parents want her to talk to a counselor who would help her think through all the ramifications of such a decision.

4. An elderly couple wants advice about how to handle their 45-year-old son, who refuses to get a job and move out of their home. The son claims his parents "owe him," and the parents are confused and upset.

5. A 50-year-old widower wants to marry a 19-year-old "free spirit" who refuses to care for the widower's 13- and 15-year-old daughters. He is upset that his daughters will not cooperate by going to boarding school.

6. A 14-year-old boy is upset about his parents' drug usage but does not want to report them because he is afraid of being sent to foster care.

7. A 16-year-old girl has been caught shoplifting. She refuses to acknowledge that she did anything wrong and is angry that she was caught. Her parents insist that she see you.

8. A 48-year-old man who has smoked marijuana most of his adult life is angry at his fiancée for insisting he not be with her when or after he smokes. He claims she is "controlling" and threatens to terminate the engagement. He wants you to explain to her that "everyone does this and there is nothing wrong about it." Now replace "marijuana" with "cigarettes" and repeat the example.

9. A single mother of Latino culture is sent to see you by her 11-year-old son's teacher. The boy and his mother live in a one-room apartment and have always shared a bed.

10. A same-gender couple is considering adopting a child. What if the two partners are men? What if they are women?

11. A 21-year-old male college senior wants to talk with you about a sex-change operation. He tells you that he has always felt feminine and he knows he would be happier if he could have surgery to become a woman.

Sexism

In the past 35 years, changes in the economic, social, and legal position of women have resulted in dramatic shifts in the traditional values, expectations, and life goals of both men and women. These changes are reflected in our educational and child-rearing practices as well as in different types of family structures.

Today's generation of adolescents and young adults is making very different career, family, and lifestyle choices from those of their parents and grandparents. For example, many more women have not only entered but advanced in professions and occupations that were heretofore the domain of men (such as law, computers, finance, government leadership, aviation, medicine, management, high technology, and the military). There are increasing numbers of dual-career couples (some even commute to see each other), single men and women choosing to have children naturally or by adoption, single parents as a result of divorce or widowhood, same-gender couples, and men and women single by choice, all of whom struggle to balance individual, career, and family needs and demands. Another emerging family trend is for the wife to be the major breadwinner and the father to remain at home as the primary parent.

Today, there is more acceptance and understanding of gender differences due to biological and socialization variables, and there is a continuous demand for equal treatment of and power for both genders. The work of Gilligan (1982) and Miller (1986) has been crucial for understanding that women are socialized to be more relational and attached than men, who are socialized to be more autonomous and separate. Technology now enables us to learn about sex differences in the brain, which may be associated with gendered differences in human behavior. Throughout the life span, women deal with issues and transitions from a nondominant perspective in a male-dominant culture. These different developmental paths have a profound impact on individual, couple, and family experiences.

All helpers need to understand nonstereotypic career development, the gender issues of life-span development, and more complex family and couples' difficulties as people deal with dual-career pressures, divorce, widowhood, being single, gay and lesbian relationships, and single parenting. In addition, such issues as unplanned pregnancy, abortion, adoption, infertility, rape, sexual abuse and harassment, and decisions about sexual orientation may become important topics in counseling.

Despite the progress that has been made in the past decades, stereotypes have not yet been totally erased. Recent economic downturns and tensions about "family" and "family values" have unleashed a resurgent backlash of sexism (along with racism, ethnocentrism, and heterosexism). Regional, generational, and ethnic variables affect the degree and pervasiveness of sexism in our personal and professional lives. Studies still indicate a widespread incidence of sexist counseling (Klonoff, Landrine, & Campbell, 2000). In fact, the danger is more insidious than before in that many helpers believe they are open-minded and *not* sexist while their actual helping reflects basic stereotypic beliefs and values. A classic study by Broverman and his colleagues (1970), clinical psychologists known for their research into sex roles, indicated that mental health workers had different standards of mental health for men and women. The research found that many mental health workers perceived males as "healthier" than females in general and "healthy" women as more submissive, less independent, less adventurous, less competitive, more easily influenced, less aggressive, more excitable in minor crises, and more emotional than "healthy" men. A study by O'Malley and Richardson (1985) has updated the Broverman study, finding that while counselors' standards are a reflection of sex stereotyping in society as a whole, counselors now perceive both typically feminine and typically masculine characteristics as appropriate for the normal adult. Current work (Barnett & Rivers, 2004; Enns, 2004; Green, 2003; Hyde, 2005; Mirkin, Suyemoto & Okun, 2005) focuses on the clinical implications of gender similarities and differences.

While covert and overt sexism still exist, we are now recognizing that gender bias cannot be separated from other sociocultural forms of discrimination (particularly classism and racism) as significant biases affecting the helping relationship. Sexual harassment and abuse by helpers are serious concerns of the mental health profession. Although the number of complaints has risen in recent years, the problem is thought to be vastly underreported (Corey & Herlihy, 1997; Gartrell, Herman, Olarte, Feldstein, & Localio, 1987; Herlihy & Corey, 1997; Peterson, 1992; Pope, 1988; Pope, Sonne, & Holroyd, 1993; Pope & Vetter, 1992). There is no equivocation by the mental health professions that such abuse is unethical and harmful. Codes of ethics address this issue directly. While some states have legislation making this action a civil and/or criminal infraction, unless the helpee is willing to bring charges against the helper who violates this ethical code, little can be done formally. One of us (REK) was the therapist for a woman who had been involved sexually with her previous therapist. The client was unwilling to either press charges or report the prior therapist's ethical violations to the professional association. Due to rules of confidentiality, I had to respect my client's wishes. Because of the increasing number of complaints, professional associations and state legislatures are paying more attention to this issue, hoping to have an impact on the incidence rate. As with all kinds of sexual and power abuse, media coverage and legal means of redress empower victims and may deter perpetrators.

Sexist counseling occurs when gendered stereotypical roles and behaviors are encouraged, as when boys are discouraged from becoming elementary or preschool teachers or nurses, discouraged from expressing emotions and feelings, or chastised for not being athletic. Perhaps a more insidious example is the helper who suggests that a woman is not a "true feminist" if she enjoys staying home with her family and homemaking and who urges her to seek a career to "fulfill" herself. Single men who choose to adopt a child often find adoption workers leery about a man's parenting capabilities compared to a woman's.

In addition to those mentioned previously, sexist counseling practices reported by professional association task forces include fostering prolonged dependency relationships; having sexual contact with clients; encouraging women to submit to oppressive and stereotyped sex-role behaviors within marital, sexual, career, and employment situations; blaming the woman who is a victim of assault or of sexist practices by others; interpreting women's problems in terms of sexist theoretical concepts; providing a husband with unauthorized information about his wife; and failing to use appropriate community referral resources.

Sexism exists in most organizations and is often subtle and difficult to identify. Okun and Ziady (2005) discuss the relatively high degree of sexism in hierarchically organized corporate cultures as opposed to newer (high-technology) collaboratively organized corporate cultures. Aside from obvious sexist practices, such as paying different salaries for the same job functions and practicing discriminatory promotion, many so-called progressive organizations assign women to leadership tasks involving human relations because "women are better at that kind of stuff." Women are also subtly discouraged from applying for positions supervising men and from behaving assertively in staff meetings and at conferences.

We now recognize the impact of sexual discrimination on men, as well; they are often discouraged from entering traditionally feminine occupations. Men who value family over career and participate in primary or coparenting often experience discrimination from female primary parents as well as schools and other community organizations.

Nonsexist occupational, family, and lifestyle choices are just as necessary for men as for women. Although it is possible that sex-role stereotyping may be changing as a result of affirmative action programs, the women's movement, and the economic necessity for more and more women to enter the labor market, it is important for helpers to deal with their own biases, the biases of others in their work settings, and the biases present in testing and informational materials in order to expand, rather than restrict, options for both males and females.

Feminist theorists emphasize the importance of social change as a key component of individual change. Social change attempts to remedy the problems brought about by power differentials, as well as to make systemic changes to create equality. Thus, if you want to combat sexism, you need to go beyond your work with individual clients. You can work actively in organizations and in human relations to promote day-care facilities for women in your setting; promote flexible hours and jobs for women with families; actively agitate for the opening of jobs, courses, programs, and activities to both males and females in your work setting and community; and help reduce sex discrimination in recruitment and hiring as well as in training and placement. In other words, you can practice what you preach. Also, whenever possible, you can initiate group discussion among men and women within your organization and community about current gender-role ideologies and possibilities for expansion into personal, family, and work lifestyles. If you have children, you can help them reach their full potential by not imposing traditional gender roles. These activities will have a ripple effect on your actual helping relationships; greater awareness results in more open, fairer helping relationships.

The following exercises will help you discuss gender-role ideologies within your training group.

EXERCISE 10.3 ■ Divide your group into women and men. First, each individual ranks men and women in general from 1 (low) to 5 (high) on the characteristics in the following list. After each person has completed his or her rating, men and women compile group ratings, which they post on the board or on a large piece of paper, using the following form:

Men				Women	
Men	**Women**			**Men**	**Women**

    1. Serious intellectual pursuit

    2. Aggressiveness

    3. Emotionality

    4. Physical strength

    5. Nurturance

    6. Humor

Compare the results and discuss them as a large group. Are there greater differences *between* the men and the women than between the ratings of men and women *within* each group? How do you explain these differences? What helped or hindered reaching a consensus in each group? Does the consensus agree closely with your individual scores? How did you feel about sharing your views with the others in your group? How much pressure, either externally or internally, did you feel to be "politically correct" about your values?

EXERCISE 10.4 ▪ First decide how you feel about each of the following statements. Then, in small mixed groups, discuss them as freely as possible, remembering to practice responsive listening, to listen closely to the views of others, and to express your own values without imposing them on others.

1. Most women are capable of performing well as both worker and homemaker.
2. Women are not capable of becoming police officers or firefighters.
3. Women should not make more money than their husbands.
4. Women with children under 5 years old should not work.
5. There is something wrong with women who are not married by the age of 35.
6. There is something wrong with men who are not married by the age of 35.
7. No man wants to work for a female boss.
8. No woman wants to work for a female boss.
9. Women are better suited to parenting than men.
10. Men have more leadership capabilities than women.
11. Men and women should not have close friendships with someone of the opposite gender if they are in a significant heterosexual relationship.
12. Men and women should not have close friendships with someone of the same gender if they are in a significant homosexual relationship.
13. Women who are assertive and successful in their careers lose their femininity and their attractiveness to men.

Racism and Ethnocentrism

Like sexism, racism exists in our society. Biased counseling exists when helpers ignore factors such as the impact of poverty and a history of cultural oppression and allow their prejudices about different racial, ethnic, and foreign groups to contaminate helping relationships.

The most common form of biased counseling is a result of stereotypical assumptions and leads to lower expectations for nondominant (in terms of color, religion, or ethnicity) populations. Blatant examples of biased counseling in schools occur when minority children are discouraged from enrolling in college preparatory programs, from pursuing white-collar career exploration and postsecondary education, and from joining school clubs and seeking office. The same discrimination and prejudice occur in work settings of all varieties, where nondominant or minority groups are denied access to certain jobs or where tokenism is practiced. Counseling that is influenced by institutional racism also surfaces in family service agencies when white middle-class helpers act on false assumptions about minority groups' family roles, when people of color are assigned only to counselors of color, or when a higher no-show rate for families of color is considered evidence of their unwillingness to change or ignorance, rather than as a sign that the agency may not be meeting their needs.

Ethnocentrism refers to the assumption that one's own cultural values are universal or can be applied universally. When, for example, we assume that a helpee of another culture is being "resistant" because he is not sharing his feelings with us, we are being ethnocentric in that we are not considering that our notion of client behavior may be at odds with this particular client's cultural values and beliefs. As the demographics in our country continue to change, we need to learn to value others' worldviews. Atkinson (2004) and Corey (2005) suggest that we work toward a shared worldview and learn communication strategies, such as perspective-taking skills and behavioral flexibility, that enhance our ability to arrive at mutually shared perspectives.

Racism and ethnocentrism can be combated only with ongoing consciousness raising, study, exposure to different cultural value systems, continued professional development training, and training of more minority helpers (see Okun, Fried, & Okun, 1999). It is important that helpers support equality for people of all races, ethnicities, and nationalities and that a concerted effort be made to train more diverse people for the helping professions so that heterogeneous groups of helpers can learn from each other to deal with their own and others' biases and stereotypes. In this way, helpers can remove racism and ethnocentrism, among other "isms," from the counseling relationship.

The issue of how effective white helpers can be with minority helpees or how effective minority helpers can be with white helpees has been raised over and over again during recent years. We have seen many examples of minority counselors effectively helping white clients and vice versa. It is our belief that a skilled, competent helper who is conscious of his or her biases and values can work effectively with a wide variety of clients. However, conclusive research findings do not exist. We base our views on the belief that all people have the same kinds of psychological needs, problems, and physical sensations despite the obvious differences in circumstances and societal opportunities, and on our collaborative experiences with helpers of different backgrounds. Helpers' skills and specialized knowledge are more important than factors such as race, ethnicity, religion, or gender.

It is important for helpers to seek out unbiased information and tests, to provide for group interaction among people of different backgrounds, and to attempt to expand horizons for all people. Likewise, it is useful for helpers at all levels to keep up with the current literature and research regarding racism and ethnocentrism and to continue to expand their consciousness.

Horror stories illustrating discrimination in counseling abound. One Mexican American student recently reported her feelings of dismay when her high school counselor said she should not attempt to go to college because her father disapproved and it was "important to stick to her heritage." A very talented

African American graduate student was told "kindly" by his university counselor that he would have difficulty entering an area of study dominated by white men and was advised to change his major. Many white helpers report they feel uneasy when working with minority clients, fearing they will be considered racist if they challenge the client in any way. African American and white helpers who work with minority clients recommend that helpers bring up the issue of race or ethnicity during the initiation/entry stage of helping. An example might be "You're probably wondering how I, as a white person, can possibly understand you and your experience as an African American." If the helpee is concerned about the race or ethnicity of the helper, then it can be discussed and explored at the outset. If the client is surprised by the introduction of this topic and states that it is not an issue, the helper can proceed to the concerns presented by the helpee.

A more subtle form of prejudice exists when helpers modify the helping process in any way based on unsubstantiated attitudes and assumptions about race or ethnicity rather than on the nature of the helpee's problem. Some helpers have been heard to say that responsive listening is not effective with African American helpees, that directive behavioral techniques are more effective; however, responsive listening has been found to be effective in developing helping relationships with helpees who possess normal verbal skills.

As international boundaries continue to blur, we will be interacting with more people from different cultures than ever before. As helpers, we need to become aware of our own values, acquire knowledge of whatever cultural groups we are working with, and learn whatever helping strategies and approaches may be applicable to members of that group, while at the same time remembering that there is a great deal of variation within groups.

Pedersen (2003) suggests that helpers need to be eclectic so as to deliver services appropriate to a variety of cultural groups. He urges helpers to figure out which of their basic values are shared by everyone, regardless of culture, and how cultures differ along a continuum. For example, styles of interpersonal communication range from direct to indirect, expectations of authoritarian figures range from powerful to weak, and degrees of individual control and responsibility range from high to low. Das (1995) suggests that counselors need to focus on the social and political contexts of counseling, highlighting such phenomena as social stratification, unequal power relationships among racial and ethnic groups, economic disadvantage experienced by some minority groups, changing demographics, social change, and acculturation. Sue and Sue (2002) also stress how important it is for a helper to understand clients' views of the social environment so as to evaluate problems from their perspective. This will enable helpers to understand clients' cultural attitudes toward helping relationships and the helping process.

Obviously, further research is needed so that counselors can continue to expand their understanding of how best to help a diverse clientele. The main points to remember are that you bring your own cultural values and perspectives to the helping process and that there are many differences in values, attitudes, and beliefs both among groups and among individuals within groups. We need to become increasingly sensitive to clients' struggles to integrate multiple cultures into their identities rather than assimilating into a dominant culture at the expense of part of their cultural heritage. It is also important to consider the different effects of such factors as gender, generation, class, and assimilation experiences and opportunities within diverse cultures.

Thus, our theories and techniques, as well as the profession itself, are cultural phenomena reflecting our culture's history, beliefs, and values. Our norms are not necessarily applicable to other cultural groups, and we need to continually reassess our assumptions.

EXERCISE 10.5 ■ This is a much-used exercise, with many variations, that helps you recognize discrimination. Divide into two groups—they may or may not be the same size. The class leader arbitrarily assigns one group to be the "privileged" and the other group to be the "underprivileged." The underprivileged use armbands or some other means to distinguish themselves from the privileged. For the next 30 minutes, the privileged are to practice every form of discrimination they can conceive of, such as placing all the underprivileged together in a corner of the room, eating and having fun in front of them without letting them participate, taunting them, whispering about them, and so forth. At the end of the 30 minutes, without any processing, switch the group roles for an additional 30 minutes. After this, process your experiences: How did you feel as a privileged and as an underprivileged person? What was easy and difficult for you? What kinds of leadership emerged in each of the groups? With whom did you find yourself allying? Did you stay away from certain people? What did you do or not do?

EXERCISE 10.6 ■ In small groups, see if you can agree on at least five basic values that apply to all human beings regardless of racial, ethnic, and cultural differences. Then share your findings in the large group. After group discussion, rank each value SD (strongly disagree), D (disagree), A (agree), or SA (strongly agree). What did you learn from this exercise? Did you change your mind about any of the values listed?

EXERCISE 10.7 ■ When you have completed Exercise 10.6, discuss what attitudes may arise in the following counseling dyads: (1) white client/ethnic minority counselor; (2) Latino counselor/Native American client; (3) gay counselor/heterosexual female client. How might you overcome these attitudinal differences? How do they interface with the five basic values you arrived at in Exercise 10.6?

Ageism

Ageism—perhaps a less obvious "ism"—is defined as imposing on other people our own beliefs and values about what can or should be done at different ages. We know that age discrimination exists in the labor market in that some people are considered too old for a job and some too young. Age discrimination also exists in human services in that some helpers believe that older people cannot really be helped, and therefore avoid working with them. (Ageism usually refers to the problems of being old rather than to the problems of being too young.)

Helpers should try to understand that there are wide varieties and differences in individual development and that restricting opportunities by age may not be valid. Likewise, each developmental stage or age has something unique to contribute to society, and we should begin to think more about the positive aspects of old age than about the problematic aspects.

The number of healthy, actively functioning people over the age of 70 has been steadily increasing in the past decades, and this trend will continue in the 21st century. As a result, people in many societies are learning to revise negative, restrictive expectations and attitudes about late adulthood. (It must be noted that negative attitudes about the elderly are not universal; in certain cultures, elders have long been respected and revered.) The meanings of life and possibilities for gratification in later years are limitless. Yet many people over 70 are poor and face health, housing, and economic problems, with limited social supports and resources.

Helpers need to study the age-linked changes that occur in sensory, cognitive, motor, and affective areas, and the effects of environmental, social, and health factors on older people. For example, older people often feel inadequate because they can no longer support themselves financially. We as helpers can let them know that their poverty is not of their making and that we understand that their problems often result from inappropriate societal opportunities.

Again, we need to become conscious of our own attitudes and beliefs, to examine our stereotypic assumptions about different age groups. An example of ageist helping occurred when a 69-year-old woman told her 40-something therapist that she wanted to go to school to obtain an M.S.W. degree. The therapist told her she was "past that stage of life" and should focus on volunteer work. It would not have been "ageist counseling" if the therapist, by using responsive listening, had led the woman to arrive at her own conclusions.

Current research (Birren & Schaie, 1996; Hepple, 2004; Trotman & Brody, 2002; Weiss & Bass, 2002) focuses on the plasticity of the aging brain. This research enables helpers to understand cognitive processes in late adulthood and to recognize the variables contributing to "successful aging." Effective helping relationships for the elderly require time, patience, and empathic communication skills. In addition, reminiscing is an important strategy in the work with many older adults. Reviewing with the elderly all they have done with their lives and focusing on the positive (as in crisis intervention strategies) can be helpful.

Advocacy seems to be one of the best strategies for working with the elderly. Helpers need to learn about the services and resources for the aged within their communities, identify key people within helping organizations, and familiarize themselves with bureaucratic procedures (for example, Medicaid and Social Security practices).

Helpers can educate families and members of the community about the facts of old age and options for dealing with aged relatives. It is hoped that such education will help reduce discrimination and segregation due to age in schools and work settings as well as in facilities for the aged, and increase incorporation of the aged into the mainstream of society. For example, senior citizens are increasingly participating in activities in the community, such as reading to children and volunteering in preschools, public schools, nursing homes, and rehabilitation settings. More and more community programs for the elderly are focusing on physical fitness, social engagement, and cognitive stimulation.

An emerging career path for professional helpers is to provide direct and indirect services to the elderly and their families. These helpers coordinate services, arrange for home visits, find transportation to doctors, and consult regularly with distant family members. They also help determine the appropriateness of nursing home or assisted living placement.

EXERCISE 10.8 ■ Think about all the older people you have known, in your own family and in your friends' and neighbors' families. What 10 words that come to mind to characterize these people and your attitudes toward them? Give three examples of age-related discrimination. How would you want your parents to experience the ages between 65 and 85? Over 85? What would you like your own experiences to be? What kinds of dependence issues can you foresee? What kinds of social policies do you think we need?

Other Issues

Other values that may affect the counseling process relate to economic and social status (class), dress and physical appearance, physical ability, sexual orientation (homophobia), language, religion, and health status. These factors may represent deviations from mainstream cultural norms and, therefore, are sometimes mistaken as indicative of mental illness. During the past two decades, the mental health professions have paid more attention to the effects of stress related to societal stigmatization and oppression of differences (such as homosexuality, bisexuality, socioeconomic class, disability, ethnicity, race, and gender) on the psychological functioning of nondominant groups. Helpers should deal with these issues, as with those discussed in the preceding pages, by clarifying and expressing their values in a nonjudgmental manner and by collecting valid new information on the topics.

During the 1970s, social and legislative attention was paid to issues of discrimination. The 1980s brought fiercer competition for more limited funding and a backlash reaction to social programs that were even more discriminatory than pre-1970 attitudes. Examples include the hysteria about allowing children with AIDS to attend school and the widespread anger over the costs of providing special building access and education programs for people with physical disabilities.

In the 1990s, the hysteria continued. Now, in the first decade of the 21st century, as we struggle with the ups and downs of the economy, prioritizing our social issues has become more complicated. In the United States there are sharp disagreements about such values as the right to life; the right to die; the right of homosexuals to marry; the right to health care; the civil rights of prisoners, homosexuals, and AIDS patients; birth technology; bilingual education; organ transplants; immigration; and fighting wars. In particular, the culture wars of the 2000s are challenging hard-won civil rights legislation and social service program gains achieved in the late 1990s. In such an atmosphere, helpers need to be more socially aware and more flexible than ever before to make the most of the limited resources available to them and their clients.

ETHICAL CONSIDERATIONS

A critical task for helping professionals is to guide trainees in their development as moral thinkers, appropriate role models, and safe interventionists. An important teaching tool is the code of ethics relevant to the trainees' particular disciplines. Most ethical codes are based on five fundamental ethical principles: respect autonomy, do no harm, benefit others, be fair, and be faithful (Kitchener, 1988, 2003). Professional organizations—such as the American Counseling Association (which includes the American Mental Health Counselors Association and the American Rehabilitation Counseling Association), the American Psychological Association, and the National Association of Social Workers—continue to update their codes of ethics to protect helpers from the public and vice versa.

Modern codes of ethics, in addition to providing standards—obligations that are the basis for punitive action—also provide or promote discussion of a more social constructionist model of virtue ethics. *Virtue ethics* refers to a set of ideals (shared worldviews and views unique to each culture) to which helping professionals aspire. Examples of such ideals include integrity, respectfulness, fairness, trustworthiness, and benevolence (kindness) (Shanahan & Hyman, 2003). These models overlap, and both acknowledge the impact of ethnicity and culture on ethical behavior (Cottone, 2001). Understanding and tolerating our own and others' values underlie the standards and virtues of ethical helping behavior.

Ethical dilemmas are increasingly common, complicated, and complex, and it is impossible for this brief introduction to fully prepare students to handle such situations. We suggest that helpers read relevant codes of ethics and take courses and professional development workshops on this important topic. Furthermore, we believe that those helpers whose behavior is consistent with their definition of helping, who are committed to examining their own behaviors and motives, and who seek consultation from others are less likely to function unethically than those who are closed to such reflections. Ethical helpers do not participate in institutional biases, do not administer tests without norms for the client group being tested, respectfully utilize the services of an interpreter when needed, and respectfully protect human and civil rights.

Ethical issues that appear to be especially relevant today are (1) privileged communication and sharing of confidential information, particularly in this era of managed care and high technology; (2) conflicts of interest; (3) record keeping; (4) use of tests and computerized programs; (5) dual or multiple relationships; and (6) misrepresentation. Successful handling of these issues requires awareness of appropriate boundaries and multicultural sensitivity. The managed care movement has added a complex dimension to these ethical issues, creating challenges for agencies, helpers, and helpees. Decisions must be made about who provides and who receives services, as well as how ethical dilemmas are resolved.

Privileged Communication and Confidentiality

Most helpers do not have privileged communication, which means they can be called on to testify in a court of law about the nature of their discussions with helpees, and their records can be subpoenaed. In some states, certified counselors and certified psychologists do have privileged communication, but laws relating to this issue are not uniformly applied.

There are two kinds of confidentiality: legal and personal. The former depends on the laws of your state. The latter is of your own making, regardless of the policies of your work setting. In other words, if because of your setting (such as in a school or correctional institution) you are unable to treat information obtained in a helping session confidentially, you *must* make this clear to the helpee in advance of his or her sharing concerns with you. Then the helpee can choose whether to tell you anything that is controversial. If you are able to promise personal confidentiality, you must maintain it; under no circumstances should you reveal to anyone what has been told to you in confidence unless the client is a danger to himself or someone else. When you are working with children or adolescents, you must tell them what kinds of information you will and will not share with their parents or teachers.

Remember not to discuss helpees with anyone in their family or with another staff member of your organization, such as a teacher, supervisor, or employer, without the helpee's specific verbal permission. This precaution is necessary to ensure trust and to communicate helper interest in helpee welfare.

Recent court cases indicate that professional helpers can be held accountable if they do not warn potential victims of violence. Since each state has different legislation, mental health professionals encounter legal as well as ethical dilemmas in their attempts to determine whether a client is likely to do psychological or physical harm to another person. Generalist human services workers and nonprofessional helpers are also affected by this dilemma. Should they report legitimate concerns about the welfare of a helpee to another person, whether a family member, a helping professional, or an official? For example, if they know that someone is contemplating suicide, should they tell someone? Who? Under what circumstances?

EXERCISE 10.9 ▪ You are working as an assistant counselor in a high school, and one of your students (sent to you by her parents) tells you that she needs to smoke pot several times a day in order to get to class. Her grades have fallen dramatically, and her teachers and parents are concerned. She insists that she does not want to change her behaviors and that she will never talk to anyone again if you tell anyone what she has revealed. Discuss all the ethical issues, and brainstorm in a group how you might want to deal with this situation.

Current issues concerning confidentiality involve the kind of information shared with third-party payers who require access to client information stored on computer. Most clients do not realize when they sign up for health care insurance that they are signing away their right to absolute confidentiality with a counselor or therapist. The helper may be obliged by the third-party payer to reveal details of each session in order to justify authorization for further services. It seems to us that the best way for counselors and clients to be protected is for clients to sign an informed consent form (see Appendix B) and for the counselor and client to discuss openly what diagnosis will be used, what information must be shared, how, and with whom. As computer security breaches in hospitals and clinics have come to light, the federal government has imposed regulations (HIPAA) about confidentiality of records, and organizations have been required to change their practices about access to this information. Helpers are ethically responsible for ensuring that their employer organization's policies are congruent with their own professional and personal ethical codes.

Conflict of Interest

There are times when you may experience a conflict of interest between your obligations to your organization and your obligations to your helpee. There are no blanket solutions for such cases. Each person must find an answer that he or she can live with. For example, a mental health counselor was asked by her employer to refer a quota of patients to group counseling. In many cases, this was helpful to the clients, but there were some for whom group counseling was not suitable, and the counselor wanted to have the latitude to make the referral case by case. When she was unable to resolve this dilemma with her employer, she elected to leave. She ended up taking a lower-paying position, even though it affected her lifestyle as a single parent.

It is important for helpers to remember that their primary responsibility during the helping process is to the helpee, not to any other individual or group. Thus, if a conflict of interest arises, helpers must make sure that they do not breach a helpee's confidentiality because of their own ignorance, insecurity, or ineptness, or for the good of some organization or group. The only justification for a breach of confidentiality is that the welfare of the helpee or some other human being is at stake.

Conflicts of interest may also pose ethical dilemmas for workers in settings concerned with census count. One mental health worker in a psychiatric hospital reported discomfort when the director of the hospital suggested to the staff that they "treat all the patients as if they were at home, as it's important to keep them here until their insurance runs out." Another mental health worker decided to leave his HMO employer because he was offered a financial bonus for every case he was able to counsel in fewer than five sessions. These types of stories abound in today's cost-conscious climate and are of concern to all the professional associations.

Record Keeping

Each state has different requirements regarding the nature of records, the disposition of records, and the length of time records must be kept. The purpose of record keeping is to provide documentation of a helpee's progress and continuity of treatment. Opinions differ among legal and risk management advisers as to how detailed and complete records should be. You may find it a good idea to write down only objective, behavioral information and to exclude subjective material such as your values, attitudes, and, above all, interpretations. You should also be sensitive to potentially damaging effects of any information you write. Some helpers keep certain personal information and coded personal notes in their office files. If tape recordings are used, it should be with the full knowledge of the helpee, a full explanation of the intentions and purposes of the recordings, and the helper's guarantee that the tapes will be destroyed after they fulfill their purposes. If third-party (for example, insurance) payments are involved, discuss what specific information is provided to that party. Remember, the overriding objective is the helpee's welfare.

Recently, a client who worked in the hospital that managed his health care (his supervisor was the mental health reviewer) consulted me (BFO) about a serious personal problem. I was reluctant to write down the accurate diagnosis for fear it would jeopardize his employment. Yet he was entitled to his health benefits. After discussion with the consulting psychopharmacologist and attempts to get the mental health reviewer changed, I discussed my dilemma at length with the client. Together we decided that I would see him privately at a reduced fee in order to avoid disclosure of his diagnosis to his employer. It was highly stressful for me, the client, and the consulting psychopharmacologist.

Testing

Some human services workers are involved in testing helpees. They may employ interest, aptitude, or achievement tests or a paper-and-pencil personality inventory that could be used for screening, placement, or some other kind of classification. It is ethical for helpers to administer tests only if they have had sufficient training and supervision in the administration of the particular test. In addition, helpers are ethically bound to determine and explain clearly to helpees the rationale for and purposes of the testing process. They must discuss culture fairness of the instruments as well as known limitations.

A related issue concerns the use of test data—who receives these data and what use will be made of them. Does the helpee receive feedback in order to increase self-understanding? Is the helper able to interpret test data accurately and explain them to the helpee, along with the meaning and validity of the test? In these cases, each helper must determine the extent of his or her ethical responsibility.

Dual- or Multiple-Role Relationships

A troublesome concern of ethics committees has been the potential harm of dual or multiple relationships between professional helpers and students, supervisees, clients, employees, or research subjects. Different roles involve different expectations of behavior, power, and obligations. There is likely to be conflict between these role expectations if the helper engages in any role other than that of the professional helper (Lazarus & Zur, 2002). Examples of dual or multiple relationships are forming a social or sexual relationship with a helpee, having a business relationship with a helpee, becoming a student's or supervisee's therapist, or entering into a professional helping relationship with a friend or family member.

Clear boundaries between the helper and the helpee, and clarification of the nature and process of the helping relationship, will mitigate against possible abuses of power. For example, if professional helpers conduct counseling or therapy with their students or supervisees, confidentiality may be compromised and the students' or supervisees' autonomy may be impaired. Furthermore, the helping process is nonevaluative, and teachers and supervisors are usually required to evaluate their students and supervisees, so objectivity will be damaged. The point is that dual or multiple relationships have a high potential for exploiting the helpee, who is in a less powerful position than the helper, regardless of the circumstances. If this power differential is not acknowledged and both parties consent to another kind of relationship, the damage may be more insidious.

Misrepresentation

Misrepresentation can occur when a helper directly claims or indirectly implies knowledge, training, experience, and/or expertise with a particular type of client or a particular type of problem. This could be an issue for nonprofessional, generalist human services, or professional helpers who are uncomfortable with or unable to acknowledge their personal and helping limitations. Helpees are often too confused and eager for assistance when they seek help to check the qualifications and experience of the helper and assume that the helper has a level of experience and expertise greater than what he or she actually possesses.

Professional codes of ethics specifically require helpers to acknowledge their limitations and to seek supervision or consultation. For example, a colleague came to me (BFO) to discuss her dilemma when it became evident that one of her clients had multiple personalities. My colleague had never experienced this kind of case. She discussed her limitations with the client and offered her three options: (1) continue their work together, given the effectiveness of their helping relationship, with supervision and consultation from an outside expert; (2) refer the client to an expert for direct treatment; or (3) use cotherapy with an expert.

Failing to consider other forms of assessment and treatment, such as not giving a referral for a physical examination, psychopharmacology, or testing, is another ethical issue. For example, many clients experience psychological distress that turns out to be related to underlying medical conditions. Psychological and sociocultural variables may compound symptoms, but it should never be assumed that there is only one etiology of symptoms of stress. A pluralistic approach ensures multifaceted perspectives of assessment and treatment.

One of the major issues of the 21st century concerns the quality of services and information that are and will be provided via the Internet. As stated by Russ Newman, practice director of the American Psychological Association, "The need for ethical standards, laws or regulations is seriously complicated by the exponential development of the technology" (cited in Rabasca, 2000). Little is known about whether self-help and other kinds of online helping services are effective (Foxhall, 2000; Rabasca, 2000). In addition to lack of data on quality of treatment and outcome, we need to be concerned about confidentiality, accurate assessment and diagnosis, and the practice of pharmacotherapy via the computer. Nevertheless, more and more health care is likely to be delivered directly to consumers via the Internet, and managed care companies have a great incentive to go online.

No code of ethics can cover all situations and all circumstances. Ethical issues involving the use of computers for assessment as well as record keeping are now being addressed by professional associations. How do we guard against the release of information from computers? How do we maintain a humanistic, socially conscious perspective as we become more reliant on high technology and psychopharmacology in the helping process? How do we deal with the fear of litigation? Appendix B contains a sample policy statement that we use with our clients. You will have to decide for yourself what course of action is right for you.

OTHER ISSUES THAT AFFECT THE COUNSELING PROCESS

We will touch briefly on other issues that frequently arise in helping relationships. The readings at the end of the chapter will provide more in-depth coverage of these areas.

Reluctant Clients

A frequent concern of helpers in certain institutions centers on the reluctant client, the individual who is told he or she must seek help. This may cause an ethical dilemma for helpers who believe in the self-determination of helpees. After all, if people have the right to determine for themselves whether they want to be helped or "get better," how can we force our services on them? If you feel this way, you can inform the helpee, communicating empathy and concern for his or her position while explaining your own. Confrontation of

resistance (see Chapter 4) is more likely to engage reluctant clients than eva-
sion. Sometimes the reluctant client is testing you, waiting to see how committed you are. And he or she may have all the time in the world to wait.

Self-Disclosure

Self-disclosure, the technique in which helpers talk about themselves with
helpees, is another controversial issue. At one time it was considered disastrous
and unethical, but now many helpers believe that judicious self-disclosure can
enhance the helping relationship, help balance the power in the relationship,
and aid in problem solving. The guiding principle is that the helper's self-
disclosure should be for the helpee's benefit. This means the helper does not
burden the client with his or her problems but instead regulates the quality and
timing of self-disclosure to help the client focus more on his or her concerns.

If the helper's self-disclosure is used to further the helpee's exploration and
self-understanding, it allows the helper to become a positive role model, because
it both reveals the helper's humanness and provides a look at the possibility of
coping effectively with whatever the issue is. It neither distracts the helpee from
pressing concerns nor adversely affects the relationship by showing up the
helper's flaws. Rather, it aids the helpee in focusing on the central issues and
teaches him or her that, although all human beings have problems and can
make mistakes, one can learn from mistakes and work through those problems.

An example of inappropriate self-disclosure occurred when a client was
crying about her difficulty maintaining sobriety. The helper ignored the client's
emotions and for the next 20 minutes talked about her own success attaining
sobriety and how much better her life was now. The client felt as if her emotional
experience was unimportant to the helper. An instance of useful self-disclosure
occurred in a pregnancy advisory service. A volunteer helper was discussing the
possibility of abortion with a 19-year-old single woman. The helpee was hesitant
about considering abortion, but she felt trapped and unsure about having a child.
When she began to contemplate the guilt feelings that might result from an abortion, the helper shared her own painful, guilty feelings from a similar experience
and explained that there would most likely be guilt and discomfort resulting from
any of the options being considered. The helpee seemed relieved to be talking to
someone who had experienced those feelings and lived through them.

It is important that helpers have the capacity to share themselves intimately
with other people, although they must carefully choose the people for such
personal revelations and the appropriate time for them. We expect helpees to
share themselves, and we need to experience and understand that same process
of sharing and relating. The underlying principle here is that we do not ask
others to do what we cannot or would not do.

Advocacy and Change Agentry

When helpers take active roles in bringing about political and institutional
changes to combat discrimination and inequality, they are acting as change

agents, or advocates. (The sections on sexism and racism in this chapter gave some examples of change agentry/advocacy.) Increasing numbers of people in the helping fields are taking active stands against racism, sexism, heterosexism, and ageism; against poverty and other forms of inequity; and against discrimination toward those who are politically active, such as union organizers and "whistleblowers." Consistency between what one practices and what one preaches is necessary for changes to occur within systems and for the development of effective helping relationships

As helpers, we are becoming more and more aware of the problems that systems and institutions impose on helpees, which subsequently become labeled as the helpees' problems. As helpers become frustrated struggling against the limitations imposed by institutions, they may become more politicized and radicalized. This does not mean that they revolt or seek destruction of the institution; rather, they try to foster systemic, innovative change within the institution.

Change agentry strategies may be directed at program control and budgets or the political process involved in staffing, organizational decisions, and public policies. Techniques include generating public support by disseminating written materials; organizing support groups; training staff; providing public education; mobilizing local, state, and national election task forces; pressuring elected officials; writing legislators; and participating in confrontations such as boycotts, demonstrations, and strikes when they are part of a total strategy or campaign.

Effective change agents plan strategies, determine goals, and design a structure to reflect those goals, as well as make tentative implementation and evaluation plans. Although change agents or innovators may assume initial leadership, a frequent priority in institutional change is a more broadly based sharing of power among all members of the institution. If the number of facilitative helpers, rather than "authoritarian experts," can be increased as a result of staff recruitment and training in human services agencies, then the needs of helpees will assume a higher priority than the needs of helpers or the organization.

As an example, let's consider a federally funded mental health agency that experienced a great deal of chaos a few years ago. This chaos was reflected in high staff turnover, a large number of written and verbal client complaints and no-shows for appointments, and resistance to the agency from other community groups. Staff believed that the agency was not being run to meet the needs of the community it was supposed to serve. Two staff helpers became so frustrated with the bureaucratic red tape they encountered every time they brought up the idea of change that they finally recruited support from members of the clerical and volunteer staff, as well as from members of the community. As a task force, they prepared a written report of what they perceived to be problems of the community and of the agency, as well as conflicting directives and policies, and presented it to their director and senior staff. The report included a written proposal for a pilot project that would change the staff loads and include members of the community and some representative helpees at regular agency meetings.

Because their proposal was fully documented and specific, the director agreed to a two-month trial. At the end of the trial period, modifications were suggested, and some changes in leadership occurred when some senior staff members realized they would be unable to muster the support necessary to revert to the previous way of operating. The new leaders encouraged members of the community to participate in agency policy making and decision making and were successful in effecting many of the changes recommended in the original proposal.

Dedicated helpers are increasingly aware that communities must have a hand in the development of their own institutions and that these institutions must become more responsive to their client population. This means that services must be provided to meet the unique needs of a particular community, not to provide research data for an erudite report or to provide training for generalist human services workers and professional helpers from other communities. You must decide for yourself, as you consider your helping role and your own personal and professional ethics, just how involved you will become in systemwide changes.

The following exercises are designed to help you become more familiar with the issues just discussed.

EXERCISE 10.10 ■ This exercise should help you experience the feelings of both a reluctant client and the helper of a reluctant client. In pairs, assign roles of helper and helpee. Engage in a role play in which the helpee knows that he or she does not want help and the helper is trying to establish a helping relationship. (It might be helpful for the helpee to keep in mind something that he or she would not want to share under any circumstances, in order to play the role of reluctant client well.) After each person has played both roles, process your experiences, feelings, and reactions. In this exercise, most students learn that there is no way someone can make helpees reveal what they do not choose to reveal.

EXERCISE 10.11 ■ What are the issues in the following cases? What would you do as the helper in each case? Role-play these situations and discuss them in small groups.

1. You are a youth street worker, and you overhear a gang of boys talk about a burglary they committed yesterday. Later, one of the boys tells you that this gang is having trouble fencing some of the loot and asks you to help. He offers you a free color TV. It's taken you a long time to gain the trust of this boy.

2. You are working as a volunteer in a crafts program for the aged. An 85-year-old man with whom you've established a helping relationship tells you that he wants to marry a 78-year-old woman in the program. His children are raising strenuous objections and want to pull him out of the program to keep him away from "foolish temptation." He wants your help.

3. You are a white generalist human services worker in a community school. You act as a vocational counseling aide. An African American couple comes in with their

11th-grade son. They have just received notice from the guidance department that on the basis of an IQ test, their son is being sent to trade school for the rest of the year. The parents are very upset. They want him in a college-bound track.

4. You are a personnel worker, and Ms. Jones, a very competent administrative assistant in the advertising department, comes in to complain that a male administrative assistant with less background and experience has been promoted over her.

5. You are a helper in a drop-in center for teens. A 14-year-old girl tells you she thinks she is pregnant and that she was seduced by her employer. She says that her parents "will kill her" if they find out.

6. You are a male supervisor in a factory, supervising 14 male forklift operators. A woman is hired because of your factory's affirmative action plan. Your men are angry and upset and come to see you to plan how to stop this invasion of their territory.

7. You are an African American helper in a youth activities program. A 15-year-old African American youth who is bussed to a suburban school tells you he wants to ask a white girl to the school dance but is somewhat nervous about it.

8. You are a school counselor in an upper-middle-class community. The parents of one of the students have come to see you and are very angry with you for encouraging their son in his interest in shop. They had always planned for him to go to medical school. The boy is a C student and is very talented in shop work.

9. You are a helper in a community center. Drugs are not allowed on the premises, but you find a youngster with whom you have been working smoking a joint.

10. You are an African American counselor in a prison. You notice that only African American prisoners are placed in behavior modification programs and that selection is arbitrarily determined by the prison administration. Subjects have no choice and are penalized if they do not cooperate.

11. You are a helper in a college counseling center. A 19-year-old girl comes in, terrified by the sexual attraction she feels toward her roommate.

12. You are a non-Asian counselor at a public school. Sue, the only Asian American at the school, has been sent to you by her teacher because of her C grade in the first quarter. Her teacher said that something must be wrong with Sue because Asians always did very well in math.

COMMON PROBLEMS YOU MAY ENCOUNTER AS A HELPER

Regardless of the amount of training and experience you have had, you will often feel insecure and doubt your adequacy as a helper. Perhaps this type of self-doubt is one of the necessary qualities of an effective helper; it keeps us on our toes, prevents us from becoming cocky and overconfident, and constantly reminds us of our own frailty as human beings. Working with people in a helping relationship is awesome and often frightening in that we become aware of the importance and vulnerability of human life. However, self-doubt can protect us from getting in over our heads, from attempting to work with people and problems beyond the scope of our training and capabilities.

Another problem that beginning helpers often experience is becoming too emotionally involved with helpees, wanting to take responsibility for them and do for them rather than teach them to do for themselves. It is because of this problem that we spend time developing our own self-awareness and examining our apparent and underlying motivations for becoming helpers as we study the helping process. As we learn about ourselves and the helping process, we can learn to take care of ourselves and allow others to take care of themselves.

Helper **burnout** is an increasing problem in the pressured human services field. You may be suffering from burnout when you feel exhausted and are unable to pay attention to what someone is saying; you find yourself reacting more impatiently and intolerantly than you have in the past; your sleeping and eating habits change or you experience a new physical symptom; or you find yourself dreading the beginning of the workday and lacking enthusiasm, motivation, and interest.

Perhaps you will be able to make some changes in your work life to restore your energy and interest. For example, teachers can change the grade level or subject they teach, and school counselors can change their grade level. A clinical colleague of ours volunteered for major administrative and committee responsibilities to seek relief from full-time clinical practice. She intends to return to her clinical work but recognizes her need for temporary relief and distance from other people's emotional problems. Some helpers use burnout as an entry into their own personal therapy or regular peer consultation. Others undertake stress reduction activities, such as aerobic exercise, yoga, new hobbies or activities, or a vacation. Group work has been found to be effective, allowing helpers to share their concerns with each other or to associate with new, different people from other fields.

The point is to recognize beginning symptoms so that you can take steps to prevent the further effects of burnout. We need to recognize our own limitations, to learn how to say "no" to others and feel OK about it. We need to reassess our expectations in accordance with the changing realities of our work.

In other words, like helpees, we need to take care of ourselves, to make time for our own inner selves so as to replenish and renew our energies and enthusiasm for living. An additional problem you may encounter is that of total frustration with the limitations your organization or some of your community institutions impose on you and others. Learning what your options are and deciding what you want to do about them, what risks you can incur, and what resources you can muster can be painful and difficult and cause you to feel lonely and isolated from others. Along the same line, you will often feel anger and frustration with other members of the human services professions. You will question the quality and methods of some of the services provided. This kind of skepticism can occur in any area of endeavor associated with human beings and their welfare; eliminating it requires using your communication skills and knowledge to consult effectively with other human services workers to see if you can bring about change. The problem-solving model is especially applicable here in that it can show you how to team up with others to identify problems and brainstorm for alternative solutions.

A final problem we want to mention is your own resistance to changes and new ways of delivering services. People sometimes get so used to doing things in a certain way that, without realizing it, they become very set in their ways. Keeping open channels of communication with peers in your setting and others, attending meetings and conferences, reading new materials, and taking advantage of in-service training whenever possible will help you keep abreast of new developments and opportunities in your field.

EXERCISE 10.12 ▪ Take a few minutes to write yourself a personal contract for the coming week. What will you do to be good to yourself, to be your own helper? Try to contract for at least one way of reducing stress each day, one way of taking time for your own inner self.

RECENT TRENDS

There is evidence that the helping skills and strategies we have discussed can be effectively implemented by all levels of helpers—lay, generalist human services, and professional. Often, trusting, understanding human contact alone is sufficient to begin the helping process.

For example, telephone crisis intervention services report that short telephone calls using the communication skills we've discussed can provide sufficient help to callers to avert a pending crisis, such as a suicide or a crime. A recently developed telephone career-education counseling project demonstrated that vocational counseling can be effectively delivered by trained lay helpers via telephone. In many early intervention, school, and mental health settings, a team approach involving professionals, lay helpers, and generalist human services workers has proven to be an effective way to provide human services. These mental health teams have also been helpful in the coordination and delivery of needed services after disasters.

Human resource staffs are increasingly providing helping services to employees in the business sector, although this staff is often the first to be let go when downsizing occurs. HR staffs often consist of professional counselors or social workers who have knowledge of organizational behavior, as well as counseling theory and application. Some companies contract with outside helpers for employee assistance programs. Organizations that provide a range of services, such as health counseling, outplacement and retirement counseling, career counseling, and alcoholism and drug abuse counseling, usually have higher retention and productivity rates.

Another trend is the use of helpers in traditional health settings, providing such services as nutrition, stress reduction, or mindfulness programs and other preventive health measures. Holistic health programs, focusing on prevention, and behavioral medicine, examining mind–body connections, are other approaches using interdisciplinary teamwork.

However, in spite of changes in the delivery and accessibility of counseling services, the helping process needs to be demystified. Professional helpers must learn how to be effective supervisors and consultants so they can provide supervisory services as well as more intensive care when necessary. Community-based and in-service training opportunities should be expanded. Increasing numbers of human services and community workers are required to deliver services on their own "turf," so that vital human services can be provided to all who need them. Every community possesses indigenous helping resources that can be identified and utilized.

We need to recruit volunteer helpers from within the community to assist their neighbors in accepting people who have traditionally been isolated. We need trained workers to assist the ill, impoverished, homeless, substance-abusing, and otherwise disabled persons who already live in our communities. Adequate levels of services should be offered to returning veterans and their families, as well as to refugees and immigrants from all over the world who are moving to our neighborhoods. Never before has the need for effective helpers been so critical to our healthy survival as a society.

The nature and delivery of helping services are in upheaval as we struggle with cost containment and new models of delivery. The paradigm shifts required for helpers require attention to (1) good problem formulation, leading to clear focus and specification of helping objectives; (2) alliance with as many members as possible of the helpees' contexts (family as well as relationship and work/school networks) and other helpers (teachers, doctors, clergy); (3) flexibility of format (individual, group, family, organizational consulting, and community education); (4) working with, rather than against, resistance; (5) treatment goals, so that you can stay on course and change strategies as needed; and (6) developing new roles that include more expert consultant, rather than direct treatment provider, skills. This new paradigm may result in intermittent consultation over a long period of time, rather than brief, focused helping. The new school counseling model expands the counselor role to include leading small and large groups, teaching in the classroom, and consulting with parents, teachers, and administrators. There is no one way that will be suitable to all helping situations.

SUMMARY AND CONCLUSIONS

In this chapter, we have discussed some of the major personal values and professional issues that affect helping relationships. As helpers we must be aware of our values and be careful not to impose them on clients. We can use responsive listening and send "I" messages to communicate respect for helpees and their values. Three issues discussed at some length were sexism, racism/ethnocentrism, and ageism. There are no absolute answers to the challenges raised by these issues in developing effective helping relationships, but we can keep informed and maintain heightened sensitivity by continuing to discuss them. This process is as important as learning communication skills and understanding the stages of the helping relationship.

This chapter also discussed personal, professional, and ethical considerations, and recent trends in counseling. The ways we resolve the problems of privileged communication, confidentiality, conflicts of interest, record keeping, testing, dual or multiple relationships, and misrepresentation will determine our effectiveness as helpers. Another important component in our ability to provide competent, ethical help is how we take care of ourselves.

Using the written and verbal exercises in this book, you have had the opportunity to apply communication skills, expand your understanding of the steps in the helping relationship stages, and implement strategies. These exercises have provided you the opportunity to personally experience and react to the material in the text. They were designed to increase your awareness of your behaviors, thoughts, and feelings, as well as to give you a chance to integrate conceptual material with experience.

Whether the case material has been appropriate to your setting and level of helping, it illustrates the stages of helping and many of the issues discussed. Most of the examples and case studies are from our own, our trainees', and our colleagues' practices. This material does not favor any particular approaches or strategies over others.

Now that you have a foundation, you can decide whether to further develop your skills and your understanding of the helping process and the use of strategies. If you wish to become a more effective helper, it is essential for you to receive supervised field experience as well as pursue academic courses in helping and the social sciences. Only by continual practice and application, however, can you improve your communication skills.

Strategy application can be learned in coursework, fieldwork, and specialized training institutes and workshops. There are many opportunities for continuing education, since evidence of professional development is required for professional licensure. Although the quality varies, carefully selected programs can offer excellent training opportunities. These workshops are often sponsored by professional associations and are held at local, regional, and national conferences. Some are sponsored by human relations groups in your community or by professional institutes. Local announcements and human services bulletins will alert you to available opportunities.

The implementation of certain approaches requires more advanced training and experience than others. However, this requirement does not preclude you from having a basic understanding of all the major theories. Your interest in a certain area may serve as a stimulus, either now or in the future, for you to pursue further education. There are opportunities for lay helpers to become generalist human services workers and for generalist human services workers to become professionals. One need only look at the students enrolled in different levels of training programs to recognize that people are coming into human services fields at all ages, with all kinds of experiences and backgrounds. The need for effective helpers is great, and we welcome the expansion of the field.

REFERENCES AND
FURTHER READING

Alinsky, S. (1972) *Rules for radicals.* New York:Vintage Books.

American Association for Marriage and Family Therapy. (1998). *AAMFT code of ethics.* Washington, DC: Author.

American Counseling Association. (1995). *Code of ethics and standards of practice.* Alexandria, VA: Author.

American Psychological Association. (2002). *Ethical principles of psychologists and code of conduct* (rev. ed.). Washington, DC: Author.

Atkinson, D. R. (2004). *Counseling American minorities* (6th ed.). New York: McGraw-Hill.

Ballou, M., & Brown, L. S. (Eds.). (2002). *Rethinking mental health and disorder: Feminist perspectives.* New York: Guilford Press.

Ballou, M., & Gabalac, N. W. (1985). *A feminist position on mental health.* Springfield, IL: Charles C. Thomas.

Barnett, R., & Rivers, C. (2004). *How gender myths are hurting our relationships, our children and our jobs.* New York: Basic Books.

Bates, C. M., & Brodsky, A. M. (1989). *Sex in the therapy hour.* New York: Guilford Press.

Birren, J. E., & Schaie, K. W. (1996). *Handbook of the psychology of aging.* San Diego: Academic Press.

Broverman, I., Broverman, D., Clarkson, F., Rosenkrantz, P., & Vogel, S. (1970). Sex-role stereotypes and clinical judgments of mental health. *Journal of Consulting and Clinical Psychology, 34,* 1–7.

Cohen, E. D., & Cohen, G. S. (1999). *The virtuous therapist: Ethical practice of counseling and psychotherapy.* Pacific Grove, CA: Brooks/Cole.

Corey, G. (2005). *Theory and practice of counseling and psychotherapy* (7th ed.). Belmont, CA: Brooks/Cole.

Corey, G., Corey, M. S., & Callanan, P. (2003). *Issues and ethics in the helping professions* (6th ed.). Belmont, CA: Brooks/Cole.

Corey, G., Corey, M., & Haynes, R. (2003). *Ethics in action: CD-ROM.* Belmont, CA: Brooks/Cole.

Corey, G., & Herlihy, B. (1997). Dual/multiple relationships: Toward a consensus of thinking. In *Hatherleigh guide to ethics in therapy* (pp. 193–205). New York: Hatherleigh Press.

Cottone, R. (2001). A social constructivism model of ethical decision making in counseling. *Journal of Counseling and Development, 79*(1), 39–45.

Das, A. K. (1995). Rethinking multicultural counseling: Implications for counselor education. *Journal of Counseling and Development, 74,* 45–52.

Enns, C. Z. (2004). *Feminist theories and feminist psychotherapies: Origins, themes and variations* (2nd ed.). Binghamton, NY: Haworth.

Enns, C. Z., & Hackett, G. (1990). Comparison of feminist and nonfeminist women's reactions to variants of nonsexist and feminist counseling. *Journal of Counseling Psychology, 37,* 33–40.

Enns, C. Z., & Hackett, G. (1993). A comparison of feminist and nonfeminist women's and men's reactions to nonsexist and feminist counseling: A replication and extension. *Journal of Counseling and Development, 71,* 499–509.

Farber, B. A. (1983). *Stress and burnout in the human service professions.* New York: Pergamon Press.

Foxhall, K. (2000). How will the rules of telehealth be written? *Monitor on Psychology, 31*(4), 38–41.

Gartrell, N., Herman, J., Olarte, S., Feldstein, M., & Localio, R. (1987). Reporting practices of psychiatrists who knew of sexual misconduct by colleagues. *American Journal of Orthopsychiatry, 57,* 126–131.

Gilligan, C. (1982). *In a different voice.* Cambridge, MA: Harvard University Press.

Glaser, B., & Kirschenbaum, H. (1980). Using values clarification in counseling settings. *Personnel and Guidance Journal, 58,* 569–576.

Green, S. (2003). *The psychological development of girls and women: Rethinking change in time.* New York: Routledge.

Hepple, J. (2004). Ageism in psychotherapy and beyond. In J. Hepple & L. Sutton (Eds.), *Cognitive analytic therapy in late life: A new perspective in old age.* Hove, UK: Brunner-Routledge.

Herlihy, B., & Corey, G. (1997). *Boundary issues in counseling: Multiple roles and responsibilities.* Alexandria, VA: American Counseling Association.

Hyde, J. S. (2005). The gender similarities hypothesis. *American Psychologist, 60*(6), 581–593.

Kenyon, P. (1999). *What would you do? An ethical case workbook for human service professionals.* Pacific Grove, CA: Brooks/Cole.

Kilburg, R. R., Nathan, P. E., & Thoreson, R. W. (Eds.). (1986). *Professionals in distress: Issues, syndromes, and solutions in psychology.* Washington, DC: American Psychological Association.

Kitchener, K. S. (1988). Dual role relationships: What makes them so problematic? *Journal of Counseling and Development, 67,* 217–221.

Kitchener, K. S. (2003). *Foundations of ethical practice and research in teaching psychology.* New York: Erlbaum.

Klonoff, E., Landrine, H., & Campbell, R. (2000). Sexist discrimination may account for well-known gender differences in psychiatric symptoms. *Psychology of Women Quarterly, 24,* 93–99.

Lazarus, A. A., & Zur, O. (2002). *Dual relationships and psychotherapy.* New York: Springer.

Lomranz, J. (Ed.). (1998). *Handbook of aging and mental health: An integrative approach.* New York: Plenum Press.

Miller, J. B. (1986). *Toward a new psychology of women* (2nd ed.). Boston: Beacon Press.

Mirkin, M. P., Suyemoto, K. L., & Okun, B. F. (2005). *Psychotherapy with women: Exploring diverse contexts and identities.* New York: Guilford Press.

National Association of Social Workers. (1998). *Code of ethics.* Washington, DC: Author.

National Board for Certified Counselors. (1998). *Code of ethics.* Alexandria, VA: Author.

National Organization for Human Service Education. (1995). *Ethical standards for the National Organization of Human Service Education.* Philadelphia: Author.

Okapaku, S. (Ed.). (1998). *Clinical methods in transcultural psychiatry.* Washington, DC: American Psychiatric Association Press.

Okun, B. (1984). *Working with adults: Individual, family, and career development.* Pacific Grove, CA: Brooks/Cole.

Okun, B. F. (1989). Therapist blindspots related to gender socialization. In D. Kantor & B. F. Okun (Eds.), *Intimate environments: Sex, intimacy, and gender in families* (pp. 129–163). New York: Guilford Press.

Okun, B. F., Fried, J., & Okun, M. L. (1999). *Understanding diversity: A learning-as-practice primer.* Pacific Grove, CA: Brooks/Cole.

Okun, B. F., & Ziady, L. G. (2005). Redefining the career ladder: New visions of women at work. In M. P. Mirkin, K. L. Suyemoto, & B. F. Okun (Eds.), *Psychotherapy with women: Exploring diverse contexts and identities* (pp. 215–236). New York: Guilford Press.

O'Malley, K. M., & Richardson, S. (1985). Sex bias in counseling: Have things changed? *Journal of Counseling and Development, 63,* 294–300.

Parker, G. (1967). Some concomitants of therapist dominance in the psychotherapy interview. *Journal of Consulting Psychology, 31,* 313–318.

Pedersen, P. (2000). *A handbook for developing multicultural awareness* (3rd ed.). Alexandria, VA: American Counseling Association.

Pedersen, P. (2003). Increasing the cultural awareness, knowledge and skills of culture-centered counselors. In F. D. Harper & J. McFadden (Eds.), *Culture and counseling: New approaches* (pp. 31–46). Needham Heights, MA: Allyn & Bacon.

Peterson, M. R. (1992). *At personal risk: Boundary violations in professional–client relationship.* New York: W. W. Norton.

Pope, K. S. (1988). How clients are harmed by sexual contact with mental health professionals: The syndrome and its prevalence. *Journal of Counseling and Development, 67,* 222–226.

Pope, K. S., Sonne, J. L., & Holroyd, J. (1993). *Sexual feelings in psychotherapy: Explorations for therapists and therapists-in-training.* Washington, DC: American Psychological Association.

Pope, K. S., & Vetter, V. A. (1992). Ethical dilemmas encountered by members of the American Psychological Association. *American Psychologist, 47,* 397–411.

Rabasca, L. (2000). Self-help sites: A blessing or a bane? *Monitor on Psychology, 31*(4), 28–30.

Rogers, C. (1967). The necessary and sufficient conditions of therapeutic personality change. *Journal of Consulting Psychology, 21,* 95–103.

Rosewater, L. B., & Walker, L. E. A. (Eds.). (1985). *Handbook of feminist therapy: Women's issues in psychotherapy.* New York: Springer.

Rubin, L. B. (1985). *Just friends: The role of friendship in our lives.* New York: Harper.

Ryff, C. D., & Marshall, V. W. (Eds.). (1999). *The self and society in aging processes.* New York: Springer.

Shanahan, K. J., & Hyman, M. R. (2003). The development of a virtue ethics scale. *Journal of Business Ethics, 42*(2), 197–228.

Sheridan, K. (1982). Sex bias in therapy: Are counselors immune? *Personnel and Guidance Journal, 61,* 81–83.

Simon, S., Howe, L., & Kirschenbaum, H. (1972). *Values clarification.* New York: Hart.

Sinacore-Guinn, A. L. (1995). The diagnostic window: Culture- and gender-sensitive diagnosis and training. *Counselor Education and Supervision, 35,* 18–31.

Smith, M. L. (1980). Sex bias in counseling and psychotherapy. *Psychological Bulletin, 87,* 392–407.

Sue, D. W., & Sue, D. (2002). *Counseling the culturally different: Theory and practice* (4th ed.) New York: Wiley.

Tjeltveit, H. C. (1999). *Ethics and values in psychotherapy.* London: Routledge.

Tobin, S. (1999). *Preservation of the self in the oldest years with implications for practice.* New York: Springer.

Trotman, F. K., & Brody, C. M. (Eds.). (2002). *Psychotherapy and counseling with older women: Cross-cultural, family, and end-of-life issues.* New York: Springer.

Weiss, R. S., & Bass, S. A. (Eds.). (2002). *Challenges of the third age: Meaning and purpose in later life.* London: Oxford University Press.

Welfel, E. R. (1998). *Ethics in counseling and psychotherapy: Standards, research, and emerging issues.* Pacific Grove, CA: Brooks/Cole.

Visit the book companion site at www.thomsonedu.com to access tutorial quizzes.

Appendix A

Observer's Guide
to Rating
Communication Skills

This observer's guide can be used in conjunction with the exercises on communication skills in Chapters 3 and 4. The helper will not use all the behaviors listed for every role play, but over a period of time the ratings will indicate verbal and nonverbal behaviors that need further development as well as those that the helper is already using effectively. This guide will help both observer and helper understand and recognize the communication behaviors that are necessary to make helping relationships effective.

Rate the helper's behaviors on a scale of 0 to 3: 0 = did not occur, 1 = occurred but needs improvement, 2 = occurred and is adequate, 3 = helper especially strong on this point.

NONVERBAL BEHAVIORS

1. The helper maintained eye contact with the helpee.

    0   1   2   3

2. The helper varied facial expressions during the interview.

    0   1   2   3

3. The helper responded to the helpee with alertness and facial animation.

    0   1   2   3

4. The helper sometimes nodded his or her head.

   0   1   2   3

5. The helper had a relaxed body position.

   0   1   2   3

6. The helper leaned toward the helpee to encourage the helpee.

   0   1   2   3

7. The helper's vocal pitch varied when talking.

   0   1   2   3

8. The helper's voice was easily heard by the helpee.

   0   1   2   3

9. Sometimes the helper used one-word comments, such as "mm-hm" or "uh-huh," to encourage the helpee.

   0   1   2   3

10. The helper communicated warmth, concern, and empathy by smiling and using other gestures.

    0   1   2   3

VERBAL BEHAVIORS

11. The helper responded to the most important theme of each of the helpee's statements.

    0   1   2   3

12. The helper usually identified and responded to the feelings of the helpee.

    0   1   2   3

13. The helper usually identified and responded to the behaviors of the helpee.

    0   1   2   3

14. The helper verbally responded to at least one nonverbal cue from the helpee.

    0   1   2   3

15. The helper encouraged the helpee to talk about his or her feelings.

    0   1   2   3

16. The helper asked questions that could not be answered in a yes-or-no fashion.

    0   1   2   3

17. The helper confronted the helpee with any discrepancies between behavior and communication.

    0   1   2   3

18. The helper shared his or her feelings with the helpee.

    0   1   2   3

19. The helper communicated understanding of the helpee.

    0   1   2   3

20. The helper responded in ways that communicated liking for and appreci-
    ation of the helpee.

    0   1   2   3

21. The helper summarized statements and themes to clarify issues for the
    helpee.

    0   1   2   3

22. The helper sent "I" messages when confronting the helpee or expressing
    lack of understanding.

    0   1   2   3

YOUR SUMMARY OF SUGGESTIONS
FOR THE HELPER

Appendix B

Sample Psychotherapy
Policies

Please read this information carefully. It describes my policies and the related practices to be followed as part of the therapy services I will provide you. Be sure to raise any questions you may have. I would appreciate your returning a signed copy the next time we meet.

APPOINTMENTS
AND CANCELLATIONS

Every effort will be made to schedule appointments that are mutually convenient. If it becomes necessary for you to cancel, at least 24 hours' notice must be given. If less than 24 hours' notice is given, you will be expected to pay for that appointment. (Insurance companies will not reimburse for canceled or missed sessions.) There is no need to confirm appointments unless you have a question.

PAYMENT AND INSURANCE

Please know your insurance coverage. Pay special attention to annual limits, deductible amounts you must pay yourself, percentages of charges your insurance pays, and any waiting period if your insurance is new.

This form is based on a model developed by Judith Birnbaum, Ph.D., Wellesley, MA.

I will complete your insurer's claim forms, but it remains your responsibility to guarantee payment and to follow up with your insurance company if there are any questions. Billing is generally by the month. It is expected that payments will be made on a timely basis—within one month of billing.

You should be aware that for claims to be processed, insurance companies require a diagnosis and, occasionally, other information. By law, such information cannot be released by insurance companies without your specific, informed consent.

CONFIDENTIALITY

Communications between my clients and me are confidential, in accord with professional ethics and in compliance with the law. However, Massachusetts law also specifies certain limitations to this confidentiality. While these limits may not be at all relevant to your particular situation, I am legally obligated to inform you about them. The following are conditions in which disclosure can be made without your consent. I must disclose information:

1. In order to protect you or others if
   a. You present a danger to yourself and refuse to accept appropriate treatment.
   b. You tell me of an actual threat to harm another person.
   c. You have a history of violence and there is cause to believe you pose a danger of physical violence to another.
2. In case of child or elder abuse, which must be reported to appropriate state agencies.
3. In order to collect debts or to protect myself in a court action.
4. In certain legal proceedings should a court of law issue an order requiring the release of confidential information.
5. With colleagues about my work with you (never revealing your identity) to provide the best services possible. In any case, only appropriate and necessary information will be provided.

Of course, whenever you wish to give expressed, written consent, I can share information about you. When I am working with you and your family (or partner), it is important that nothing anyone says during a session be used against him or her outside of the session. Likewise, I will never discuss one member of a family with another during any individual sessions that might occur adjunctively with couples or family work unless one of the above conditions is present.

(*Signed*) _____

(*Signed*) _____

(*Date*) _____

Appendix C

Sample Client Information Sheet

Name _____ Date _____

Address _____

Telephone number: Day _____ Evening _____

Cell phone _____ E-mail _____

Date of birth _____ Marital status _____ Sex _____

Health insurance _____

Occupation _____

Years of education _____ Previous counseling? _____Yes _____No

If yes, whom did you see? _____

For what reason(s)? _____

Family History:

Parent 1: Name _____ Living? _____ Age _____

       Marital status _____ Years of education _____

       Occupation _____

       Past and present health _____

Parent 2: Name _____ Living? _____ Age _____

    Marital status _____ Years of education _____

    Occupation _____

    Past and present health _____

Siblings:

Name	Age	Marital Status	Health (Past/Present)	Occupation
_____	____	_____	_____	_____
_____	____	_____	_____	_____
_____	____	_____	_____	_____
_____	____	_____	_____	_____
_____	____	_____	_____	_____
_____	____	_____	_____	_____
_____	____	_____	_____	_____
_____	____	_____	_____	_____
_____	____	_____	_____	_____

Current Family:

Partner's name _____ Age _____

Years married/cohabitated _____ Number of children _____

Partner's occupation _____

Years of education _____ Past/present health _____

Previous marriages and/or divorces (please give details):

Names and age of children/stepchildren; where is each living?

Other people living in same household? Please give name, age, and relationship.

Have you or anyone in your extended family been treated for psychiatric problems, alcoholism, or drug abuse problems? Please describe.

List any past/present legal history.

What present problems do you have that you feel you need help with?

What do you think is causing these problems?

Why are you coming for counseling at this particular time?

What are your expectations and goals for counseling at this time?

How will you know when your goals have been achieved?

Are you currently being treated for any health condition? Are you taking any prescription medication? Please indicate and explain what the medication is prescribed for.

Thank you for completing this form. All information is confidential.

Appendix D

What Is the HIPAA Privacy Rule?

The Privacy Rule, or Standards for the Privacy of Individually Identifiable Health Information, issued by the Department of Health and Human Services implements the requirement of the Health Insurance Portability and Accountability Act of 1996. It establishes a set of national standards for the protection of certain health information. The standards address the use and disclosure of individuals' health information—called protected health information (PHI)—by organizations subject to the Privacy Rule—called covered entities—for various purposes including research. It also sets standards for individuals' privacy rights to gain access to, be informed of, and control how their health information is used.

The Privacy Rule applies to health plans, health care clearinghouses, and any health care provider who electronically transmits health information in connection with certain transactions, which include claims, benefit eligibility inquiries, referral authorization requests, or other transactions for which DHHS has established standards under the HIPAA Transactions Rule.

Also see the Department of Health and Human Services website: http://www.hipaa.org.

Source: http://www.apa.org/science/research/HIPAA.html

HIPAA DE-IDENTIFYING
REQUIREMENTS

This information about HIPAA de-identifiers is for informational purposes only. It is not intended to be complete, definitive, or to be relied on without first consulting legal counsel.

To de-identify information so that it is not subject to HIPAA, a number of identifying variables must all be taken out of electronic records. The following identifiers of the individual or of relatives, employers, or household members of the individual, are removed:

(A) Names;

(B) All geographic subdivisions smaller than a State, including street address, city, county, precinct, zip code, and their equivalent geocodes, except for the initial three digits of a zip code if, according to the current publicly available data from the Bureau of the Census:

    (1) The geographic unit formed by combining all zip codes with the same three initial digits contains more than 20,000 people; and

    (2) The initial three digits of a zip code for all such geographic units containing 20,000 or fewer people is changed to 000;

(C) All elements of dates (except year) for dates directly related to an individual, including birth date, admission date, discharge date, date of death; and all ages over 89 and all elements of dates (including year) indicative of such age, except that such ages and elements may be aggregated into a single category of age 90 or older;

(D) Telephone numbers;

(E) Fax numbers;

(F) Electronic mail addresses;

(G) Social security numbers;

(H) Medical record numbers;

(I) Health plan beneficiary numbers;

(J) Account numbers;

(K) Certificate/license numbers;

(L) Vehicle identifiers and serial numbers, including license plate numbers;

(M) Device identifiers and serial numbers;

(N) Web Universal Resource Locators (URLs);

(O) Internet Protocol (IP) address numbers;

(P) Biometric identifiers, including finger and voice prints;

(Q) Full face photographic images and any comparable images; and

(R) Any other unique identifying number, characteristic, or code, except as permitted by paragraph (c) of this section; and

The covered entity does not have actual knowledge that the information could be used alone or in combination with other information to identify an individual who is a subject of the information.

Glossary

Abreaction   A Freudian term for the situation in which a helpee relives painful emotional experiences during therapy, becoming conscious of previously repressed material.

Acute stress disorder   An anxiety disorder that occurs within one month of experiencing a traumatic event. Symptoms include a sense of numbing or lack of emotional responsiveness, reexperiencing the trauma, avoidance of stimuli associated with the event, and increased arousal and anxiety.

Additive responses   Empathic verbal responses that increase the helpee's self-understanding by clarifying and providing perspective on the helpee's underlying meaning.

Advocacy   Active behaviors such as direct contact, written letters, or petitions to obtain services or benefits for clients.

Affective.   Pertaining to feelings and emotions. The affective domain comprises the feeling, emotional aspects of experience. These feelings may be conscious or unconscious.

Anal stage   In psychoanalysis, the developmental stage between 2 and 3 years of age in which the child focuses on pleasure from the anal erogenous zone. This is a pregenital phase of sexual development during which bowel training becomes important.

Anima   According to Jung, the feminine side of men and women.

Animus   According to Jung, the masculine side of women and men.

Anxiety   A state of tension that warns us of impending danger. Anxiety may be realistic, involving fear of danger from the external world; neurotic, involving fear that one's instincts will get out of control and lead to a punishable act; or moral, involving fear of one's own conscience. According to Freudian theory, anxiety results from the repression of the basic conflicts among the id, the ego, and the superego.

Approach reaction   Behavior directed toward a situation or stimulus, regardless of positive or negative emotions. This tendency to deal with whatever issues are at hand implies a positive ability to work through difficulties.

Assertiveness training   A behavioral technique whereby the client learns progressively more assertive behaviors (standing up for one's own rights without impinging on the rights of others) through such means as modeling, role playing, and instruction. Assertive behaviors include saying no without feeling guilty and learning to ask directly for what one wants.

Avoidance reaction   Withdrawal from or avoidance of a situation or stimulus that might have threatening or adverse emotional aspects. This reaction indicates a refusal to work through or check out problems and issues.

Behavioral   Pertaining to an observable physical action or performance; a concrete response one makes to a stimulus situation. Behaviors may be motor, perceptual, or glandular.

Biofeedback   A learning procedure in which sophisticated electronic instrumentation to monitor changes in physiological functioning aids the client in becoming aware of and controlling certain physiological variables.

Birth order   Adlerian concept that one's placement within the family structure (that is, whether one is the firstborn child, the second, and so on) is a major determinant of personality.

Brainstorming   A group problem-solving technique; every person's idea is considered before evaluative screening occurs. This is an important step in problem solving, allowing for all possible input before a decision is reached.

Burnout   Depletion of physical and mental resources resulting in loss of motivation, interest, and capabilities for helping relationships.

Change agentry   Action strategies designed to influence and promote change in some aspect(s) of organizations and systems.

Circular causality   The idea that there is a reciprocal connection between cause and effect, a cyclical interaction. This idea is the basis of systems theory.

Clarification   A verbal response that helps the client to better understand issues and needs through what has been said or felt.

Client-centered   Rogerian term meaning that the direction of the counseling (goals, course, and process) is wholly determined by the client, not the counselor.

Cognitive   Pertaining to thinking and knowing. Covers all modes of knowing: perceiving, remembering, imagining, conceiving, judging, reasoning. Cognition is a conscious process.

Cognitive-behavioral   Focuses both on cognition and the behavioral skills necessary for problem resolution and behavior change.

Cognitive restructuring   Rational emotive therapy technique that identifies irrational thinking and replaces it with rational thinking through didactic teaching. One is taught how to correct faulty belief systems by unlearning irrational beliefs and learning rational ones.

Compassion fatigue   The stress resulting from caring too much, particularly affecting those who deal with others' trauma. It may manifest in physical, emotional, or spiritual exhaustion, symptoms of burnout.

Compensation   In psychoanalysis, a defense mechanism whereby one substitutes a satisfying activity for a frustrating one to reduce tension. One covers up a weakness or defect by displaying in exaggerated fashion a less defective or more desirable characteristic.

Concrete reinforcement   A specific object, such as a desired piece of food, or a special event, such as watching television, used as a reward for exhibiting designated behavior.

Conditioned response   A response that is learned, as opposed to one that is instinctive.

Conditioning   A process in which a response is elicited by a stimulus, object, or situation; in other words, not a natural reflex.

Confrontation   A verbal technique whereby helpers present helpees with discrepancies between their verbal and nonverbal behaviors or between the helpee's and the helper's perceptions. Confrontation is often used to encourage approach reactions rather than avoidance reactions.

Congruence   A client-centered therapy concept indicating agreement between one's experience and one's perceptions of that experience, or one's self-awareness. In other words, one's behavior is in tune with one's values and beliefs. One is said to "practice what one preaches."

Constructivism   A cognitive-behavioral approach focusing on people's active creation of and attribution of meaning to their personal and social realities.

Content   The material or constituents of an experience, as distinct from the form or process of an experience. The "what" as opposed to the "how."

Contingency contracting   A positive behavioral contract between helper and helpee specifically stating desired behavioral outcomes and consequential reinforcements to follow performance of each stated behavior. An elaboration of the "If you do X, you will get (to do) Y" formula that is clearly stated, agreed to by all parties, and systematically applied.

Countertransference   In psychoanalysis, the positive and/or negative distortion of the analyst's interpretations of the client by the analyst's own conflicts.

Critical incident stress debriefing   A debriefing process that prevents or limits the development of posttraumatic stress in people exposed to a critical incident, an event causing unusually intense stress reactions.

Defense mechanism   Psychoanalytic construct of unconscious or involuntary strategies that one uses to protect oneself against painful negative feelings associated with a situation that is extremely disagreeable. The situation may be physical or mental and may occur frequently or infrequently.

Denial   In psychoanalysis, a defense mechanism whereby one's mind refuses to acknowledge and experience something that would cause anxiety and distress if acknowledged. It manifests itself as a firm belief that what happened did not happen or is not so.

Determinism   In psychoanalysis, the assumption that every mental event or attitude was caused by earlier psychological experiences and biological factors.

Directive therapy   A form of therapy in which the therapist guides the course, objectives, and process of therapy. The therapist is a director, a teacher, and a guide who has full control of the therapeutic relationship.

Discrimination   Learning theory term involving the ability to differentiate among slightly different stimuli. Reinforcement will have been present or stronger for some stimuli than for others.

Displacement   In psychoanalysis, a defense mechanism whereby the psychic energy (often anger or some other emotion) directed toward a particular person or object is transferred to another similar person or object. Displacement frequently occurs in dreams, in which feelings are shifted from one object or person to another object or person to which they do not really apply.

Dissonance   What occurs when two parts or aspects of experience do not blend or fuse, resulting in discrepancies and discomfort. Dissonance may occur between two behaviors, between behavior and feeling, or between inner and outer experiences.

Eclectic   The blending or integration of elements of different approaches and perspectives. Requires knowledge of the principles and methods of a range of helping approaches.

Ecological   Perspective that acknowledges the powerful reciprocal influences of sociocultural ideologies and systems on individual development and systems functioning. Ecological-based therapies focus on person/environment fit rather than on internal individual problems.

Ego   Psychoanalytic concept of the partly preconscious, partly conscious part of the personality that is in direct contact with the external world, with the reality of the world. It includes conscious perceptions of reality as given by the senses and preconscious memories, together with those selected impulses and influences from within that have been accepted and are under control.

Electra complex   According to psychoanalytic theory, the feelings during the phallic stage of psychosexual development (ages 3 to 5), when a girl experiences unconscious sexual/erotic emotions for her father and antagonism for her "rival" mother.

Empathy   The ability to see the world the way the helpee sees it, from the helpee's "frame of reference," to experience the helpee's feelings.

Empowerment   Helping strategy that encourages one to think and take action in a positive way, leading to a sense of self-efficacy.

Empty seat   Gestalt technique in which a client uses an empty chair to represent an imagined partner in a dialogue or a role play. The client sits in the "empty seat" when speaking as the person the seat represents.

Ethnocentrism   The belief by members of a specific culture that their ideas about the universe are the way things are, the way they should be, and the way others see them.

Existential   Philosophical viewpoint focusing on the here and now, the presence of time, people's freedom to choose for themselves, purposes of life, potential, and humanness. Existential psychology deals with those aspects of experience that can be observed introspectively (sensory and imaginal processes), together with feelings.

Extinguish   Behavioral technique in which any reinforcing consequences of a particular behavior are discontinued, resulting in that behavior being diminished and eventually discontinued. Extinction techniques are used to unlearn (erase) a specific behavior that is deemed inappropriate.

Extroversion   Jungian term that describes the state of being oriented toward the external and objective world. An extrovert is one who is primarily interested in things outside the self.

Eye movement desensitization and reprocessing (EMDR)   Technique that integrates a wide range of procedural elements along with the use of rhythmic eye movements and other forms of bilateral stimulation to treat traumatic stress and memories.

Free association   Psychoanalytic technique in which clients tell analysts everything that comes into their minds in response to a word or concept stimulus.

Generalization   Learning theory term for a response learned in one situation that can be used in other situations with similar but different stimuli; also refers to a general concept formed on the basis of several component ideas.

Genital stage In psychoanalysis, the adult psychosexual stage of development that occurs as a child reaches puberty and his or her interests become heterosexual rather than self-centered. At this stage, the earlier psychosexual stages are fused, and genital eroticism predominates.

Gestalt German word meaning configuration—that is, the form, pattern, structure, or configuration of an integrated whole, not a mere summation of its parts. Gestalt psychology contends that mental processes and behavior cannot be analyzed into separate elementary units because the human personality is a unified structure, a whole. Gestalt psychology is a psychology of perception.

Heterosexism The assumption that heterosexual behavior is the norm for mature adults and that homosexual behavior should be suppressed.

Hypnosis A relaxed, sleeplike, trancelike condition psychically induced by a helper in which the client loses consciousness but responds, with certain limitations, to the suggestions of the hypnotist.

Id Psychoanalytic concept of a primitive, unconscious source of psychic energy, a part of the personality that demands immediate gratification in order to reduce tension and increase pleasure. The inner determinant of conscious life.

Imagery techniques Techniques that help people to imagine other people, scenes, and events, to recall or imagine sights, smells, feelings, and thoughts as vividly as possible.

Implosive therapy A form of behavioral therapy in which the client vividly imagines intense exposure to aversive stimuli in order to extinguish anxiety about those stimuli. After repeated imaginary exposures, the client is able to deal with the aversive stimuli in real life with reduced anxiety.

Incongruence In person-centered psychology, a term that refers to a discrepancy between a person's actual experience and his or her version of the experience. If someone's behavior is incongruent, it is not in keeping with what he or she says.

Inherent inferiority Term in Adlerian psychology that refers to the belief that everyone comes into this life with built-in feelings of inferiority (based on helplessness, smallness, and dependency). This inferiority provides the ultimate driving force of humans in that they strive to overcome inferiority and achieve superiority.

Intellectualization In psychoanalytic psychology, a defense mechanism whereby one emphasizes intellectuality or cognition and neglects emotion and volition to avoid experiencing and dealing with emotional content.

Interpretation A psychotherapeutic technique that uncovers the meanings and relationships underlying the apparent verbal content of a helpee statement or behavior. This technique may involve connecting different aspects of experience for the helpee or explaining relationships and causal factors.

Intrapsychic A Freudian concept referring to the unconscious, internal conflicts among id, ego, and superego affecting personality development and behavior.

Introversion Jungian term that describes the state of being oriented toward the internal and subjective world. An introvert is concerned primarily with his or her own thoughts and feelings.

Isolation In psychoanalytic psychology, a defense mechanism used by people to detach an idea from its affective or emotional content; for example, isolation may be indicated by a blank pause between a highly unpleasant or personally significant experience and a person's reaction to it.

Latency stage   Psychoanalytic concept of the stage of psychosexual development, occurring between the age of 4 or 5 and emerging adolescence, that separates infantile from genital sexuality. During this period, there are no conscious sexual interests or activities.

Leading   A verbal skill that elicits client responses in an open-ended yet focused manner. Leads include "door openers" such as "Tell me more . . ." and "I'm wondering about . . ." as well as questions, reflections, and clarifications.

Libido   Psychoanalytic concept referring to psychic energy that includes the sexual and survival instincts. Libido is a dynamic force that includes both sexual and ego drives. It is the life force that serves to neutralize the destructive impulses in the system.

Lifestyle   In Adlerian psychology, a person's unique, directional pattern of behavior based on the process of judging both status of the self and status of the world.

Modeling   A learning theory principle whereby new modes of behavior are learned or old ones changed by observing others' actual or simulated behavior and its consequences. Modeling is based on imitation.

Neuroses   In the psychoanalytic sense, functional disorders of the nervous system that are psychological rather than organic in origin. These disorders can result in somatic and behavioral symptoms. Because the adequate satisfaction of subjective needs is the function of the ego, neurosis can be understood to be a disturbance of ego functions.

Object   In psychoanalytic object relations, an object refers to one's mental representations of significant others who are sources of sustenance, protection, and gratification.

Object relations   In psychoanalytic theory, refers to both the external and internalized relationships between self and others.

Oedipal complex   According to psychoanalytic theory, the feelings during the phallic stage of psychosexual development (ages 3 to 5), when one experiences unconscious erotic/sexual desires toward the opposite-gender parent and antagonism to the same-gender parent. Although traditionally used to describe boys' experience, this concept is now often used to refer to both boys and girls.

Operant conditioning   A principle of behavioral learning theory whereby the actual consequences of behavior, rather than the original cause (stimulus), are of concern. These consequences of a behavior "operate" on the behavior and on the environment, causing the behavior to recur.

Oral stage   Psychoanalytic term for the infantile stage of psychosexual development when pleasure is centered around the mouth, around sucking and eating activities.

Organismic   Pertaining to the individual as a whole entity; emphasis is placed on the organized system of interrelated and interdependent parts.

Paraphrase   A rewording of the thought or meaning expressed in something that has been said or written before.

Penis envy   Psychoanalytic concept describing little girls' envy of boys, and their desire to have a penis.

Persona   The Jungian term for the disguise or mask that one displays in public and that frequently differs from one's true attitude or appearance.

Phallic stage   In psychoanalysis, a developmental stage in which a child's interests shift from the anal to the genital area. According to Freud, during this stage children believe that both males and females have penises.

Phenomenological   Perceiving someone else's world through his or her eyes; emphasizing conscious experience as real experience.

Positive reinforcement   Rewards that have good significance (for example, money or good grades). Positive reinforcement may be social or concrete.

Posttraumatic stress disorder   An anxiety disorder with a duration of more than one month that develops after the experience of an extreme traumatic event. Symptoms include a sense of numbing or lack of emotional responsiveness, reexperiencing the trauma, avoidance of stimuli associated with the event, and increased arousal and anxiety.

Potency   A term used in Gestalt psychology implying that the helper or helpee has the power to do something, the expertise and credibility to deliver.

Principle of gradation   Learning theory principle whereby a sequence of intermediate or subgoals leads gradually to a more complex behavior.

Process   A series of successive but interdependent changes or events. Also refers to "how" something is happening and what the associated effects and form are, as opposed to the content, the actual facts and events.

Projection   In psychoanalytic and object relations theory, a defense mechanism whereby one unconsciously attributes feelings (for example, guilt or inferiority), thoughts, or acts unacceptable to one's own ego to other people. These projections are usually a defense against unpleasant feelings in ourselves and are means by which we can justify ourselves in our own eyes.

Projective identification   In object relations theory, projective identification occurs in relationships when the other person unconsciously accepts the projection and responds as if the projection were his or her own.

Psychodynamic   A focus on unconscious factors that motivate behavior.

Psychoeducation   Helping strategy that teaches people about areas of emotional and relationship functioning—that is, how people learn and develop.

Psychoses   Severe mental disorders, characterized by such symptoms as delusions (false beliefs), hallucinations (false sensory perceptions), and disorganized speech or behavior, which result in individuals being "out of touch" with external reality.

Psychosexual stages   Psychoanalytic developmental stages that are crucial in the child's personality development. Because the Freudian view places sexual impulses at the root of all human personality problems, sexual development and sexually oriented experiences in childhood directly affect future development.

Rationalization   In psychoanalysis, a defense mechanism whereby a person assigns a socially acceptable motive to his or her behavior. The process of rationally justifying an act helps one defend oneself against self-accusation or guilt.

Reaction formation   A psychoanalytic term for behavior that is directly opposed to unconscious wishes; this behavior represents a defense mechanism that allows the ego to keep unacceptable character traits in check. Reaction formation behavior can sometimes be excessive or violent.

Recall   A psychoanalytic term meaning to revive or reinstate a past experience in memory.

Referral   The arrangement of other assistance for a helpee when the initial helping situation is not or cannot be effective.

Reflection   Providing a response to what has been communicated after serious consideration and contemplation.

Reframing Technique that relabels behavior in a more positive framework—for example, "When you fight, you're expressing caring." This changes people's perspectives and allows new responses.

Regression Psychoanalytic term that describes the retreat to an earlier stage of development in which one felt more adequate; one expresses interests and behavior characteristic of an earlier stage. Regression is a defense mechanism used to reduce tension or anxiety.

Reinforcement Behavioral term for the environmental event that, when following certain behavior, causes that behavior to recur. May be positive or negative. Reinforcements are the environmental consequences of behavior.

Repression In psychoanalysis, a defense mechanism whereby one forces into the unconscious painful perceptions, ideas, and feelings. Impulses and desires in conflict with enforced standards of conduct are thrust into the unconscious where they can still remain active, indirectly determining behavior and experience, perhaps through dreams or neurotic symptoms. According to Freud, repression is often the cause of neurotic disorders.

Resistance Defensive behavior of the helpee that prevents him or her from participating effectively in helping relationships and process.

Responsive listening An empathic verbal response that communicates acceptance and concern.

Schedules of reinforcement Behavioral term describing reinforcement schedules used in contingency contracting: (1) continual reinforcement—reinforcement that follows each time target behavior occurs; (2) interval schedule—reinforcement that occurs after a certain period of time, such as every hour; and (3) ratio schedule—reinforcement that occurs after a certain number of responses, such as on every third response.

Secondary traumatization Also known as vicarious traumatization. Stress reactions affecting those who work directly or indirectly with survivors of trauma and who have difficulty coping with the intense emotions. Viewers of trauma, such as those watching the events of 9/11 on television, may also experience these reactions.

Self-concept According to person-centered theory, the perception we have of ourselves based on information from significant others and from our experiences; our image of who and what we are, what we are all about.

Shaping Learning theory term for the modification of behavior by reinforcing more and more refined responses that come closer and closer to the desired behavior. One can shape behavior by breaking it into its smallest parts and reinforcing one part at a time, in sequence.

Significant other A parent, relative, teacher, or other person who is especially meaningful and important to an individual. Significant others have influence over our feelings and actions.

Social reinforcement Behavioral term meaning attention from a significant other (for example, a smile, nod, physical contact, praise) that follows a particular behavior and makes that behavior more likely to recur.

Splitting Psychoanalytic object relations term for separating off an intolerable part of the self (or ego) as a polar opposite of the rest, or being oblivious to one part of the self (or ego). It is an unconscious defense mechanism for separating incompatible feelings, perceptions, or experiences.

Sublimation According to psychoanalytic psychology, a defense mechanism that gives blocked energy an alternative, socially acceptable outlet; for example, instead of seeking sexual gratification, one might help people or engage in artistic endeavors.

Successive approximation   A learning theory concept whereby a desired behavior is broken into its smallest parts, and behaviors resembling one of those parts are reinforced. For example, the act of holding a pencil in the writing hand may be the first behavioral component of learning to write. This or other resembling behaviors can be reinforced in order to shape the desired target behavior.

Superego   A psychoanalytic term for the part of the personality that interjects parental and social values. The superego is a structure in the unconscious built up by early experiences with parents and significant others. When the ego gratifies the primitive impulses of the id, the superego criticizes the ego, which results in feelings of guilt and anxiety.

Symbiotic   A mutually dependent relationship in which neither party feels complete without the other.

System   A set of components that interact with one another. Each component of the system is affected by whatever happens to the other components. The system is greater than the sum of the individual components.

Systematic desensitization   Behavioral technique of counterconditioning to reduce anxiety by associating negative stimuli with positive experiences so that the stimuli no longer arouse anxiety. Desensitization begins when a client learns complete muscle relaxation (which is antithetical to anxiety) and establishes an anxiety hierarchy. An anxiety-causing stimulus is then paired with positive mental images and the process of relaxation. The pairing continues until the entire hierarchy can be imagined without anxiety.

Third-party payer   Insurance or party other than the provider and consumer who pays for services.

Token economy   A behavioral reinforcement program in which desired behaviors are reinforced with tokens that can be exchanged for rewards. The tokens can be awarded immediately after the behavior is performed, and the exchange of tokens can occur later.

Transference   Psychoanalytic term for the situation in which the client unconsciously puts the analyst in the place of one or more significant others in his or her life and attributes to the analyst the attitudes, behaviors, and attributes of the significant person(s). Transference refers to the patient's developing a positive or negative emotional attitude toward the analyst. It may occur in other relationships.

Triage   Quick assessment of the severity and scope of need.

Unfinished business   Gestalt term for unexpressed feelings, associated with memories or fantasies, that affect current functioning.

Index

F

Facilitative responses, 66
Facilities, 91
Faded overt modeling, 189
Faded overt self-guidance, 189
Fairbairn, Ronald, 124
False self, 125
Family context, 7
Family sculpting, 202
Fantasizing, 177
Faulty thinking, 136–137, 183–184
Feelings
    exercises related to, 60–63
    major categories of, 60
Feldstein, M., 284
Feminist therapies, 151–153
    further reading on, 163–164
    implications for helpers, 153
    principles of helping, 152–153
    social change and, 285
Figley, C. R., 255
Fisch, R., 261
Follow-up process, 229–230, 261
Formal helping relationships, 26–27, 47
Forms and applications, 89–90
Foxhall, K., 297
Frankl, Viktor, 127
Free association, 126, 178, 324
Freud, Anna, 124
Freud, Sigmund, 119, 120–122
Freudian theory, 120–122
Fried, J., 3, 37, 66, 154, 287
Friends of clients, 91–92
Fromm, Erich, 119

G

Galvan, N., 154
Gartrell, N., 284
Gender issues
    awareness of, 39
    exercises related to, 285–286
    feminist therapies and, 151–153
    sexism and, 282–286
Generalist human services workers, 12
    kinds of helping relationships for, 26
    knowledge requirement for, 43
Generalization, 134, 324
Genital stage, 121, 325
Genograms, 202

Gergen, K., 150
Gestalt theory, 130–133, 325
    affective strategies and, 173–176
    exercises related to, 177–178
    further reading on, 214
    general explanation of, 130–131
    implications for helpers, 132–133
    principles of helping, 131–132
    verbal techniques, 173–174
Gilligan, C., 152, 283
Gillis, S., 152
Glaser, B., 276
Glasser, William, 138, 139
Goals/objectives, 109–112
    crisis intervention and, 260
    establishing with clients, 109–111
    exercises related to, 111–112, 219
    mutual acceptance of, 217–220
Goldfried, M. R., 150
Goodman, R., 189
Gordon, T., 13
Gradation, principle of, 134
Gray, H. J., 255
Green, S., 283
Greenberg, L. S., 150
Greene, B., 2, 3
Guntrip, Harry, 124

H

Hackett, G., 278
Hamilton, S., 254
Hartling, L. M., 153
Hartmann, Heinz, 124
Health Insurance Portability and
    Accountability Act (HIPAA), 6,
    318–320
Helpees. *See* Clients
Helpers
    burnout suffered by, 302
    categories of, 10
    changing roles/functions of, 4–6
    characteristics of effective, 37–44
    dual or multiple roles of, 296
    gender awareness by, 39, 282–286
    generalist human services workers
        as, 12
    misrepresentation by, 296–297
    nonprofessionals as, 12
    personal values of, 28–29, 276–292